OCULAR THERAPEUTICS
AND PHARMACOLOGY

OCULAR THERAPEUTICS AND PHARMACOLOGY

Philip P. Ellis, M.D.

Professor and Head, Division of
Ophthalmology, Department of Surgery,
University of Colorado Medical Center,
Denver, Colorado

FIFTH EDITION

The C. V. Mosby Company

Saint Louis 1977

FIFTH EDITION

Copyright © 1977 by The C. V. Mosby Company

Previous editions copyrighted 1963, 1966, 1969, 1973

Printed in the United States of America

Distributed in Great Britain by Henry Kimpton, London

The C. V. Mosby Company
11830 Westline Industrial Drive, St. Louis, Missouri 63141

Library of Congress Cataloging in Publication Data

Ellis, Philip P
  Ocular therapeutics and pharmacology.

  Fourth ed. published in 1973 under title: Handbook of ocular therapeutics and pharmacology.
  Includes bibliographies and index.
  1. Therapeutics, Ophthalmological. 2. Ocular
pharmacology. I. Title.
RE991.E4 1977   617.7′061   77-6320
ISBN 0-8016-1516-X

CB/CB/B 9 8 7 6 5 4 3 2 1

PREFACE to fifth edition

In this edition an effort has been made to continue the fundamental purpose of the book, that is, to present in a concise form the basic considerations of current ocular therapy and pharmacology.

Extensive revisions have been made in this edition. Two new chapters have been added: one on carbonic anhydrase inhibitors and osmotherapeutic agents and another on anesthetic agents. Many sections have been rewritten entirely. New therapeutic agents, including various antibiotics, anti-inflammatory drugs, enzyme inhibitors, autonomic nervous system agents, and antiglaucoma medications, have been added. Newly reported side reactions to local and systemic ocular therapy are described. Consideration of new techniques of therapy and drug delivery is presented. The pediatric dosage tables have been expanded.

The second section on therapeutic agents has been condensed so that groups of drugs are described together. This avoids the needless repetition that occurred with the previous system of alphabetical listing. Referral to the index will provide the reader with the location of individual drug descriptions.

It is impossible to give recognition to all those who contributed to the preparation of this revised text. I particularly wish to thank Dr. S. Lance Forstot for his help in revisions of the chapters on therapy of diseases of the conjunctiva and therapy of the diseases of the cornea, Dr. Richard Deitrich for review of the chapter on autonomic nervous system agents, Dr. Theodore Eickhoff for his help with antibiotic medications, Dr. Merritt Rudolph for his assistance on the chapter on principles of cortisone and ACTH therapy, Dr. Jerry Meislik for his assistance on the chapter on glaucoma medications, Dr. Stuart Frankel for his help on the chapter on therapy of diseases of the eyelids, Dr. W. Bruce Wilson for his assistance on the chapter on therapy of optic neuritis, Dr. Dale Johnson for his help with the pediatric dosage tables, Dr. William Roberts for his assistance with the chapter on medical agents in surgical care, and Dr. Charles Van Way for his help with the fluid and electrolyte medications. I am extremely grateful to Mrs. Toma Wilson for her considerable efforts in manuscript editing, and I am especially thankful to Miss Kit Skiby for her many secretarial activities in preparation of this edition.

Dr. Donn L. Smith, who was a coauthor of the first four editions, has withdrawn in this edition. His past contributions are most appreciated.

Philip P. Ellis

v

PREFACE to first edition

All books have purposes; some are realized, but probably more are not. Besides the obvious desires to satisfy an ego and to impress the medical school administration, this handbook has been compiled for very definite reasons. It was written to serve as a quick reference for the busy practicing ophthalmologist who may have forgotten a specific dose or side reaction of a certain medication. It will also serve as a guide in therapy for beginning residents in ophthalmology and for nonspecialists who are treating ocular disorders. In general, it was designed to present in a concise form the basic considerations of current ocular therapy and pharmacology. It is not intended to be a textbook of therapeutics and pharmacology, nor is it meant to serve as a review of all types of treatment and ocular medications.

When any handbook is compiled, it becomes necessary to be somewhat arbitrary in presentation of material. One must take the license of deciding what are the most significant, practical, and effective forms of current therapy, realizing quite well that what he presents at any particular time may rapidly become outdated. The reader will find that some rare ocular conditions have been considered in detail, whereas other rather common ocular disorders have been dealt with in a very general fashion. This variation in approach has usually been based on the assumption that the reader has a basic knowledge of therapeutics and pharmacology and is acquainted in a general sense with the use of common medications. The reader will further observe that there is frequently a duplication of the rationale and methods of administration of a certain drug for treating the same disorders in various parts of the eye. This duplication is necessary because the book was designed for quick reference to treatment of a specific condition without it being necessary to read through the entire text.

The handbook is divided into two sections. The first section, on therapeutics, is designed to present some basic considerations of treatment and also to summarize the present medical therapy of most ocular disorders. The second section, on pharmacology, presents the most commonly used medications that a practicing ophthalmologist would have occasion to administer. The actions, uses, side reactions and contraindications, preparations, and dosages of these drugs are presented. The basic pharmacology is outlined, but the emphasis has been on the clinical use of drugs in ophthalmology. Attention is directed to the fact that the dosage schedule is for adults unless otherwise stated. Methods of determining pediatric doses are given at the beginning of the section.

It is impossible to give complete recognition to all those people who contributed to the development of this book. The therapeutic approaches have been evolved from the teachings and opinions expressed by many authorities in ocular therapeutics, and listing the sources of all these references is obviously impossible. Furthermore, some of the therapeutic ideas expressed have resulted from several years of teaching ocular therapeutics to eye residents.

We would particularly like to thank Dr. George Tyner of the Division of Ophthalmology, University of Colorado Medical Center, for his contributions to the organization and preparation of the chapters on the therapy of glaucoma and the therapy of uveitis.

Dr. Herbert P. Jacobi of the Department of Biochemistry, University of Nebraska College of Medicine, and Mr. Herbert Carlin, Chief of the Hospital Pharmacy at the University of Colorado Medical Center, have been most helpful in the preparation of the section on basic considerations. We are indebted to Dr. Ralph Druckman, Division of Neurology, University of Colorado Medical Center, for his constructive criticism during the preparation of the manuscript. Finally, we should like to thank Miss Barbra Pehrson and Mrs. Janet Kelley for their valuable help in typing the manuscript.

Philip P. Ellis
Donn L. Smith

CONTENTS

OCULAR THERAPEUTICS

Basic considerations

MECHANISMS OF DRUG ACTION
Drug receptor interactions

In order for a drug to produce a pharmacological action, it must interact with a receptor and in addition induce some change in that receptor. Compounds such as acetylcholine, which do both, are called agonists. Drugs such as atropine, which interact only with the receptor but do not induce a physiological change, are called pharmacological antagonists. The term "potency" refers to how tightly the compound is bound to the receptor. A compound that is very avidly taken up by the receptor will be a very potent compound, either as an agonist or antagonist. The strength of this binding, and therefore potency, is determined by how well the molecular and electronic configuration of the drug fits into that of the receptor site. The example often used is that of a lock and key. Although definite proof is lacking, receptors probably are mainly proteins and may have enzymatic activity. For example, the adenyl cyclase receptor system is located on the cell membrane. The combination of epinephrine with this receptor system leads to activation of adenyl cyclase, which in turn catalyzes the formation of cyclic AMP (cAMP). The effect of cAMP on the cell is dependent on the cell type.

Once an agonist is bound to the receptor, it must produce a change in the receptor, which is then amplified many times to bring about an observable reaction in the system. The ability of a compound to bring about this change is referred to as the power of the drug. The most powerful compound in a group of drugs is usually taken as the standard against which all others are compared. It is not necessarily true that the most powerful drug is also the most potent one. A drug that does not produce a maximum effect is referred to as a partial agonist. Obviously it is also a partial antagonist because it diminishes the action by blocking access of more powerful drugs to receptor sites. Pilocarpine is an example of a partial agonist.

Drug interactions

The interactions between drugs are extremely important. We have already referred to one such interaction, pharmacological antagonism, in which two drugs are competing for the same receptor site. Another interaction is physiological antagonism, in which two antagonists react with their respective receptors but produce opposite end results, for example, antagonistic effects of acetyl-choline and norepinephrine on pupil size. A third type of antagonism is simple chemical antagonism. Two compounds may react chemically either within or outside the body to effectively neutralize their pharmacological action much as an acid neutralizes a base. An example is chelation of calcium by ethylene-diamine tetra-acetate (EDTA). Much more complicated drug interactions are possible.

One drug may stimulate the metabolism of another, thus decreasing its effectiveness or shortening the duration of its action. Barbiturates are classic examples of compounds capable of inducing drug-metabolizing enzymes and thus of increasing the metabolism of many other drugs. The metabolic pathway of one drug may be suppressed by another drug, and therefore a prolonged effect occurs. As an example, prolonged action of succinylcholine occurs in patients receiving echothiophate iodide drops for treatment of glaucoma. Pseudocholinesterase hydrolyzes succinylcholine, and the plasma concentration of this enzyme decreases with systemic absorption of echothiophate iodide.

Additive or synergistic drug actions occur by a variety of mechanisms. If two equally powerful drugs are given at the same relative dose and act on the same receptor, their effects will simply be additive provided that the system is not reacting maximally already. An example would be increased miosis occurring with the concurrent administration of pilocarpine and carbachol. On the other hand, if the two drugs act on different receptors to bring about the same end results, a combination may produce a greater than additive, or synergistic, effect. An example of this phenomenon is the increased improvement in aqueous humor outflow with the combined use of pilocarpine and epinephrine.

Since patients are frequently treated with multiple drugs by different physicians, the possibility of adverse drug interactions becomes of great clinical importance. For example, when aspirin is given to a patient who is taking anticoagulants orally, an increased effect of the anticoagulants occurs. It is also important to recognize that drug therapy may alter the results of clinical laboratory tests. It is beyond the scope of this book to list such reactions, but an indication of these effects may be appreciated by the following examples. Acetazolamide therapy results in elevated blood levels of ammonia, bilirubin, glucose, sodium, and uric acid and in decreased levels of potassium and decreased blood pH. Corticosteroid therapy produces elevated blood levels of glucose, sodium, and amylase and decreased levels of potassium, uric acid, and protein bound iodine. Corticosteroids may also elevate the levels of urinary glucose and proteins.

It is impossible for any physician to memorize all the potential drug interactions. Nonetheless, it is important for him to be aware of other drugs the patient is receiving and to consider the possibilities of significant drug interactions to medications he is prescribing. Some drug interactions of importance to the ophthalmologist are cited in sections related to specific uses of drugs for treatment of various ocular disorders and in the discussion of therapeutic agents in the second section of this book.

PREPARATION OF OPHTHALMIC SOLUTIONS

At the present time most of the routinely prescribed ophthalmic medications are prepared by pharmaceutical manufacturers. Although it may be argued that the physician has thus been forced to standardize his dosage, the advantages of commercial ophthalmic preparations seem to outweigh their disadvantages. Stability, uniformity, and sterility characterize these products. It is no longer necessary for the physician to be concerned with the pharmacist's knowledge of proper pH and correct buffering for ophthalmic collyria or to fear that any patient will be unable to duplicate his prescription in any part of the country. Nonetheless, since all students of ophthalmology should be aware of basic pharmacological and pharmaceutical principles in the preparation of ophthalmic medications and since all preparations are not commercially available, a brief summary is given here.

Preparation of ophthalmic solutions is largely a problem of tonicity, pH, stability, and sterility. Of these, sterility is the most important but often the most neglected. These problems have been reviewed by Riegelman and Vaughan.

Tonicity

For many years pharmacists gave considerable attention to the matter of making ophthalmic solutions isotonic with tears (initially, 1.4% sodium chloride equivalent; later, 0.9% sodium chloride equivalent). Sodium chloride equivalents of most aqueous solutions of water-soluble drugs were determined, and buffers and salts were then added as required for isotonicity. Many buffers were employed; phosphate buffer is the most commonly used.

It is now recognized that the eye easily tolerates solutions with sodium chloride equivalents ranging from 0.7% to 2%. Therefore if the ophthalmic solution has about a 0.9% sodium equivalent, as in 2% boric acid or 4% pilocarpine, no adjustment to effect isotonicity is required. In cases in which the further concentration of the drug exceeds 5%, sterile water should be used as the diluent, since the solution is already hypertonic. Although hypertonic drops are rapidly diluted by tears, it is probably desirable to achieve isotonicity in a physiologically buffered solution for certain drugs in order to reduce discomfort caused by instillation. This is true notably of pilocarpine.

pH

In most instances the pH of ophthalmic solutions is of little importance. Since the tears rapidly neutralize the small effect of the unbuffered drug, the use of buffered solutions is generally unnecessary to control pH. It should be pointed out that increasing the pH of alkaloid drugs favors penetration of the lipid barrier of the cornea but that increasing the pH decreases solubility and stability of the alkaloid substances. Certain other drug solutions, such as the sulfonamides and fluorescein sodium, remain stable only at a pH slightly above 7. (See discussions of stability and drug penetration.)

Most ophthalmic solutions with pH values varying from 3.5 to 10.5 are well tolerated by the eye. However, unbuffered solutions of pilocarpine hydrochloride, 2% and higher, are quite irritating to the eye because of their acidity. Consequently, they are usually buffered to a pH of about 6.8

Stability

The stability of ophthalmic drugs in solution is largely dependent on the temperature and pH of the solutions and on the degree of dissociation of the drug. Alkaloids and other weak bases are much more stable at a pH of 5 than at a pH of 7. This is related to the proportion of the drug that exists in the less stable undissociated form at a given pH. With decreasing pH, dissociation of the drug increases, and therefore stability increases. Decomposition of the drug occurs much more rapidly at the elevated temperatures encountered in autoclaving than at room temperature. The rate of decomposition with autoclaving is much less if the pH is 5 than if it is 6.8. Therefore the general use of 2% boric acid solution (pH 4.7) as the vehicle, slightly modified by an added drug, is desirable to ensure stability, particularly if the solution is to be autoclaved. The exception to this rule is the preparation of fluorescein sodium and sulfonamide eye solutions, since these drugs are unstable at a pH of 5 (Table 1).

Chemical deterioration producing pharmacological inactivity is characteristic of certain ophthalmic preparations. Epinephrine solutions and, to a lesser extent, phenylephrine hydrochloride (Neo-Synephrine) oxidize in the presence of air, with resultant loss of activity. Solutions of most antibiotics lose their antimicrobial effect at room temperature within a few days after preparation. Isofluorophate (DFP), which is dispensed in anhydrous peanut oil, rapidly hydrolyzes

Table 1. Stability of selected ophthalmic drugs (time for 50% decomposition)*

Drug	pH 5.0		pH 6.8	
	25° C	120° C	25° C	120° C
Procaine and tetracaine	19 yr	36 hr	—	10 min
Atropine	130 yr	60 hr	2 yr	1 yr
Pilocarpine	S†	>24 hr	66 days	34 min
Physostigmine	S	~1 hr‡	6 mo	<10 min
Phenylephrine	S	>2 hr	?	?
Chlorobutanol	40 yr	~2.5 hr	1 yr	<5 min
Homatropine	14 yr	10 hr	0.4 yr	<10 min

*From Riegelman, S., and Sorby, D. L.: EENT preparations. In Martin, E. W., editor: Husa's pharmaceutical dispensing, ed. 6, Easton, Pa., 1966, Mack Publishing Co.
†S, several years.
‡When properly buffered, methylamine is formed during the hydrolysis. It shifts the pH to more alkaline values and thereby increases the rate of hydrolysis.

on exposure to water and becomes inactive. Physostigmine solutions undergo partial oxidizations and develop a pink color. However, this partial breakdown to rubreserine does not materially interfere with the pharmacological action of physostigmine. The addition of sodium bisulfite will inhibit the formation of the "pink" rubreserine.

Sterility

Complete sterility of ophthalmic medications can be achieved by autoclaving. Whenever possible, drugs to be placed in a traumatized or "surgical" eye should be so treated. Filtration to remove bacteria is another effective method of sterilizing ophthalmic solutions. Although widely advocated in the past, this method is now less popular because the technique is time consuming and subject to chemical contamination.

Once the dispensing container is opened, the entire contents may become contaminated. Therefore single-dose dispensers are recommended for use in the "surgical" or traumatized eye. The ever-present danger of contamination of fluorescein sodium solutions with *Pseudomonas* may be avoided by the use of fluorescein-impregnated filter paper strips.

Preservatives should not be used for single-dose solutions because they may cause severe irritation. They should be employed only in multiple-dose solutions, which tend to become contaminated in time. Among the widely used preservatives are benzalkonium (Zephiran) chloride, chlorobutanol, polymyxin B sulfate, organic mercurials, phenols, and substituted alcohols.

PREPARATION OF OPHTHALMIC OINTMENTS

Preparation of ophthalmic ointment does not present the same problems as does preparation of ophthalmic solutions.

The active ingredient for an ophthalmic ointment is mixed in a bland, nonirritating base. In such a medium the drug does not ionize readily, and consequently, tonicity and pH are not factors in stability. A petrolatum base is most commonly used. Water-soluble bases are suitable for preparing some medications, but they cannot be used for any of the antibiotics, since these drugs rapidly lose their effect in an aqueous medium.

In past years little attention was given to the problem of sterility in the preparation of ophthalmic ointments. Although microorganisms do not multiply significantly or spread in ointments, they can survive. Several studies have demonstrated a significant incidence of contamination of ophthalmic ointments. In the past few years considerably more attention has been given to the sterile preparation of ophthalmic ointments. Additionally, techniques of formulation with preservatives compatible with ointment preparation have been developed.

Ophthalmic ointments in general are much more stable than are ophthalmic solutions.

METHODS OF APPLICATION
Solutions for topical application

Solutions are the most commonly used preparations in the local treatment of eye disease. They have several advantages: They are easily instilled; they do not cause interference with vision; they cause few skin reactions; and they do not interfere with the mitosis of the corneal epithelium. Their chief disadvantage is that they do not remain in contact long with the eye; 90% of aqueous solutions are eliminated from the eye within the first minute or two of application. The contact time of drops with the external surface of the eye is dependent on several factors: the amount of tearing and blinking, degree of conjunctival injection, intactness of corneal surface, and viscosity of the medication. More rapid elimination of the medication occurs with increased tearing and blinking. Conjunctival hyperemia increases the absorption of the drug. The medication may be retained longer if surface defects are present.

Aqueous solutions are still commonly used, particularly as presurgical preparations and in the dispensing of topical anesthetics. Aqueous methylcellulose solutions are now commonly prescribed. The addition of methylcellulose to water increases the viscosity of the solution and, consequently, the contact time of the drug with the eye. Methylcellulose solutions can be autoclaved. Although the methylcellulose becomes solidified at high temperatures, the mass can be dispersed by agitation as the solution approaches room temperature. Polyvinyl alcohol in a 1.4% concentration, also now employed as an ophthalmic vehicle, increases contact time of the ophthalmic medication and is easily sterilized. Agents such as polyvinylpyrrolidone, gelatin, and dextrans have been employed in ophthalmic solutions to simulate the physiological effects of mucins usually found in the tear film. It is now believed that mucus adsorbs on the epithelium of the cornea, forming a hydrophilic surface and permitting even spread of the tear film on the corneal surface.

Oily solutions are sometimes used. In the case of DFP, a hygroscopic drug, an oily solution is necessary to prevent inactivation of the drug by hydrolysis.

Ointments for topical application

Ointments have several advantages over solutions: They remain in contact with the eye much longer and thereby give a prolonged effect; they are usually quite comfortable upon initial instillation; there is less absorption into lacrimal passages; and ointments, particularly antibiotic carriers, are more stable than solutions. Disadvantages are that they produce a film in front of the eye and obstruct vision, they more frequently cause contact dermatitis reactions, and they may inhibit mitosis of the corneal epithelial cells.

Packs

Packs are sometimes used to give prolonged contact of a solution with the eye. A cotton pledget is saturated with an ophthalmic solution, and this pledget is inserted into the superior or inferior cul-de-sac. Packs are most commonly used to produce mydriasis. In this case the cotton pledget is saturated with epinephrine or phenylephrine solution.

Iontophoresis

Iontophoresis has the advantage of achieving drug penetration despite the presence of the epithelial barrier. In this instance the drug solution is kept in contact with the cornea in an eyecup bearing an electrode, and diffusion of the drug into the eye is effected by application of a difference of potential. The charge of the electrode must be the same as that of the drug in solution. Cathode iontophoresis (negative pole on the cornea) is used to drive drugs that are negative in solution, such as penicillins and cephalosporins, into the eye. Anode iontophoresis (positive pole on the cornea) is used to force drugs (such as gentamicin, kanamycin, and streptomycin) that have a positive change in solution through the cornea.

Subconjunctival (sub-Tenon's) injections

Subconjunctival injections are frequently used to introduce medications that cannot be absorbed by topical administration into the anterior portion of the eye. The drug is injected underneath the conjunctiva or Tenon's capsule and is then able to pass through the limbus and sclera and into the eye by the process of simple diffusion. Subconjunctival injections of antibiotics are often administered for severe infections of the anterior portion of the eye, including corneal ulcers and infected filtering blebs. They are also used as supplemental therapy with systemic administration of antibiotics for treatment of bacterial endophthalmitis. Subconjunctival injections of mydriatics and cycloplegics are also used to achieve good pupillary dilatation. Corticosteroids are given for the treatment of severe acute anterior uveitis and for the treatment of chronic cyclitis.

Retrobulbar injections

Anesthetic solutions are frequently administered by a retrobulbar injection technique. The needle is usually passed beneath the globe and positioned inside the muscle cone after insertion either through the lower eyelid or inside the eyelid through the lower conjunctival cul-de-sac. Repository corticosteroids may be injected retrobulbarly for the treatment of severe inflammatory disease of the posterior segment of the globe. Other medications such as vasodilators and autonomic nervous system agents were formerly injected in a retrobulbar fashion, but this technique is now seldom employed.

Periocular injections

Periocular, as the term suggests, refers to the placement of medication alongside the globe; actually the term paraocular might be more appropriate. Regardless, the term periocular is somewhat vague and overlaps with the terms subconjunctival, sub-Tenon's, and retrobulbar. Periocular injections may be made through the skin or conjunctiva. The placement of medication may be anterior to, posterior to, or at the region of the equator and may be located under the conjunctiva or beneath or outside Tenon's capsule. Periocular injections of corticosteroids and antibiotics are most often used.

Intracameral and intravitreal injections

Antibiotics and chemotherapeutic agents may be injected directly into the anterior chamber (intracameral) or into the vitreous cavity in cases of severe infection (Chapter 14). Only very low concentrations of small amounts (0.1 to 0.2 ml) should be injected since high concentrations of drugs can be quite toxic to the corneal endothelium, lens, and retina. Silicone solutions were formerly injected into the vitreous cavity as treatment supplemental to surgical procedures in certain cases of retinal detachment, but this practice has largely been abandoned because of damage to the lens and cornea. Certain gases such as sulfur hexafluoride have also been injected into the vitreous cavity as an aid to surgical treatment of certain retinal detachments.

Sustained-release devices

In recent years attempts have been made to develop drug delivery systems that permit a slow release of medication. Insertion into the eye of a hydrophilic contact lens soaked in 0.5% to 1% pilocarpine exerts a significant effect on intraocular pressure for 24 hours. A major portion of the effect, however, may be a pulsed delivery of the medication, since half of the medication escapes from the lens in 30 minutes.

A conjunctival insert (Ocusert) has been developed as a method for constant rate release of a drug over a prolonged period. The Ocusert system is a flexible elliptical unit consisting of a drug-containing core and outer copolymer membranes through which the drug diffuses at a constant rate. The rate of drug diffusion is controlled by the polymer composition, the membrane thickness, and the solubility of the drug. The devices are sterile and contain no preservatives. Two pilocarpine-Ocusert systems are now available. One is the Pilo-20, which is programmed to release 20 μg/hr for 1 week, and the other, Pilo-40, releases pilocarpine at the rate of 40 μg/hr for 1 week. See Chapter 13 for clinical use of these units in the treatment of glaucoma. Other Ocusert systems containing corticosteroids and tetracyclines are under investigation.

Irrigations

Continuous irrigation therapy may be desirable as in the treatment of *Pseudomonas* corneal ulcers, severe chemical burns of the cornea, and advanced keratitis sicca. The medication may be delivered through a catheter inserted through a stab wound incision in the upper lid into the conjunctival cul-de-sac. Continuous flow of medication also may be delivered through a scleral contact lens with attached plastic tubing (Medi-Flow lens). Miniaturized infusion pumps have also been used for continuous delivery of a drug solution via plastic tubes attached to spectacle frames.

AGENTS EMPLOYED FOR SPECIAL PHYSICOCHEMICAL EFFECTS
Bandage soft contact lenses

Soft contact lenses are frequently employed for their mechanical splinting or bandaging effect. Two types of soft contact lenses are employed for this purpose, the Sofcon lens manufactured by Warner-Lambert and the Plano-T lens produced by Bausch and Lomb. The fitting of a soft contact lens for therapeutic purposes is often on an empirical, trial-and-error basis. Frequently it is not possible to get an accurate K reading. If the base refraction is known, either from testing or from old spectacles, a more refined selection of the lens may be made after allowances for vertex distance and conversion of the refraction to spherical equivalents are completed. If K readings can be obtained, charts provided by the manufacturer can be utilized for an indication of what lens should be tried initially. Subsequently, refinement of the lens dimensions and power can be made after a trial wearing period. The soft lenses used for bandaging and other therapeutic purposes should be fitted quite tightly. One can ascertain the desirable fit of the lens by having the patient look from side to side and up and down and by observing lens movement. If the lens moves more than 1 mm, a tighter, flatter lens should be tried.

Bandage lenses have proved useful in some cases of bullous keratopathy. Soft lenses may provide relief of pain to patients with bullous keratopathy apparently by splinting the cornea and preventing bullae from rupturing. Sometimes they may improve patients' vision by overcoming the irregular astigmatism produced by epithelial edema. The lenses do not seem to improve stromal corneal edema. Five percent sodium chloride is used along with the lenses to reduce corneal edema.

Soft lenses are also used in the treatment of extremely dry eyes; normal or half-normal saline is instilled frequently to keep the lenses moist. Soft lenses are somtimes employed to promote epithelialization of the cornea either in recurrent corneal erosions or for chronic corneal ulcers; appropriate antimicrobial therapy should be used concurrently. The lenses have also been of value for the treatment of Stevens-Johnson's disease and cicatricial pemphigus. Therapeutic soft lenses have been used to treat small (less than 5 mm) corneal lacerations if the edges of the wound are in good apposition. They have been employed in the treatment of leaking surgical wounds.

The reader is referred to Chapter 11 on treatment of corneal diseases for additional information regarding uses of therapeutic soft contact lenses.

Hypertonic substances

Glycerin is used for the purpose of clearing the cornea for ophthalmoscopic examination. Hypertonic sodium chloride solutions and ointments containing 2% to 8% sodium chloride, 40% glucose, 40% sodium ascorbate, 50% isosorbide, albumin solutions, and cellulose gums are sometimes used in the treatment of corneal epithelial edema.

Lubricants

Ointments and 1% to 2% methylcellulose solutions and 1.4% polyvinyl alcohol solutions are used to lubricate the eye to prevent exposure keratitis. They are most commonly used in patients suffering from seventh nerve palsies and in unconscious patients with exposed globes. Silicone solutions are used as lubricants in the sockets of patients wearing ocular prostheses.

Epitheliolytes

Iodine and ether solutions are used to remove the corneal epithelium in corneal ulceration, particularly that caused by the herpes simplex virus. Trichloroacetic acid solutions are sometimes used to coagulate the epithelial proteins and to cause resultant epithelial slough.

Tattooing

Tattooing of corneal leucomas for cosmetic purposes is performed with gold and platinum salts. The epithelium is removed; the salts are introduced into the anterior stromal portion of the cornea with a fine needle and then are oxidized to produce a black color that conceals the unsightly corneal leukoma. Various mineral pigments may also be used for tattooing.

Staining agents

Fluorescein and merbromin solutions are dyes that are used to show corneal epithelial defects in injured or ulcerated eyes. Rose bengal solution stains devitalized epithelium and is particularly useful in demonstrating conjunctival and corneal changes in Sjögren's syndrome.

Chelating agents

Solutions of ethylenediamine tetra-acetate sodium (EDTA, disodium edetate, Versenate sodium) may be used to remove the calcium deposited in Bowman's membrane in band keratopathies. In this treatment the epithelium is removed, and the EDTA solution is kept in contact with the cornea for several minutes by the application of an eyecup containing the drug. Alternatively a Weck Cel sponge soaked in EDTA may be applied to the cornea or the solution of EDTA can be delivered with continuous irrigation for 15 minutes (see EDTA in Section 2). The calcium ions become incorporated into the inner-ring structure of the molecule. Solutions of EDTA have also been suggested as treatment for blepharitis.

Irritants

In the past certain irritants (ethylmorphine, desiccated thyroid solution, and so forth) have been used in the eye with the hope that they would produce increased vascularity. The value of such agents is quite doubtful.

DRUG PENETRATION
Topically applied drugs

To penetrate the globe when applied topically, drugs must have both fat-soluble and water-soluble characteristics. The epithelium of the cornea contains sufficient lipid material to present a barrier to all medications that are not fat soluble. The alkaloids, the corticosteroid solutions and suspensions, and many topical anesthetics are capable of entering the eye by topical administration. Other agents, including fluorescein and the sulfonamide drugs, cross the cornea in very small quantities. Most antibiotics that are topically applied do not enter the eye in therapeutic concentrations.

The mechanism of the penetration of the alkaloid drugs has been fairly well worked out. The penetration of these drugs into the eye is dependent on their dissociation constant, which in turn is dependent on the pH of the solution. As a drug undergoes dissociation (ionization), it increases in water solubility. Conversely, with decreasing dissociation, water solubility decreases and lipid solubility increases. The alkaloid drug in solution is capable of remaining both in the dissociated (ionized) and the undissociated (nonionized) forms, thus possessing both water and fat solubility properties. The higher the pH the greater will be the undissociated fraction and resulting penetrability of the lipid barrier of the cornea.

It must be recognized that alkaloid drugs exhibit decreased solubility and stability with increasing pH. With decreasing pH the proportion of the drug in the dissociated form increases, with a resulting decrease in penetrability of the lipid barrier.

$$RN \cdot HCl \rightleftarrows RNH^+ + Cl^- \rightleftarrows R_3N + H^+ + Cl^-$$
$$\text{Alkaloid} \rightleftarrows \text{Dissociated form} \rightleftarrows \text{Undissociated form}$$

Certain drugs may also penetrate the eye better if there is injury to the epithelium and, consequently, an alteration of the lipid barrier. To allow the penetration of drugs this barrier may be destroyed by the use of a wetting agent such as benzalkonium or by iontophoresis. There also appears to be a relationship between chemical structure of a drug and its corneal penetration. Nonpolar drugs are fat soluble, and polar drugs are fat insoluble.

Although under special circumstances topically applied medications have affected the posterior part of the eye (for example, macular edema after topical epinephrine therapy in aphakia), topically administered drugs reach therapeutic concentrations in the eye only as far back as the ciliary body. Therefore they should be used only for inflammation of the anterior part of the eye. For example, the use of topically administered corticosteroid preparations is indicated only for inflammations of the anterior portion of the uveal tract.

Subconjunctival injections

Certain agents can penetrate the eye if administered subconjunctivally. Drugs administered in the bulbar subconjunctival space probably cross through the limbus or sclera and enter into the cornea and globe by simple diffusion. This method of treatment is used in the management of corneal ulcers and anterior segment infections and inflammations. It would be quite possible to get the medication back farther if the drug were injected underneath Tenon's capsule in the more posterior portions of the eye.

Retrobulbar injections

Drugs administered by retrobulbar injection may enter the globe by a process of diffusion. It is also possible that the drug is picked up by the vessels and carried into the eye. Occasionally, retrobulbar injections of respository corticosteroids are used to treat posterior segment intraocular disease. However, retrobulbar injections usually are not given for the purpose of getting medications into the globe but, rather, to affect the nerves and other structures in the retrobulbar space.

Systemic administration

The eyelids and orbital structures are highly vascular. Therefore almost any drug given by the systemic route reaches these structures in good concentration. The drug enters the optic nerve, the retina, and the uveal tract because of the high vascularity of these structures, but unless it contains lipid-soluble properties it will not cross the blood-aqueous barrier into the anterior chamber. Some drugs, however, may enter the anterior chamber because they are of sufficiently small molecular size to pass through the pore capacities of the ciliary epithelium. However, they often reach the anterior chamber in less than therapeutic concentrations. Hyperosmotic agents such as glycerol and mannitol and, to a lesser extent, urea do not cross the blood-aqueous barrier and therefore are used to lower intraocular pressure; an osmotic gradient is produced in which the blood is hypertonic to the intraocular fluids.

In the normal eye most systemically administered antibiotics do not reach the anterior chamber in therapeutically significant concentrations because they do not have sufficient lipid-soluble properties and because of their molecular size. Another consideration is the degree of plasma protein binding; the greater the plasma protein binding of a drug the less it will penetrate the blood-aqueous barrier. Chloramphenicol has high lipid solubility and therefore gives effective concentration in the aqueous humor. Penicillin has a low degree of lipid solubility, and therefore very high doses must be given systemically to obtain minimal effective levels in the anterior chamber of the eye.

In the inflamed eye the blood-aqueous barrier is not intact, and therefore many antibiotic solutions reach the anterior chamber in therapeutic concentrations when given intravenously in large doses. Human studies show adequate penetration of many new antibiotics into secondary aqueous humor.

COMPLICATIONS OF DRUG THERAPY

The two major groups of complications of drug therapy are drug hypersensitivity, or allergy, and "toxic reaction."

By definition, a hypersensitivity reaction is restricted to an unexpected response of the patient to a drug. These reactions may manifest themselves in various ways, most commonly various forms of skin eruptions, but they may also produce blood dyscrasias, drug fever, serum sickness, bronchial asthma, hepatitis, and anaphylactic shock.

Toxic reactions include a variety of undesirable effects of a drug. They differ from hypersensitivity reactions in that they are not pharmacologically unexpected. They may occur in some patients after unusually small doses, but the effects are characteristic of the medication.

Ocular therapeutic agents may produce both hypersensitivity and toxic reactions. The particular side effects of the various drugs are reviewed in the section on therapeutic agents.

Complications of local treatment

The most common complication of local treatment in ophthalmology is contact dermatitis, usually localized to the mucous membrane and skin surfaces of the immediate tissues of the treated eye. Atropine, penicillin, sulfathiazole, and neomycin are agents that most commonly cause contact dermatitis. Follicular hypertrophy in the conjunctiva may occur from prolonged use of local agents such as pilocarpine or eserine. Prolonged use of silver solutions may produce argyrosis of the conjunctiva, characterized by brown discoloration. Long-term use of epinephrine may produce melaninlike deposits in the conjunctiva and cornea that may be mistaken for foreign bodies, nevi, or melanomas. Corneal epithelial changes are seen after topical administration of the anesthetics or 10% phenylephrine. Certain cholinesterase inhibitors such as DFP and echothiophate iodide may cause areas of hypertrophy of the pigment epithelium of the iris, which present at the pupillary margin as pigmentary cysts. The use of 2.5% phenylephrine as a diluent prevents iris cyst formation with echothiophate iodide therapy; intermittent use of epinephrine prevents cyst formation with DFP treatment. Prolonged use of some topically applied ophthalmic medications such as eserine, DFP, pilocarpine, or epinephrine may result in occlusion of the lacrimal puncta.

There may be systemic absorption of the topically applied drug by way of the lacrimal passages and mucous membranes in sufficient concentration to cause symptoms. An example of this is the flush seen after atropine is used for purposes of cycloplegia. Tachycardia has been reported after packs saturated with 10% phenylephrine had been inserted into the conjunctival cul-de-sac and after topical epinephrine therapy. Topical application of cyclopentolate (Cyclogyl) may produce symptoms of central nervous system toxicity such as confusion, ataxia, dysarthria, and personality changes. These symptoms are much more common when the 2% solution is used. Solutions for topical administration of neostigmine (Prostigmin), methacholine (Mecholyl), and echothiophate iodide have caused excessive parasympathomimetic stimulation and symptoms of nausea, vomiting, gastrointestinal cramping, and sweating. Plasma pseudo-cholinesterase levels are depressed in patients receiving topical echothiophate iodide and demecarium therapy. The administration of succinylcholine during general anesthesia to patients with depressed pseudocholinesterase may produce prolonged apnea.

The topical administration of corticosteroids, particularly those with good intraocular penetrability and high anti-inflammatory activity, such as dexamethasone and betamethasone, for a period of 3 to 4 weeks produces a significant rise in intraocular pressure in approximately one third of the patients. Topical corticosteroids and echothiophate iodide have also been thought to be responsible for subcapsular lens opacities.

Complications of systemic therapy

Medications administered systemically for eye disease may, of course, cause various generalized adverse effects such as hypersensitivity reactions, blood dyscrasias, changes in the gastrointestinal flora, renal calculi, and perforated ulcers.

Ocular complications may also occur from the systemic administration of medications. Pupillary dilatation and cycloplegia may follow the use of certain belladonna and atropinelike drugs given as preanesthetic agents or for treatment of peptic ulcer, Parkinson's disease, or other maladies. Corneal epithelial edema, opacities of the corneal epithelium and subepithelium, retinal edema and pigmentation, and optic atrophy may occur after chloroquine therapy. Long-term gold therapy for arthritis may produce deposition of the metal in the deep layers of the cornea. Indomethacin has been reported to cause punctate opacities in the corneal epithelium and fine pigmentary changes in the macula. Loss of accommodation may occur after the use of acetazolamide and other sulfonamide derivatives. Prolonged use of the corticosteroids may produce posterior subcapsular lens opacities and ocular hypertension (glaucoma). Conjunctival and corneal scarring has been reported with several drugs including phenylbutazone, practolol, oxyprenolol, and sulfonamides.

Phenothiazine tranquilizers may produce oculogyric crises and blurred vision. Long-term chlorpromazine (Thorazine) may produce golden brown pigmentation of the bulbar conjunctiva in the exposed interpalpebral area, light golden brown dust opacities in the cornea and anterior part of the lens, and anterior stellate cataracts. Thioridazine (Mellaril) may produce pigmentary retinopathy when given in large doses.

Optic neuritis has been produced by countless drugs. Antibiotics and chemotherapeutic agents such as chloramphenicol, streptomycin, ethambutol, and isoniazid have produced optic neuritis and optic nerve atrophy.

Transient visual impairment, including disturbance of form and color vision, may result from an overdosage of various medications. Digitalis produces a disturbance in color vision, most commonly xanthopsia, or yellow color vision; the drug may also cause blurred vision and central scotomas. Chronic bromide intoxication may produce blurred color and form vision and diplopia. Trimethadione (Tridione) may induce photophobia and dazzled vision. Barbiturates and meprobamate can cause blurred vision and diplopia. Blurred vision has been associated rarely with the chlorothiazide (Diuril) and hydrochlorothiazide (Hydrodiuril). Acute loss of vision occurs with quinine overdosage.

Form and color visual hallucinations are a common effect of *d*-lysergic acid diethylamide (LSD-25). Phenytoin (Dilantin) may produce diplopia, nystagmus, and visual hallucinations. The heavy metals, particularly the arsenicals, may cause optic atrophy.

Oral contraceptives have been indicted as a cause of ocular migraine and retinal vascular disorders; this relationship has not been fully established. Quinine therapy can result in retinal damage and secondary vascular disturbances. Excessive doses of vitamin D can produce calcium deposits in the cornea and conjunctiva, and excessive intake of vitamin A may result in papilledema and retinal hemorrhages.

REFERENCES

Barza, M., and Baum, J.: Penetration of ocular compartments by penicillins, Surv. Ophthalmol. **18:**71, 1973.

Chin, N. B., Gold, A. A., and Breinin, G. A.: Iris cysts and miotics, Arch. Ophthalmol. **71:** 611, 1964.

Dohlman, C. H., Doane, M. G., and Reshmi, C. S.: Mobile infusion pumps for continuous delivery of fluid and therapeutic agents to the eye, Ann. Ophthalmol. 3:126, 1971.

Ellis, P. P., editor: Side effects of drugs in ophthalmology, Int. Ophthalmol. Clin. 11, 1971.

Ellis, P. P.: Subconjunctival therapy. In Leopold, I. H., editor: Symposium on ocular therapy, vol. 5, St. Louis, 1972, The C. V. Mosby Co.

Fraunfelder, F. T., and Hanna, C.: Ophthalmic drug delivery systems, Surv. Ophthalmol. **18:** 292, 1974.

Gasset, A. R., and Kaufman, H. E.: Therapeutic uses of hydrophilic contact lenses, Am. J. Ophthalmol. **69:**252, 1970.

Grant, W. M.: Toxicology of the eye, ed. 2, Springfield, Ill., 1974, Charles C Thomas, Publisher.

Haddad, M.: Adverse effects of ophthalmic agents in pediatrics. In Leopold, I. H., editor: Ocular therapy, complications and management, vol. 2, St. Louis, 1966, The C. V. Mosby Co.

Hansten, P. D.: Drug interactions, ed. 3, Philadelphia, 1975, Lea & Febiger.

Hardy, R. G., Jr., and Paterson, C. A.: Ocular penetration of ^{14}C-labeled chloramphenicol following subconjunctival or sub-Tenon's injection, Am. J. Ophthalmol. **71:**1307, 1971.

Kaufman, H. E., and others: The medical use of soft contact lenses. Trans. Am. Acad. Ophthalmol. Otolaryngol. **75:**361, 1971.

Kennedy, R. E., Roca, P. D., and Landers, P. H.: Atypical band keratopathy in glaucoma patients, Trans. Am. Ophthalmol. Soc. 69:124, 1971.

Lemp, M. A., Dohlman, C. H., and Kuwabara, T.: Dry eye secondary to mucus deficiency, Trans. Am. Acad. Ophthalmol. Otolaryngol. **75:**1223, 1971.

Leopold, I. H., and Gordon, B.: Drug interactions. In Leopold, I. H., editor: Symposium on ocular therapy, vol. 6, St. Louis, 1973, The C. V. Mosby Co.

Morgan, L. B.: Plastic scleral lens help to end pain in injured eyes and promote healing, J.A.M.A. **214**:835, 1970.

Moses, R. A.: Adler's physiology of the eye: clinical application, ed. 6, St. Louis, 1975, The C. V. Mosby Co.

Mullen, W., Shepherd, W., and Labovitz, J.: Ophthalmic preservatives and vehicles, Surv. Ophthalmol. **17**:469, 1973.

Norn, M. S.: Role of vehicle in local treatment of eye, Acta Ophthalmol. **42**:727, 1964.

Podos, S. M., and others: Pilocarpine therapy with soft contact lenses, Am. J. Ophthalmol. **73**:336, 1972.

Richardson, K. T.: Ocular pharmacodynamics. In Symposium on ocular pharmacology and therapeutics, Transactions of the New Orleans Academy of Ophthalmology, St. Louis, 1970, The C. V. Mosby Co.

Richardson, K. T.: Ocular microtherapy: membrane-controlled drug delivery, Arch. Ophthalmol. **93**:74, 1975.

Riegelman, S., and Sorby, D. L.: EENT preparations. In Martin, E. W., editor: Husa's pharmaceutical dispensing, ed. 6, Easton, Pa., 1966, Mack Publishing Co.

Riegelman, S., and Vaughan, D. G.: A rational basis for the preparation of ophthalmic solutions, part I, J. Am. Pharm. Assoc. **19**:474, 1958; part II, J. Am. Pharm. Assoc. **19**:537, 1958; part III, J. Am. Pharm. Assoc. **19**:665, 1958.

CHAPTER 2

Principles of cortisone and ACTH therapy

The development of cortisone and ACTH, with their subsequent use in the treatment of certain diseases of the eye, has undoubtedly been the greatest recent single contribution to ophthalmology. Corticosteroids have been employed in the treatment of ocular disease for over 25 years. In no other field of medicine are more dramatic effects obtained with these hormones than in the treatment of inflammatory and allergic ocular disorders. However, as with other potent drugs, corticosteroid therapy may produce many undesirable side effects. Therefore it is important for the physician to assess the potential benefits of treatment against the likelihood of harmful results for each patient being considered as a candidate for corticosteroid therapy.

Corticosteroids produce both physiological and pharmacological effects, depending on the dosage and the health of the individual. Normally, 10 to 25 mg of hydrocortisone (cortisol) is secreted daily; the amount varies somewhat with the health and activities of the individual. Under stressful conditions the adrenal gland secretes much larger amounts of cortisol, up to 300 mg daily. Many diversified physiological functions are maintained by this hormone. A pharmacological effect will be achieved when the physiological dose is exceeded. In the normal subject any dose of corticoid will have a pharmacological effect. In patients with adrenal insufficiency (which may result from corticoid therapy), pharmacological effects are achieved only with doses larger than necessary to preserve homeostasis.

PHYSIOLOGY

Adrenal cortical function is essential for life. Removal of the adrenal glands results in death within a short time because of disturbed fluid and electrolyte metabolism unless substitute hormone therapy is given. Adrenal insufficiency results in excessive loss of sodium and chloride in the urine and increased tubular reabsorption of potassium. With the increased salt loss resulting from failure of tubular reabsorption of sodium, there is an increased loss of water and a decreased blood volume. Such decreased blood volume leads to hypotension. In addition, adrenal insufficiency causes hypoglycemia, muscle weakness, gastrointestinal disturbances, leukopenia, eosinophilia, lowered basal metabolism, increased skin pigmentation, and retention of nitrogenous products.

Many hormones have been isolated from the adrenal gland, and some of these have been synthesized. Analogues of the naturally occurring hormones that possess high degrees of desirable therapeutic effects have been developed. All adrenal hormones are steroids and closely resemble the estrogens and androgens in structure. The corticoadrenal hormones are classified into three groups according to their predominant action:

1. The mineralocorticoids, among which are desoxycorticosterone, aldosterone, and fludrocortisone, are chiefly concerned with fluid and electrolyte metabolism. Desoxycorticosterone has no anti-inflammatory activity, and aldosterone has little anti-inflammatory activity. Fludrocortisone has significant anti-inflammatory action, but because of its high sodium retention activity it is not used for therapy of inflammatory diseases. The mineralocorticoids are used for the treatment of adrenal insufficiency, often in combination with the glucocorticoids.

2. The glucocorticoids have their predominent effect on the metabolism of carbohydrate, fat, and protein. They also possess anti-inflammatory effects, as well as many other actions. Examples of glucocorticoids are the naturally occurring hydrocortisone and cortisone and the synthetic steroids—prednisolone, methylprednisolone, triamcinolone, betamethasone, and dexamethasone.

3. The androgens are concerned with the development of sex characteristics, but their general physiological role is not understood.

Of these groups of adrenal hormones, the glucocorticoids are of greatest interest to the ophthalmologist.

Anabolic steroids, which are similar to androgens, have been suggested for the treatment of diabetic retinopathy, but this therapy has not proved to be beneficial. Aldosterone has been reported to support aqueous humor formation, and aldosterone inhibitors (spironolactone [Aldactone]) have been tried without much success as therapeutic agents to lower intraocular pressure.

Normal adrenal cortex function is controlled by hypothalamic-pituitary-adrenal interactions. Cortisol secretion by the adrenal is governed by the blood concentration of ACTH, the adrenocorticotropic hormone of the anterior pituitary gland. The secretion of ACTH is, in turn, regulated by the corticotropic release factor (CRF), which is a product of the anterior hypothalamus and is blood borne to the anterior pituitary gland. Hypophysectomy results in adrenal atrophy, whereas continued ACTH treatment causes adrenal hypertrophy. The output of ACTH is largely governed by the blood level of cortisol. With elevated blood levels of cortisol the ACTH output is decreased, whereas with decreased blood levels of adrenal steroids the output of ACTH is increased. This feedback mechanism does not completely explain ACTH regulation, because in certain conditions elevated cortisol levels can coexist with a continued high output of ACTH. Stress situations and thyroxin and estrogen hormones also play a role in ACTH production. The hypothalamic-pituitary-adrenal axis is not appreciably affected by mineralocorticoids or androgens.

The metabolism of steroids occurs primarily in the liver. The steroid molecule is conjugated to form a glucuronide that is water soluble. This permits urinary excretion of the previously insoluble steroid molecule. These chemical transformations do not produce any pharmacological effects by themselves. The rate of metabolic removal may be altered in certain disease states such as hypothyroidism, where clearance of steroids is slowed and the pharmacological effect prolonged.

EFFECTS OF GLUCOCORTICOIDS

Although the glucocorticoids are given by the ophthalmologist for their anti-inflammatory effect, they produce many other metabolic, physiological, and pharmacological effects. The mechanism of the anti-inflammatory effect remains unknown. However, there is evidence that corticosteroids potentiate vasoconstrictive effects of epinephrine, retard macrophage movement, stabilize membranes of lysosomes (packets of proteolytic enzymes in cytoplasm that may be released during inflammation), prevent release of kinins (one of the chemical mediators in inflammation), decrease chemotaxis of neutrophils, inhibit the mitotic activity of lymphocytes, reduce the number of circulating lymphocytes, and decrease antibody production. Whatever the precise mechanisms of action, it is quite certain that the usual inflammatory response—redness, swelling, capillary dilatation, exudation, cellular infiltration, fibroblastic proliferation, collagen deposition, and cicatrization—is inhibited. The inflammatory response is suppressed, whether it is caused by trauma, chemicals, or an immune phenomenon.

The mechanisms of metabolic actions of glucocorticoids are somewhat better understood. The steroid molecule is lipid soluble and therefore passes readily through cell membranes. Inside the cell membrane steroid combines with receptor protein in the cytosol. Subsequently this hormone receptor complex migrates into the cell nucleus, where it attaches to nuclear chromatin. As a result, gene activity is altered to produce new ribonucleic acid (RNA). This new RNA results in production of new cell proteins (enzymes) that regulate cellular activity such as maintenance of cell structure or replication. The glucocorticoids affect fat, protein, and carbohydrate metabolism. Gluconeogenesis, particularly from protein breakdown, is promoted, often with resulting hyperglycemia and glycosuria. Liver glycogen storage is increased. Peripheral oxidation of glucose is inhibited. Protein synthesis is decreased. Reduction in tissue fat usually occurs, particularly in the extremities, although increased deposition of fat may occur in the back of the neck, supraclavicular area, and face. Tubular reabsorption of sodium is increased, and reabsorption of potassium is decreased, thus leading to sodium retention and potassium excretion. The glucocorticoids induce negative nitrogen balance. Urinary excretion of creatine and uric acid is increased. The excretion of creatinine is unaltered. Lymphopenia and a decrease in the size of the lymph glands occur after glucocorticoid administration. There are several cardiovascular effects, including increased blood volume, exaggerated pressor effects of epinephrine and norepinephrine, and increased peripheral vascular resistance and hypertension. Clotting time of venous blood is decreased, and thromboembolic phenomena may result. ACTH secretion is inhibited, and the function of the adrenal gland is depressed. Thyroid function is inhibited. Wound healing is somewhat delayed. Skeletal muscle function is decreased, possibly from increased potassium loss and partially from altered protein metabolism. Central nervous system changes such as euphoria, psychoses, and alterations in the electroencephalographic pattern may result. Hypercorticism often produces an elevated mood, whereas hypocorticism most often produces depression. Variable suppression of antibody formation occurs. Increased secretion of gastric acid and pepsin occurs. A reduction in circulating eosinophils occurs, whereas there is a rise in red blood cells, platelets, and neutrophils.

Prolonged systemic use of the glucocorticoids may result in Cushing's syndrome, water and salt retention, mental disturbances, pseudotumor cerebri, hypertension, increased sweating, generalized weakness, wasting of skeletal muscle, osteoporosis with fractures, thrombophlebitis, ecchymosis, delayed wound healing, menstrual irregularities, acne, increased blood glucose levels, hypopotassemia, adrenal insufficiency, peptic ulcer, decreased renal function, negative nitrogen balance, or decreased resistance to infection and retardation of growth in children. Ocular effects include decreased resistance to infections (especially to virus and fungus infections), possible delayed wound healing, papilledema, edematous eyelids, ptosis, mydriasis, exophthalmos, and cataract formation. Cataract formation appears dependent on the total and daily dosage of steroids, the age of the patient, and the basic underlying disease for which the drug was administered.

Increased intraocular pressure (glaucoma) may occur after topical corticosteroid therapy. The glaucoma is more likely to occur with preparations possessing good intraocular penetration and high anti-inflammatory activity (such as 0.1% betamethasone or dexamethasone); however, glaucoma may occur with weaker corticosteroid preparations in a small number of patients. Occasionally glaucoma is observed after systemic therapy. Glaucoma may also occur after subconjunctival administration of corticosteroids. The rise in pressure results from decreased aqueous outflow, and the glaucoma has features of the open-angle variety. A significant rise (6 mm Hg or greater) in intraocular pressure occurs in one third of the patients treated with topical 0.1% betamethasone and dexamethasone for 3 to 4 weeks. Approximately 10% of patients develop an elevation of pressure greater than 12 mm Hg. Such patients have open-angle glaucoma or an inherited tendency to develop this disease. It should be pointed out that some patients may develop glaucoma within a week if potent topical steroids are used eight to twelve times a day. Furthermore, some patients will develop glaucoma only after 5 or 6 weeks of topical steroid therapy.

Other side effects to topical steroid therapy besides glaucoma include increased incidence and exaggeration of corneal infections (herpes simplex, fungal, and bacterial), delayed healing, ptosis, and mydriasis. With prolonged high dosage, cataracts and systemic effects may occur. Mild iritis has occurred in a few patients treated with topical steroids; many of these patients have had a positive serologic test for syphilis.

Except for the salt-retaining effects, all glucocorticoid preparations have the same side effects when used in the same relative anti-inflammatory doses. The more recently developed glucocorticoids (methylprednisolone, triamcinolone, and dexamethasone) are much more potent in their anti-inflammatory effects per weight unit than are cortisone and hydrocortisone. Fortunately, the salt-retaining activity per weight unit does not parallel the anti-inflammatory activity. The result is that salt and water retention are much less likely to occur at effective therapeutic doses with the newer corticoids than will cortisone or hydrocortisone. All corticosteroid preparations appear to have similar effects on carbohydrate metabolism. Claims are also made that the likelihood of inducing peptic ulcer activity by steroid therapy is decreased with these newer compounds.

EFFECTS OF ACTH

The administration of ACTH produces essentially the same effects and toxic reactions as does the systemic administration of the glucocorticoids. For these effects to occur, however, there must be a normally functioning adrenal cortex. No beneficial anti-inflammatory effects have been attributed to ACTH, which itself is allergenic. Whereas glucocorticoids suppress adrenal function by suppressing endogenous ACTH secretion, ACTH administration stimulates the adrenal cortex. Since ACTH works indirectly through release of adrenal hormones, it is given parenterally rather than topically. ACTH produces secretion not only of hydrocortisone and cortisone but also of a large number of other adrenal corticosteroids, many of which have not been identified by structure or by physiological or pharmacological actions. ACTH is said to be more likely to cause hypertension and hirsutism than are the corticosteroids.

THERAPEUTIC USES IN OCULAR DISEASE

The glucocorticoids are effective against a large number of eye diseases, including the following:

Contact dermatitis of the eyelids and
    conjunctiva
Allergic blepharitis and conjunctivitis
Vernal conjunctivitis
Phlyctenular conjunctivitis and keratitis
Ocular pemphigus
Mucocutaneous conjunctival lesions
Acne rosacea keratitis
Insterstitial keratitis
Sympathetic ophthalmia
Herpes zoster
Episcleritis and scleritis
Pseudotumor of the orbit
Temporal arteritis (giant cell arteritis)
Sclerosing keratitis

Nonspecific keratitis
Certain chemical burns of the cornea
Superficial punctatate keratitis
Juvenile xanthogranuloma
Marginal (sensitivity) corneal ulcers
Disciform keratitis
Iritis and iridocyclitis
Most forms of posterior uveitis
Optic neuritis (various acute forms
    and dysthyroid types)
Immune reaction after keratoplasty
Progressive thyroid (malignant) exoph-
    thalmos
Neonatal hemangioma of eyelids

ADMINISTRATION AND DOSAGE

The therapeutic approach to the treatment of ocular disease with gluco-corticoids depends on the location and extent of the disease. For disorders of the eyelids, conjunctiva, cornea, and anterior segment of the globe, topical administration of the hormones is usually satisfactory. However, in severe forms of anterior uveitis, it may be desirable to supplement the local application with subconjunctival and systemic administration, as in the treatment of anterior sympathetic ophthalmia. For external inflammatory ocular disease it is advisable to employ agents that are unlikely to produce ocular hypertension (glaucoma) by virtue of their poorer penetration into the eye and less pronounced anti-inflammatory activity. Hydrocortisone and hydroxymesterone (medrysone) apparently do not produce the same degree of ocular hypertension as that of 0.1% betamethasone and dexamethasone but are sufficiently effective against most external inflammatory disorders. Weaker solutions of dexamethasone (0.01% to 0.05%) and prednisolone (0.12%) do not usually produce ocular hypertension. Fluorometholone, as a 0.1% suspension, has proved effective in the treatment of some intraocular inflammations without producing significant increases in intra-ocular pressure in most patients. For treatment of the more severe forms of iritis, stronger topical preparations such as 0.1% dexamethasone or 1% prednisolone are usually necessary. In all cases the frequency of application should be titrated to the severity of the inflammation. For mild reactions a satisfactory

Table 2. Relative anti-inflammatory activity, sodium-retaining activity, and equivalent doses of the glucocorticoids

Generic name	Trade name	Relative anti-inflammatory activity	Relative sodium-retaining activity	Equivalent dose	
Cortisone acetate	Cortone Acetate	0.8	0.8	25	mg
Hydrocortisone	Cortef, Cortril, Hydrocortone	1.0	1.0	20	mg
Prednisone	Delta-Dome, Deltasone, Lisacort, Meticorten, Orasonel, Paracort, Servisone	4.0	0.8	5	mg
Prednisolone	Delta-Cortef, Meticortelone, Nisolone, Paracortol, Prednicen, Prednis, Sterane	4.0	0.8	5	mg
Triamcinolone	Aristocort, Kenacort	5.0	0.0	4	mg
Methylprednisolone	Medrol, Stemex	5.0	0.0	4	mg
Paramethasone acetate	Haldrone	10.0	0.0	2	mg
Fluprednisolone	Alphadrol	13.5	0.0	1.5	mg
Fludrocortisone	Florinef	20.0	125.0	0.1	mg
Dexamethasone	Decadron, Deronil, Dexameth, Gam-macorten, Hexadrol	25.0	0.0	0.75	mg
Betamethasone	Celestone	25.0	0.0	0.6	mg

response sometimes is obtained with applications as infrequent as once or twice a day or occasionally even less. For more severe reactions it may be necessary to use the medications every 2 hours or so. Once improvement occurs, the dosage can be tapered.

Recently experimental evidence has been presented to indicate increased bio-availability and effectiveness of topically administered corticosteroids that utilize the acetate and alcohol forms of the drug. (In solution corticosteroid acetate and alcohol preparations in therapeutic concentrations form suspensions, whereas corticosteroid phosphate and succinate preparations form true solutions.) It is somewhat difficult to know exactly how meaningful these findings are in clinical ophthalmology, where variabilities abound. Certainly clinical improvement, as well as side effects such as glaucoma, occurs with the use of corticosteroid solutions. The practitioner should familiarize himself with several of the different commercially available topical steroid preparations and individualize his product selection for each patient.

Subconjunctival injections of corticosteroids are employed to treat various forms of anterior uveitis, corneal inflammations and to reduce postoperative inflammation. They are frequently used as supplemental treatment to topical or systemic therapy. High local tissue levels of corticosteroids can be achieved with subconjunctival injections. Repository preparations such as methylprednisolone acetate (Depo-Medrol) and triamcinolone acetonide (Kenalog) provide effective concentrations of the drug in the anterior segment of the eye for 1 to 5 weeks. In some clinical situations such a long-term effect may be undesirable. In such cases subconjunctival corticosteroid solutions may be used. Preparations are available that have both acetate and phosphate forms. In theory the phosphate solution portion of this combination provides short-term high tissue steroid levels, while the acetate suspension portion provides a prolonged effect. Subconjunctival steroids may also produce glaucoma.

For diseases of the posterior segment of the globe, the optic nerve, or the orbit, the systemic administration of glucocorticoids or ACTH may be used. Retrobulbar injection of repository corticoids has also proved effective in selected cases of posterior segment disease. The advantages of retrobulbar (probably better termed periocular) injection are high local concentration of the drug and absence of systemic effects. One of the problems of injecting retrobulbar steroids is the placement of the drug in close apposition to the sclera or optic nerve without damage to these structures. If the drug is not in close apposition, its penetration is significantly decreased. Accidental intraocular injection has occurred.

Although the choice of the particular drug is an individual decision, the tendency is to use compounds other than cortisone and hydrocortisone to avoid the salt-retaining effects of these drugs. Some ophthalmologists still prefer to use ACTH intravenously rather than a glucocorticoid in very severe forms of uveitis. It is unlikely that the intravenous use of ACTH has more to offer than the glucocorticoids if the glucocorticoids are used in sufficient concentration.

Significant systemic allergic reactions to ACTH are seen in a significant number of patients receiving long-term therapy.

The dosage of the glucocorticoids should be individualized to each patient, with minimal effective doses employed for the shortest possible period of time to effect the desired response. If the disease under treatment is acute and severe, daily doses of 40 to 80 mg of prednisone or its equivalent should be used. In severe cases of progressive thyroid exophthalmos, doses of 120 to 140 mg of prednisone may be required to control the critical phases of the disease. Dosage should be reduced within 3 to 4 days, since severe complications may develop with continued high doses. Reduction should be in gradual decrements (10 mg for large initial doses and 2.5 to 5 mg for smaller initial doses) over a period of days or weeks, depending on the total length of treatment. If the disorder is of only moderate severity, initial doses of 30 to 40 mg of prednisone or its equivalent may be employed. Again, gradual reduction of the dosage should be accomplished as soon as possible. In mild disorders an initial dose of 20 mg of prednisone is usually sufficient.

It has been suggested recently that therapeutic effects without many of the side effects could be achieved if the total calculated 48-hour dose were given at one time without additional medication until 48 hours later. Advocates of this schedule suggest that stopping steroid therapy for 48 hours permits metabolic recovery and prevents toxic effects from being cumulative. Under this regimen, a somewhat higher total dosage is required than when divided dosage therapy is used. For example, a total of 100 to 120 mg of prednisone should be given at

Table 3. Topical glucocorticoid ophthalmic preparations

Generic name	Trade name	Strengths available
Cortisone acetate ointments	Cortone Acetate	1.5%
Hydrocortisone acetate suspensions	Hydrocortone Acetate	2.5%
	Eye-Cort	0.5%
Hydrocortisone solution	Optef drops	0.2%
Hydrocortisone acetate ointment	Hydrocortone Acetate	1.5%
Hydrocortisone ointment	Cortril	0.5% and 2.5%
Hydrocortisone sodium phosphate solution	Corphos	0.5%
Prednisolone sodium phosphate solution	Hydeltrasol, Optival	0.5%
Prednisolone sodium phosphate ointment	Hydeltrasol	0.25%
Prednisolone acetate suspension	Prednefrin Forte	1.0%
	Pred Mild	0.12%
	Econopred	0.12%
	Econopred Plus	1.0%
Prednisolone sodium phosphate	Inflamase	0.125%
Prednisolone sodium phosphate	Inflamase Forte	1.0%
Dexamethasone sodium phosphate solution	Decadron	0.1%
Dexamethasone phosphate ointment	Decadron	0.05%
Dexamethasone suspension	Maxidex	0.1%
Fluorometholone	FML	0.1%
Medrysone	HMS	1.0%

48-hour intervals if used as a substitute for the administration of prednisone, 10 mg four times a day. The medication is usually given about 8 AM, when the endogenous secretion of cortisol is at a relatively low level. Other modifications have been offered, such as giving the calculated 24-hour dose (plus a 25% increase) as a single daily dose. Although high blood levels of steroids cannot be maintained by these techniques, there is some indication that tissue levels may remain in the therapeutic range for 12 to 24 hours.

The alternate-day approach to treatment has been endorsed where long-term steroid therapy is indicated, as in the management of the nephrotic syndrome, collagen vascular disorders, and some cases of asthma. However, this method of drug administration has not had universal acceptance. Some workers believe that

Table 4. Injectable glucocorticoids

Generic name	Trade name	Strengths available
Cortisone acetate suspension USP	Cortone Acetate	25 mg and 50 mg/ml
Dexamethasone sodium phosphate	Decadron Phosphate	4 mg/ml
	Hexadrol Phosphate	4 mg/ml
Hydrocortisone for injection (as the sodium succinate)	Solu-Cortef	100 mg 250 mg, 500 mg, and 1,000 mg vials
Hydrocortisone injection	Cortef aqueous suspension	50 mg/ml
Hydrocortisone suspension	Cortef intramuscular	50 mg/ml
Hydrocortisone acetate	Cortef Acetate	50 mg/ml
	Hydrocortone Acetate	25 mg and 50 mg/ml
	Cortril Acetate	25 mg/ml
Hydrocortisone sodium phosphate	Hydrocortone	50 mg/ml
Methylprednisolone acetate suspension	Depo-Medrol	20 mg, 40 mg, and 80 mg/ml
Methylprednisolone sodium succinate	Solu-Medrol	40 mg, 125 mg, 500 mg, and 1,000 mg vials
Prednisolone acetate suspension	Durapred	100 mg/ml
	Meticortelone soluble	25 mg/ml
	Nisolone aqueous	25 mg/ml
	Savacort	25 mg, 50 mg, and 100 mg/ml
	Sterane intramuscular and intra-articular	25 mg/ml
Prednisolone butylacetate suspension	Hydeltra-TBA	20 mg/ml
Prednisolone sodium phosphate	Hydeltrasol	20 mg/ml
	Savacort-S	20 mg/ml
	Sodasone	20 mg/ml
Prednisolone (phosphate and acetate combination)	Prednalone	100 mg/ml
Triamcinolone diacetate suspension	Aristocort lesional	25 mg/ml
Triamcinolone diacetate suspension	Aristocort Forte	40 mg/ml
Triamcinolone acetonide suspension	Kenalog parenteral	10 mg/ml 40 mg/ml
Betamethasone (acetate and disodium phosphate combination)	Celestone Soluspan	6 mg/ml

adrenal pituitary suppression occurs less readily with this modification of dosage, but other side reactions still occur. It would appear that the alternate-day dosage would be acceptable for the long-term management of chronic smoldering uveitis, and it would be particularly valuable in children. However, when very rapid suppression of an acute inflammatory process is desired, the divided dosage schedule is advisable. When the alternate-day routine is used, short-acting steroids such as prednisone, prednisolone, and methylprednisolone should be used. Long-acting steroids such as dexamethasone and betamethasone may continue to produce adrenal suppression on the off day of treatment and therefore produce similar toxic effects as if given on a divided-dosage schedule.

The intramuscular dose of ACTH is 40 to 50 USP units in four divided doses. Larger doses (up to 100 USP units) may be given if satisfactory response is not obtained with smaller amounts. For intravenous use, 20 to 40 USP units are dissolved in 500 to 1,000 ml of 5% dextrose in water and given over a period of 8 to 12 hours. The intramuscular dose of the purified gel form of ACTH is the same as that of regular ACTH; injections are given at 24-hour intervals.

When long-term therapy is necessary, it is important to maintain the patient on as small a dose as possible. Frequently the dose of systemically administered corticosteroids in continued therapy can be reduced if local steroids are used in conjunction with the systemic drug, as in the treatment of sympathetic ophthalmia. Whenever prolonged therapy is required, it is imperative that the patient be observed regularly for the onset of any side effects so that therapeutic corrective measures may be taken immediately. Since the problems of prolonged hormone therapy are complex, it is advisable for the ophthalmologist to have early and repeated consultation in these cases.

The time for a clinical effect from systemic steroid therapy varies with the mode of administration. A clinical effect is noticed within an hour after intravenous therapy. Oral corticosteroids and intramuscular injections of aqueous solutions produce an effect in about 4 hours; this effect lasts for about 4 hours. Intramuscular injections of cortisone acetate suspension begin to take effect in 12 hours, reach a maximal effect in 24 hours, and continue to have some clinical action for 48 to 96 hours. Injections of methylprednisolone produce clinical effects for 1 to 5 weeks.

CONTRAINDICATIONS TO CORTICOSTEROIDS

Contraindications to the use of corticosteroids are relative. A history of the patient's general health should be obtained before systemic corticosteroid therapy is started. If the ocular disorder is so severe that without steroids total blindness is inevitable, the systemic disorder that contraindicates steroid therapy can usually be satisfactorily "overtreated" while the hormone therapy is given. For example, if a patient has a severe uveitis and also a peptic ulcer, the steroids can probably be given safely if the peptic ulcer is treated vigorously at the same time. Systemic disorders that are generally considered to be relative contraindications to parenteral or oral corticosteroid therapy include active tuberculosis, thrombophlebitis, osteoporosis, severe diabetes mellitus, peptic ulcers, and generalized infections not satisfactorily controlled by drug therapy. Local steroid therapy to the eye can usually be safely employed, however, since the blood levels reached by this form of treatment are usually not sufficient to induce systemic complications.

The glucocorticoids, administered either topically or systemically, are contraindicated in herpes simplex infections of the cornea. The possible exception is a disciform type of corneal involvement. The incidence and severity of herpes simplex keratitis is much greater in patients receiving corticosteroids. The presence of any viral infection of the eye except herpes zoster and superficial punctate keratitis is a contraindication to corticosteroid therapy. Corticosteroids should not be used if fungus infections are present. Neither should they be used in the presence of bacterial infections if the activity of the bacteria is not controlled by antibiotics.

In the doses usually employed, corticosteroids do not appear to interfere significantly with wound healing after ocular surgery. Recent ocular surgery is not a contraindication to steroid therapy, although it should be appreciated that wound healing may be delayed.

OTHER CONSIDERATIONS

Since the discontinuation of systemic corticosteroid therapy may result in adrenal hypofunction that may persist for several months, certain precautions must be taken. If a patient who has received corticosteroids systemically in the past 6 months is to undergo general anesthesia, corticosteroids should be administered either preoperatively or at the time of surgery to avoid adrenal collapse. Patients who have recently been given corticosteroids systemically should not be given intravenous typhoid vaccine, since the pituitary adrenal axis may not be capable of responding to the stimulus produced by the typhoid therapy.

Disagreement exists among endocrinologists concerning whether ACTH therapy should be given concurrently with corticosteroids or during reduction of corticosteroid therapy. Advocates of such therapy believe ACTH therapy produces adrenal stimulation and prevents adrenal cortical atrophy. Others believe that anterior pituitary unresponsiveness is the principal cause of adrenal cortical suppression occurring with corticosteroid therapy, but recent evidence indicates that pituitary function returns spontaneously several months before normal adrenal responsiveness. ACTH treatment, however, may actually worsen pituitary insufficiency. Supplementary ACTH therapy is more often used in children on long-term corticosteroid therapy where stimulation of adrenal androgen production and prevention of adrenal cortical atrophy are more important.

Patients on prolonged systemic corticosteroid therapy frequently develop hypopotassemia to such a degree that muscle cramps and weakness occur. Further-

Table 5. Results of corticosteroid therapy in combination with other drugs

Drug	Effect
Barbiturates	Increased corticosteroid metabolism
Estrogens	Enhancement of corticosteroid anti-inflammatory activity
Indomethacin	Increased gastrointestinal disturbances
Salicylates	Decreased salicylate blood levels
Vitamin A	Effect of corticosteroids on wound healing decreased
Phenytoin	Increased steroid metabolism
Antibiotics	Increased possibility of superinfection; development of resistant strains of microorganisms
Potassium depleting drugs (thiazides, and so forth)	Increased hypokalemia

more, these patients are frequently given chlorothiazides (Diuril or Hydrodiuril) to relieve retention edema. This diuretic also increases potassium loss. It is often advisable to supplement the potassium intake of these patients with bananas or orange juice. A 4-ounce glass of fresh orange juice contains approximately 200 mg of potassium. Potassium chloride such as K-Lor packets of fruit-flavored powder containing 15 or 20 mEq of potassium to be added to water or juice can be given in divided doses to achieve 40 to 80 mEq daily (20 mEq = 1.5 gm potassium chloride). Potassium chloride is also marketed as slow-release 8 mEq tablets (Slow-K). Potassium Triplex, a liquid preparation containing 0.5 gram of potassium acetate, 0.5 gram of potassium bicarbonate, and 0.5 gram of potassium citrate in each 5 ml, may be prescribed in a dose of 1 teaspoonful three times a day. Enteric-coated oral potassium medications have been incriminated as producing ulcers in the small bowel and can cause diarrhea in some patients when given in ordinary form. Effervescent tablets (K-Lyte) administered in a glass of water often avoid these complications, but may not be effective in raising the serum potassium if diuretics are being administered concurrently.

To prevent the possible development of peptic ulcers during corticosteroid therapy, antacids are frequently used concurrently. This is particularly important if there is a previous history of ulcers. However, since ulcers may develop in patients receiving corticosteroids who previously never had ulcer symptoms, the use of antacids should always be considered when systemic use of corticosteroids is prescribed.

Many drug interactions have been reported with corticosteroid therapy (Table 5).

REFERENCES

Byyny, R. L.: Withdrawal from glucocorticoid therapy, N. Engl. J. Med. **295**:30, 1976.
Feldman, D., Funder, J. W., and Edelman, I. S.: Subcellular mechanisms in the action of adrenal steroids, Am. J. Med. **53**:545, 1972.
Harter, J. G., Reddy, W. J., and Thorn, G. W.: Studies on an intermittent corticosteroid dosage regimen, N. Engl. J. Med. **269**:591, 1963.

Haynes, R. C., Jr., and Larner, J.: Adrenocorticotropic hormone; adrenocortical steroids and their synthetic analogs; inhibitors of adrenocortical steroid biosynthesis. In Goodman, L. S., and Gilman, A., editors: The pharmacologic basis of therapeutics, ed. 5, New York, 1975, Macmillan, Inc.

Kaufman, H. E., editor: Symposium on ocular anti-inflammatory therapy, Springfield, Ill., 1970, Charles C Thomas, Publisher.

Leibowitz, H. M., and Kupferman, A.: Bioavailability and therapeutic effectiveness of topically administered corticosteroids, Trans. Am. Acad. Ophthalmol. Otolaryngol. 79:78(OP), 1975.

Leopold, I. H.: Treatment of eye disorders with anti-inflammatory steroids, Ann. N.Y. Acad. Sci. 82:939, 1959.

Leopold, I. H., and Barnett, A. H.: Steroids in ophthalmology, Adv. Ophthalmol. 18:1, 1967.

Liddle, G. W.: The adrenal cortex. In Williams, R. H., editor: Textbook of endocrinology, ed. 5, Philadelphia, 1974, W. B. Saunders Co.

Nozik, R. A.: Periocular injection of steroids, Trans. Am. Acad. Ophthalmol. Otolaryngol. 76:695, 1972.

Podos, S. M., and Becker, B.: Intraocular pressure effects of diluted and new topical corticosteroids. In Leopold, I. H., editor: Symposium on ocular therapy, vol. 5, St. Louis, 1972, The C. V. Mosby Co.

Richardson, K. T.: Pharmacology and pathophysiology of inflammation, Arch. Ophthalmol. 86:706, 1971.

Schwartz, B., editor: Corticosteroids and the eye, Int. Ophthalmol. Clin. 6:753, 1966.

Shin, D. H., Kass, M. A., Kolker, A. E., and others: Positive FTA-ABS tests in subjects with corticosteroid-induced uveitis, Am. J. Ophthalmol. 82:259, 1976.

Steroid therapy and the adrenals, editorial, Lancet 2:537, 1975.

Werner, S. C.: Prednisone in emergency treatment of malignant exophthalmos, Lancet 1:1004, 1966.

CHAPTER 3

Principles of antibiotic therapy

The basic question in the decision as to whether antibiotics should be employed is relatively simple: Does the probability of a desirable therapeutic effect outweigh the possibility of an undesirable effect? For the ophthalmologist the answer is quite obvious in severe bacterial infections of the eyelids, globe, or orbit. However, the answer is not so apparent in consideration of the routine use of prophylactic antibiotics in uncomplicated ocular surgery or the treatment of self-limited, low-grade external infections of doubtful bacterial origin. The purpose of this chapter is to discuss the basic principles in the use and selection of antibiotics.

Antibiotics are chemical substances produced by microorganisms that have the capacity to inhibit growth of or even destroy bacteria and other microorganisms in dilute solution. The chemical structures of most therapeutic antibiotics have been identified, and a few are now commercially synthesized. The mechanism of action of antibiotics is somewhat variable. Generally, they achieve their effects by disturbing the metabolic activities of the bacteria. Most antibiotics disturb cell wall synthesis of bacteria, some interfere with protein synthesis of bacteria, and others produce alteration in bacterial membrane permeability. At the same time they may also produce unfavorable effects on the cellular processes of the patient. Antibiotics may be either primarily bactericidal (those that kill organisms) or bacteriostatic (those that inhibit bacterial multiplication). Agents such as the penicillins are both bacteriostatic and bactericidal in relatively the same concentrations. Other agents such as the tetracyclines are usually considered primarily bacteriostatic; however they may become bactericidal in very high concentrations, not usually achievable in patients.

Bactericidal agents in current use are the penicillins (including the semisynthetic penicillins), cephalosporins, streptomycin, bacitracin, neomycin, kanamycin, vancomycin, gentamicin, polymyxin B, and colistin. Bacteriostatic agents in current use include the tetracyclines and related compounds, chloramphenicol, erythromycin, novobiocin, lincomycin, clindamycin, and the sulfonamides.

The antibacterial spectrum of the antibiotics is given in Table 7. A simple way to remember the essentials of the antibacterial spectrum is as follows: Pathogens can be divided into rods and cocci, gram positive and gram negative. Most pathogenic cocci are gram positive, and most pathogenic rods are gram negative. Bactericidal drugs that kill cocci are the penicillins, bacitracin, and vancomycin. Those that destroy rods are streptomycin, polymyxin B, gentamicin, and colistin. Other bactericidal agents such as neomycin and kanamycin are variably effective against both rods and cocci. The cephalosporins, ampicillin, and carbenicillin are active against cocci and a limited number of gram-negative organisms. Bacteriostatic agents that affect only cocci are erythromycin, novobiocin, and lincomycin. Clindamycin is effective against cocci and most anaerobes. The broad-spectrum antibiotics and the sulfonamides are variably effective against both rods and cocci.

SYNERGISM AND ANTAGONISM

Antibiotics may be classified into two large groups: group I includes bactericidal agents such as penicillins, streptomycin, bacitracin, polymyxin, neomycin, cephalosporins, and gentamicin; group II includes bacteriostatic agents such as the tetracyclines, erythromycin, chloramphenicol, and the sulfonamides. It is thought that the antibiotics in group I are frequently synergistic and never antagonistic. Antagonism or synergism may occur if antibiotics of groups I and II are employed concomitantly. Antagonism may occur if the bacteria are relatively sensitive to bactericidal agents; synergism occurs when the bacteria are relatively insensitive to bactericidal agents. The effect varies with the exact nature of the infections and the concentration of the drug used. Members of group II usually exhibit neither antagonism nor synergism toward each other but are simply additive in their effect.

In the concentrations in which antibiotics are presently used in systemic disease, it is quite doubtful that antagonism is important clinically, except in rare instances. Synergism, however, may result when combinations of antibiotics are employed in sufficient doses.

DANGER OF OVERUSE

The major dangers in the overuse of antibiotics are (1) hypersensitivity, (2) drug toxicity, (3) the development of resistant strains of bacteria, and (4) alterations of normal bacterial flora.

Hypersensitivity to antibiotics is a frequent occurrence, most often with penicillin therapy but also common with sulfonamide and streptomycin therapy. Skin eruptions often occur when penicillin is given to a sensitive patient. Similar skin reactions have been noted after sulfonamide, streptomycin, and tetracycline therapy. Other less common allergic reactions to penicillin therapy include painful swollen joints, asthma, and drug fever. Anaphylactic shock with death has been reported after streptomycin and penicillin injections.

Toxic reactions to the antibiotics are numerous, as summarized in Table 6. Attention is called to the aplastic anemia that may develop as an idiosyncratic reaction to chloramphenicol therapy, particularly in children, since this drug is frequently used by the ophthalmologist for the treatment of intraocular infections.

Text continued on p. 40.

Table 6. Chemotherapeutic and antibiotic agents

Drug	Systemic dose (adult)		
	Oral	IM	IV*
Amphotericin B (Fungizone)			0.05 to 0.1 mg/kg body weight daily, gradually increasing to 1 mg/kg body weight
p-Aminosalicylic acid (PAS)	3 to 4 grams q6h		15 grams in 3% solution in 2 doses 4 h apart; 5 mg heparin added to each liter of solution
Bacitracin	40,000 to 120,000 units in divided doses for 5 to 20 days		2,500 to 20,000 units q6h
Cefazolin (Ancef, Kefazol		1 gram q6 to 8h	1 gram q6 to 8h
Cephalexin (Keflex)	250 to 1,000 mg q6h		
Cephaloridine (Loridine)		1 gram 4 times daily	1 gram 4 times daily
Cephalothin (Keflin sodium)		500 to 1,000 mg q4 to 6h	500 to 2,000 mg q4 to 6h
Cephapirin (Cefadyl)	500 to 1,000 mg q6h		
Cephradine (Anspor, Velosef)	500 to 1,000 mg q6h		
Chloramphenicol (Amphicol, Chloromycetin, Mychel)	50 mg/kg body weight; daily 250 to 500 mg q4 to 6h	1 gram q8 to 12h	500 mg q6h
Clindamycin (Cleocin)	150 to 300 mg q6h	600 to 1,200 mg/day divided into 2 to 4 doses	600 to 1,200 mg/day divided into 2 to 4 doses
Colistin (Coly-Mycin)		1.5 to 5 mg/kg body weight/day, divided into 2 to 4 doses	
Erythromycin (Erythrocin, Ilotycin, Ilosone)	0.2 to 0.5 gram q6h		0.5 gram q12h
Flucytosine (Ancobon)	50 to 150 mg/kg/day divided into 4 doses		
Gentamicin (Garamycin)		3 to 5 mg/kg/day, divided into 3 doses	3 to 5 mg/kg/day, divided into 3 doses
Griseofulvin (Fulvicin, Grifulvin, Grisactin)	1 to 2 grams daily in 1 to 4 doses		

*See instructions accompanying drug for type and amount of diluent advised and rate of administration.

Topical eye (a) solution (b) ointment	Systemic toxic side effects
a) 1 to 5 mg/ml	Chills, fever, kidney damage, thrombophlebitis, hepatitis, hypokalemia
	Drug rash, nausea, vomiting, diarrhea, fever, hematuria, crystalluria
a) 250 to 1,000 units/ ml b) 500 units/gram	Kidney damage, albuminuria, cylindruria, systemic use rarely necessary
	Drug rash, neutropenia, leukopenia, nausea, vomiting
	Diarrhea, nausea, vomiting, drug rash, neutropenia
	Renal tubular necrosis with daily doses of 4 grams or more; drug rash, blood dyscrasias
	Drug rash, neutropenia with bone marrow depression
	Same as cephalexin
	Same as cephalexin
a) 2.5 to 5 mg/ml b) 10 mg/gram	Skin rashes, fever, abdominal cramps, bone marrow depression, gray baby syndrome, aplastic anemia
	Diarrhea, colitis, depression of blood elements, jaundice
a) 1.5 to 3 mg/ml	Drug rash, paresthesias, dizziness, kidney damage, apnea
a) 5 mg/ml b) 5 mg/gram	Nausea, vomiting, diarrhea; rarely, allergic hepatitis
a) 1 to 1.5 mg/ml	Depression of blood elements, hepatic dysfunction, skin eruptions
a) 3 to 10 mg/ml	Renal damage, eighth nerve toxicity
	Drug rash, epigastric distress, nausea, diarrhea; possible leukopenia

Table 6. Chemotherapeutic and antibiotic agents—cont'd

Drug	Systemic dose (adult)		
	Oral	IM	IV*
Isoniazid	5 to 10 mg/kg body weight daily in 2 to 3 doses	Same as oral	
Kanamycin (Kantrex)		7.5 mg/kg body weight q12h	
Lincomycin (Lincocin)	500 mg q6h	500 mg q12h	600 mg q8 to 12h
Neomycin	1 gram q4h for 24 to 72 hr		
Nitrofurantoin (Furadantin)	100 mg 4 times daily		
Nystatin (Mycostatin, Nilstat)	500,000 units 3 times daily		
Penicillin G	100,000 to 400,000 units 4 to 5 times daily	300,000 to 1.2 million units daily	300,000 to 1 million units q3 to 6h
Penicillin V	250 to 1,000 mg q6h		
Semisynthetic penicillins			
1. Methicillin sodium (Staphcillin)		1 to 2 grams q4 to 6h	1 to 2 grams q4 to 6h (larger doses in severe infections)
2. Oxacillin sodium (Bactocil, Prostaphlin)	500 to 1,000 mg q4 to 6h	500 to 1,000 mg q4 to 6h	500 to 1,000 mg q4 to 6h
3. Ampicillin (Amcill, Omnipen, Pen A, Polycillin, Penbritin, Pensyn, Principen, Procillin, QIDamP, Supen)	500 to 1,000 mg q6h	500 to 1,000 mg q6h	500 to 1,000 mg q6h
4. Amoxicillin (Amoxil, Larotid, Polymox)	250 to 500 mg q8h		
5. Nafcillin sodium (Unipen)	500 to 1,000 mg q4 to 6h	500 to 1,000 mg q4 to 6h	500 to 1,000 mg q4h
6. Dicloxacillin (Dynapen, Pathocil, Veracillin)	500 to 1,000 mg q4 to 6h		
7. Cloxacillin (Tegopen)	500 to 1,000 mg q4 to 6h		
8. Carbenicillin (Geopen, Pyopen)		2 grams q4 to 6h	25 to 35 grams/day

*See instructions accompanying drug for type and amount of diluent advised and rate of administration.

Topical eye (a) solution (b) ointment	Systemic toxic side effects
	Albuminuria, pyridoxine deficiency, anemia, eosinophila, constipation, dysuria, hypotension, hepatic dysfunction, hepatitis
mg/ml	Kidney damage, deafness
	Diarrhea, abdominal aches, skin rash
) 2.5 mg/ml) 5.0 mg/ml	Few side effects after topical or oral dosage; poorly tolerated by injection
	Drug rash, nausea, vomiting
) 25,000 to 100,000 units/ml) 100,000 units/gram	Occasional gastrointestinal disturbances
ould not be used except for treatment of specific bacterial corneal ulcers) 100,000 to 300,000 units/ml	Least toxic of all antibiotics; most serious effect is incidence of allergy or hypersensitivity; less likely with oral dosage, most likely after topical application; manifested as rash, fever, urticaria; occasional anaphylactic reaction
ould not be used	Same as penicillin G
ould not be used	Same as penicillin G
ould not be used	Same as penicillin G
ould not be used	Same as penicillin G
	Same as penicillin G
ould not be used	Same as penicillin G
ould not be used	Same as penicillin G
ould not be used	Same as penicillin G
ould not be used except for treatment of Pseudomonas corneal ulcers) 4 mg/ml	Same as penicillin G

Table 6. Chemotherapeutic and antibiotic agents—cont'd

Drug	Systemic dose (adult)		
	Oral	IM	IV*
Polymyxin B (Aerosporin)	75 to 100 mg 3 to 4 times/day	1.5 to 2.5 mg/kg. body weight daily	1.5 to 2.5 mg/kg body weight daily
Rifampin (Rifadin, Rimactane)	600 mg 1 time/day		
Streptomycin		1 to 2 grams daily	
Sulfacetamide (Sulamyd Sodium)			
Sulfadiazine or sulfamerazine; mixed sulfonamides	Initial dose 2 to 4 grams; maintenance 1 gram q6h		
Sulfadimethoxine (Madribon)	1 to 2 grams initially; then 0.5 to 1 gram daily		
Sulfamethoxypyridazine (Midicel, Acetyl)	Initially 1 gram; then 0.5 gram daily		
Sulfa-trimethoprim and sulfamethoxazole combination (Bactrim, Septra)	160 mg trimethoprim and 800 mg sulfamethoxazole q12h		
Sulfisoxazole (Gantrisin)	Initial dose 2 to 4 grams; maintenance, 1 gram q6h		
Tetracycline group (Aureomycin, Terramycin, Achromycin, Tetracyn, Mysteclin, Sumycin, Panmycin)	250 to 1,000 mg qid	250 mg q8 to 12h	250 to 500 bid
Tetracycline group Doxycycline (Doxy-II, Vibramycin)	200 mg single dose first day; 100 mg single dose daily thereafter		200 mg single dose initially; 100 to 2C mg/day thereafter
Minocycline (Minocin, Vectrin)	200 mg initially; 100 mg q12h thereafter		200 mg initially; 10C mg q12h thereafter
Tobramycin (Nebcin)		3 to 5 mg/kg/day in 3 to 4 divided doses	3 to 5 mg/kg day in 3 to 4 divided dose
Vancomycin (Vancocin)			2 grams given slowly in 2 to 4 divided doses

*See instructions accompanying drug for type and amount of diluent advised and rate of administration.

Topical eye (a) solution (b) ointment	Systemic toxic side effects
a) 10,000 to 25,000 units/ml b) 20,000 units/gram (10,000 units = 1 mg)	Paresthesias, fever, vertigo, renal irritation
	Gastrointestinal disturbances, headache, drowsiness, skin reactions, leukopenia
a) 50 mg/ml	Hypersensitivity reactions, vertigo, tinnitus; deafness uncommon with low dosage and short periods of administration
a) 100 to 300 mg/ml b) 100 mg/gram	
	Rash, fever, stomatitis, diarrhea, crystalluria, hematuria, oliguria, bone marrow depression
	Rash, gastrointestinal disturbances, blood dyscrasias, hepatic dysfunction
	Rash, blood dyscrasias, stomatitis
	Same as sulfadiazine
a) 40 mg/ml b) 40 mg/gram	Rash, fever, stomatitis, diarrhea, crystalluria, hematuria, oliguria, bone marrow depression
a) 5 mg/ml b) 5 to 10 mg/gram	Occasional hypersensitivity, nausea, vomiting, diarrhea, pruritus; incidence of side effects is low; superinfection by resistant organisms in intestinal tract; dental defects in children, photosensitivity
	Same as other tetracyclines
	Same as other tetracyclines
a) 1 to 10 mg/ml	Renal damage, eighth nerve toxicity
0 mg/ml	Drug rash, fever, renal damage, deafness

The problem of bacterial resistance is in a constant state of flux. The popularity of individual antibiotics in a certain locality has much to do with the number of resistant strains of bacteria to a given agent. In hospitals in which erythromycin had been employed as a substitute for penicillin, the usefulness of penicillin in the treatment of staphylococcic infections increased over a period of several months, while the number of strains of staphylococci resistant to erythromycin was increasing.

Penicillin-resistant strains of staphylococci are now frequently encountered. This is particularly true of staphylococci recovered in hospitals. These resistant organisms produce penicillinase, an enzyme that inactivates penicillin. Fortunately, new penicillin products (methicillin, oxacillin, cloxacillin, dicloxacillin, and nafcillin), cephalosporins, lincomycin, and clindamycin are effective against most penicillin-resistant staphylococci. A few strains of resistant staphylococci are unaffected by new penicillins or by the cephalosporins. Many of these strains are susceptible to vancomycin and kanamycin. Despite the development of strains of staphylococci resistant to penicillin, no highly resistant strains of beta-hemolytic streptococci, pneumococci, or meningococci have been identified. Strains of gonococci have been encountered that were less susceptible to penicillin; many of these organisms are susceptible to oxytetracycline or to higher doses of penicillin.

Bacterial resistance to streptomycin and dihydrostreptomycin develops easily. A resistant mutant to these drugs develops sometimes within the first week of therapy. Bacterial resistance to the sulfonamides and many of the broad-spectrum antibiotics is common. When a new antibiotic is introduced, it is usually very effective, but resistant strains of bacteria may develop as the drug is used more commonly. Fortunately, new antibiotics are continually being introduced. Furthermore, as mentioned previously, older antibiotics, which have not been widely used recently, may again become clinically effective.

Tetracyclines and related compounds have strong suppressive effects on the normal bacterial flora of the gastrointestinal tract. Because of this, there may be an overgrowth of yeastlike organisms, particularly *Candida*. Similar changes occur in the flora of the normal conjunctiva after the use of the broad-spectrum antibiotics. Increased mycotic flora of the conjunctiva has been reported after prolonged use of topical broad-spectrum antibiotics.

SELECTION AND ADMINISTRATION OF ANTIBIOTICS

The selection of an antibiotic and the method of administration are dependent on several criteria. These considerations include (1) the nature of the offending organism and its sensitivity to antibiotics; (2) the nature of the disease, its seriousness, and location; and (3) the general health, sensitivities, and allergies of the patient.

It is helpful and often important to identify the offending organism and to establish its sensitivity to antibiotics. This is sometimes quite impractical for the ophthalmologist, and needless and serious delays in therapy could result; therefore treatment with antibiotics usually is started empirically. Minor self-limited infections such as many cases of blepharitis and conjunctivitis do not justify the expense of cultures and sensitivity tests. With empirical treatment the disease is often cured before laboratory investigations can be completed.

For local treatment it is advisable to employ antibiotics that are seldom used systemically or antibiotics that are unlikely to create a sensitivity. Neomycin, bacitracin (or gramicidin), and polymyxin B are seldom used systemically, and a mixture of these agents is frequently used in the treatment of conjunctivitis. The spectrum thus obtained is much wider than that which can be obtained when these agents are used singly. Unfortunately, neomycin frequently produces local sensitivity reactions. The tetracyclines, chloramphenicol, gentamicin, sulfacetamide, and sulfamethoxazole (Gantanol) are also effective agents and seldom produce sensitivities. The effectiveness of gentamicin as a topical ophthalmic agent has been established, but this agent should be reserved for the treatment of serious infections caused by gram-negative organisms. In persistent conjunctivitis, cultures should be obtained, and the organisms found should be tested for antibiotic sensitivity (Chapter 9).

In the management of the more severe ocular infections—corneal ulcers, orbital cellulitis, endophthalmitis, and the like—an attempt should always be made to identify the organism by culture. In some instances, identification of the organism can be made by microscopic examination of a smear of material obtained from the lesion. When this cannot be done, initial treatment must be empirical. There are only two guides in such treatment. The first is the likelihood of a certain type of organism producing certain lesions. For example, postoperative intraocular infections are usually caused by staphylococci or gram-negative rods, and central bacterial corneal ulcers are usually caused by pneumococci, streptococci, or gram-positive rods. The second criterion that can be used in empirically determining the type of antibiotic therapy is the clinical response of the patient. If no improvement is noted in 48 to 72 hours with sufficient doses of one antibiotic, a switch should be made to another antibiotic.

In patients with renal insufficiency, antibiotics with nephrotoxic effects should be avoided if possible; these include tetracycline, kanamycin, gentamicin, tobramycin, polymyxin B, colistin, amphotericin B, and sulfonamides. In patients with hepatic insufficiency, antibiotics inactivated by the liver such as erythromycin, chlortetracycline, and chloramphenicol should not be used.

The individual treatment of specific ocular infections is considered in the discussions on the therapy of the various diseases. The management of intraocular infections is considered in Chapter 14.

Combinations of antibiotics may be rationally administered if there is a mixed infection to prevent resistant mutants from developing or for their synergistic effects. If a combination of antibiotics is employed, each should be used in sufficient doses to prevent drug antagonism. In prescribing antibiotics for systemic

Table 7. Sensitivity of common pathogens to chemotherapeutic agents (Because of problems of resistance, sensitivity tests should be performed.)

Pathogen	Penicillin	Streptomycin	Tetracycline group	Chloramphenicol	Erythromycin*	Cephalosporins*	Gentamicin	Miscellaneous effective agents
Actinomyces	1		2					Sulfonamides
Borrelia	2		1	2	2			Bacitracin, neomycin
Brucella		2†	1†	2	2			Neomycin, sulfonamides
Clostridium	1		2	2	2	2		Sulfonamides
Corynebacterium diphtheriae	2		2	2	1			Diphtheria antitoxin
Escherichia coli		2	2	2		2	1	Kanamycin, ampicillin
Entamoeba histolytica			2‡		2‡			Diiodohydroxyquin, metronidazole
Erysipelothrix rhusiopathiae	1			2	2	2		
Hemophilus ducreyi		2	1	2				Ampicillin, sulfonamides
Hemophilus influenzae		1†	2	2†	2	2		Ampicillin, sulfonamides
Herpes simplex virus								Idoxuridine, Vidarabine
Inclusion conjunctivitis virus			1	2	2			Sulfonamides
Klebsiella pneumoniae		2	2	2		1	1	Colistin, sulfonamides
Lymphogranuloma venereum virus			1	2	2			Sulfonamides
Mycobacterium tuberculosis		2†						Isoniazid, PAS, ethambutol, rifampin
Neisseria gonorrhoeae	1	2	2	2	2	2		Spectinomycin, sulfonamides
Neisseria meningitidis	1		2	2	2			Sulfonamides
Pasteurella tularensis		1	2	2				Neomycin, sulfonamides
Pasteurella pestis		1†	2†	2†				Neomycin, sulfonamides
Pneumococci	1		2	2	2	2		Bacitracin, sulfonamides

1 = Drug or drugs of choice; 2 = drug or drugs clinically effective.
*Drugs used frequently in therapy of patients sensitive to penicillin.
†Used in combination with other agents.
‡Intestinal forms only.
§Either methicillin, oxacillin, nafcillin, cloxacillin, or dicloxacillin.
‖Hospital acquired.

Table 7. Sensitivity of common pathogens to chemotherapeutic agents—cont'd

Pathogen	Penicillin	Streptomycin	Tetracycline group	Chloramphenicol	Erythromycin	Cephalosporins	Gentamicin	Miscellaneous effective agents
Proteus mirabilis	2					2	2	Ampicillin, kanamycin
Proteus vulgaris				2			1	Kanamycin, neomycin
Psittacosis virus	2		1	2	2			
Pseudomonas aeruginosa							1	Polymyxin B, colistin, tobramycin, carbenicillin
Rickettsia			1	1	2			
Salmonella typhosa				1		2		Ampicillin, sulfonamides
Shigella		2	2	1		2		Ampicillin, sulfonamides
Staphylococci non-penicillanse producers	1		2	2	1	1		Vancomycin, bacitracin, sulfonamides
Staphylococci penicillinase producers	§			2	2	1		Lincomycin, vancomycin
Streptococcus hemolyticus	1		2	2	2†	2		Vancomycin, bacitracin
Streptococcus viridans	1	2†	2	2	2†	2		Vancomycin, bacitracin
Trachoma virus			1	2	2			Sulfonamides
Treponema pallidum	1		2		2			

use, the physician should order the antibiotics individually rather than rely on the commercial preparations of fixed combinations to assure the desired balance and effectiveness. For topical administration the commercial combination antibiotics are quite effective.

There are countless possible antibiotic drug interactions. Drug incompatibilities with intravenously administered antibiotics abound. One antibiotic may have an inhibitory effect on the other, such as carbenicillin on gentamicin. Drugs such as probenecid that decrease renal clearance may prolong the activity of many antibiotics, among which are the penicillins. Antibiotics that have a renal toxic effect may affect renal clearance of other drugs; antibiotics such as chloramphenicol that are metabolized in the liver may decrease metabolism of such drugs as phenytoin. Some chemotherapeutic and antibiotic drug interactions are listed in Table 8.

Table 8. Some chemotherapeutic-antibiotic drug interactions

Drug	Effect
Carbenicillin	Inhibits antibacterial activity of gentamicin when drugs mixed together for intravenous use
Cephalosporins	Additive nephrotoxic effects with gentamicin
Neomycin	Decreases absorption of penicillin V
Amphotericin B	Potassium depletion exaggerated when used with corticosteroids
Chloramphenicol	Interferes with metabolism of ethyl alcohol
	May interfere with action of folic acid and iron in erythrocyte maturation
	May interfere with penicillin activity
Erythromycin	May interfere with penicillin activity
Lincomycin	Cyclamates and kaolin-pectin (Kaopectate) interfere with absorption of lincomycin
Penicillin	Antacids may increase absorption of oral penicillins
	Sulfonamides inhibit gastrointestinal absorption of penicillin
	Tetracyclines may inhibit activity of penicillin
Polymyxin B	Enhances neuromuscular blockade of skeletal muscle relaxants
Rifampin	Enhances metabolism of estrogens and reduces effectiveness of oral contraceptives
	May increase incidence of hepatotoxicity with halothane anesthesia
Sulfonamides	Local anesthetics (derivatives of para-aminobenzoic acid) may antagonize antibacterial activity of sulfonamides
	May reduce dosage needed for thiopental anesthesia
	May enhance methotrexate toxicity and effects of paraldehyde
	Antibacterial activity of sulfonamides decreased with para-aminobenzoic acid
Tetracyclines	Antacids containing certain ions (calcium, magnesium, aluminum) impair tetracycline absorption from gastrointestinal tract
	Barbiturates may enhance hepatic metabolism of some tetracyclines
	Oral ferrous sulfate and sodium bicarbonate impair absorption of tetracyclines

METHODS OF ADMINISTRATION OF ANTIBIOTICS

Antibiotics may be administered topically, subconjunctivally, intracamerally, or systemically for the treatment of ocular disorders. Topical administration is usually sufficient for the treatment of most conjunctivitis and superficial corneal ulcers. Systemic administration is necessary in the treatment of intraocular infections and infections of the orbit; it may also be valuable in the treatment of severe conjunctivitis such as trachomatous and gonococcal conjunctivitis, or in severe corneal ulcers. Subconjunctival injections in addition to systemic administration are indicated in severe intraocular infections and some corneal ulcers.

Intravitreal injections of antibiotics have been advocated again recently for the treatment of bacterial endophthalmitis. Only very low concentrations of small amounts (0.1 to 0.2 ml) should be injected since high concentrations are quite toxic to the lens and retina (Chapter 14). Therapeutic drug levels persist in the vitreous for up to 72 to 96 hours.

Irrigation of the anterior chamber with antibiotics may be resorted to if the infection is unresponsive to other methods of antibiotic administration, but in my experience this technique offers little advantage, if any, over systemic and subconjunctival methods of administration.

When an antibiotic is selected and the best method of administration is determined, the rate of penetration into the infected tissues must be considered. This is particularly true in intraocular infections, since many antibiotics do not penetrate the blood-aqueous barrier when given topically or systemically. Chloramphenicol, ampicillin, and cephaloridine are probably the antibiotics that penetrate most satisfactorily into the ocular fluids after systemic administration. The sulfonamides penetrate into the aqueous humor in satisfactory levels. Very large doses of penicillin products given intravenously produce therapeutic levels of drug concentration. It should be pointed out that in infected eyes the blood-aqueous barrier is broken down, and consequently the concentration of antibiotics in the ocular fluids is increased considerably.

Antibiotics given by the subconjunctival route probably enter the cornea and anterior chamber of the eye by simple diffusion across the sclera or limbus. By utilizing a subconjunctival technique rather than systemic administration, one can get antibiotics into the eye. Very high concentrations of antibiotics in aqueous humor can be obtained in this way, but therapeutic levels are usually gone by the end of 6 to 8 hours. Therapeutic levels of antibiotics remain in the cornea up to 24 hours after subconjunctival injection. However, the number of subconjunctival injections of antibiotics that can be given is somewhat limited. The injections may be painful, depending on the antibiotic used; for example, cephaloridine is quite painless whereas neomycin is painful. Injections produce severe inflammatory reactions in themselves. Occasionally, the conjunctiva may slough from repeated subconjunctival injections of antibiotics. Nonetheless, such treatment is indicated for severe anterior intraocular and corneal infections and has probably saved the sight of many eyes. Subconjunctival antibiotics are employed by many surgeons at the end of intraocular procedures for prophylaxis against bacterial endophthalmitis. Antibiotic dosages for systemic and topical administration are given in Table 6. Sensitivity of common pathogens to chemotherapeutic agents is presented in Table 7. Subconjunctival and intracameral dosages are given in Chapter 14. Treatment of specific infections is presented later in the book.

REFERENCES

Bloome, M. A., Golden, B., and McKee, A. P.: Antibiotic concentration in ocular tissues, Arch. Ophthalmol. 83:78, 1970.

Farrar, W. E., Jr., Boring, J. R. III, and Shulman, J. A.: Chemotherapy of bacterial infections. IV. Mechanism of action of antibiotics. In DiPalma, J. R., editor: Drill's pharmacology in medicine, ed. 4, New York, 1971, McGraw-Hill Book Co., Inc.

Handbook of antimicrobial therapy. The Medical Letter on Drugs and Therapeutics, revised edition, New York, 1976.

Hansten, P. D.: Drug interactions, ed. 3, Philadelphia, 1975, Lea & Febiger.

Leopold, I. H.: Problems in the use of antibiotics in ophthalmology. In Leopold, I. H., editor: Symposium on ocular therapy, vol. 5, St. Louis, 1972, The C. V. Mosby Co.

Moellering, R. C., and Swartz, M. N.: The newer cephalosporins, New Engl. J. Med. **294:** 24, 1976.

Peyman, G. A., Vastine, D. W., Crouch, E. R., and others: Clinical use of intravitreal antibiotics to treat bacterial endophthalmitis, Trans. Am. Acad. Ophthalmol. Otolaryngol. **78:**862(OP), 1974.

Records, R. E.: The cephalosporins in ophthalmology, Surv. Ophthalmol. **13:**345, 1969.

Records, R. E.: The penicillins in ophthalmology, Surv. Ophthalmol. **13:**207, 1969.

Weinstein, L.: Antimicrobial agents. In Goodman, L. S., and Gilman, A., editors: The pharmacological basis of therapeutics, ed. 5, New York, 1975, Macmillan, Inc.

Williams, J. D., and Geddes, A. M., editors: Chemotherapy, vol. 4, Pharmacology of antibiotics, New York, 1976, Plenum Publishing Corp.

Williams, J. D., and Geddes, A. M., editors: Chemotherapy, vol. 5, Penicillin and cephalosporins, New York, 1976, Plenum Publishing Corp.

CHAPTER 4

Autonomic nervous system agents

BASIC CONSIDERATIONS

The autonomic nervous system consists of two subsystems: the parasympathetic, or cholinergic, and the sympathetic, or adrenergic. Both innervate the eye. The ocular parasympathetic fibers exit the central nervous system through the third cranial (oculomotor) nerve, synapse in the ciliary ganglion, enter the globe via the short ciliary nerves, and run in the suprachoroidal space to reach the ciliary body and iris sphincter. The sympathetic fibers originate in the hypothalamus, pass through the brain stem via the cerebral peduncles, and run in the spinal cord to reach the centers of Budge located in the lateral column of the spinal cord at the junction of the cervical and thoracic regions. Fibers leave the cord via the white rami connections of C_7, C_8, T_1, and T_2. They run up the cervical sympathetic chain to the superior cervical ganglion, then run with the sympathetic plexus around the internal carotid artery to reach the gasserian ganglion. They pass into the orbit via the nasal ciliary nerve and reach the dilator fibers of the iris by way of the long ciliary nerves.

Acetylcholine is the neurotransmitter (chemical mediator) for the postganglionic parasympathetic fibers. Additionally, it is the neurotransmitter in all autonomic ganglia and plays an important role in central nervous system synaptic transmission. The actions of acetylcholine on smooth muscle, cardiac muscle, and various glands are called the muscarinic effects; the actions of acetylcholine on skeletal muscle and ganglia are referred to as the nicotinic effects.

Acetylcholine is synthesized from choline and acetylcoenzyme by the enzyme choline acetylase (choline acetyl transferase). Once formed, acetylcholine is held in the terminal nerve fibers and ganglia in small vesicles until it is released into the postsynaptic space upon membrane depolarization by a nerve action potential. The enzyme acetylcholinesterase rapidly inactivates acetylcholine by hydrolyzing it to acetic acid and choline.

The muscarinic action of acetylcholine may be simulated with the administration of certain alkaloids (such as pilocarpine) or congeners of acetylcholine (such as carbachol or methacholine). The administration of anticholinesterase agents such as physostigmine (eserine) and echothiophate (Phospholine) iodide produce indirect cholinergic effects by preventing the normal rapid destruction of acetylcholine and permitting a prolonged and accumulated effect of acetylcholine.

Drugs such as atropine and scopolamine block the muscarinic activity of acetylcholine by combining with the receptor sites and blocking their access to acetylcholine. The effect of acetylcholine on striated muscle is blocked by curarelike drugs, and ganglion blockade occurs with administration of agents such as hexamethonium and pentolinium. The various sites of parasympathetic nervous system stimulation and blockade are presented in Table 9.

There are several chemical neurotransmitters for the sympathetic nervous system. Both norepinephrine and epinephrine are known to be present in vivo and act as neurotransmitters for the sympathetic nervous system. The synthesis of these substances is as follows: phenylalanine $\rightarrow$ tyrosine $\rightarrow$ 3,4-dihydroxy-phenylalanine (DOPA) $\rightarrow$ dopamine $\rightarrow$ norepinephrine $\rightarrow$ epinephrine. Separate enzymes catalyze each step of this synthesis. Norepinephrine is stored in vesicles in the terminal sympathetic axons and released upon membrane depolarization by a nerve action potential. Once released from the vesicle, norepinephrine pours into the synaptic space, and some of it combines with receptor sites. A major portion of the norepinephrine that does not combine with the receptors is taken back up into the nerve terminals. Norepinephrine is also enzymatically inactivated. Two enzymes, catechol-o-methyl-transferase (largely extraneuronal) and monoamine oxidase (both extra- and intraneuronal), are involved in this process. The sequence of enzymatic inactivation of norepinephrine varies somewhat with the anatomic site and the mechanism of release, whether from nerve action potential or from the action of certain drugs.

There are two types of receptors for the sympathetic effector substances, the alpha and beta receptors. Stimulation of the alpha receptors causes vasoconstriction and related reflex effects on cardiac contraction and output, pupillary dilatation, and decreased resistance to aqueous humor outflow. Beta receptors are responsible for smooth muscle relaxation, cardiac acceleration, vasodilatation,

Table 9. Parasympathetic pharmacology of the eye

Stimulators	Site of action	Blockers
	Ciliary ganglion	
Acetylcholine (inactivated by acetyl-cholinesterase)		Hexamethonium
		Pentolinium
Tetramethylammonium		Nicotine (low concentration)
Nicotine (low concentration)		
	Effector cell	
Acetylcholine (inactivated by acetyl-cholinesterase)		Atropine
		Scopolamine
Pilocarpine		Homatropine
Methacholine		Eucatropine
Carbachol (also stimulates release of acetylcholine from nerve fiber terminals)		Cyclopentolate

bronchial dilatation, inhibition of uterine and intestinal motility, and probably decreased aqueous humor secretion. In recent years the beta receptors have been further subdivided into two groups: beta$_1$ (which is concerned with the effects on the heart, uterus, and lipolysis) and beta$_2$ (which is associated with vasodilatation and bronchodilatation). It appears that adenyl cyclase is intimately associated with the beta receptor.

Norepinephrine is the transmitter that primarily stimulates the alpha receptors. Epinephrine stimulates both alpha and beta receptors; it is generally held that in small doses it stimulates the beta receptors but in larger doses stimulates the alpha receptors. Isoproterenol (Isuprel) stimulates only beta receptors; this substance is not produced in vivo.

Adrenergic effects may be achieved by the administration of agents acting in quite different pharmacological manners. Drugs such as phenylephrine (Neo-Synephrine) combine directly with the receptor site; ephedrine and hydroxy-amphetamine (Paredrine) cause release of norepinephrine from the vesicles in the nerve terminal; cocaine and protriptyline block the reuptake of norepinephrine into the sympathetic nerve terminals and thus potentiate its adrenergic effect.

Table 10. Sympathetic pharmacology of the eye

Stimulators	Site of action	Blockers
	Superficial cervical ganglion	
Acetylcholine (inactivated by acetyl-cholinesterase)		Hexamethonium
Tetramethylammonium		Pentolinium
Nicotine (low concentration)		Nicotine (high concentration)
	Terminal nerve	
Release norepinephrine		Block synthesis, storage,
Hydroxyamphetamine		or release of norepi-
Ephedrine		nephrine
Block reuptake of norepinephrine		Guanethidine
Cocaine		Methyl dopa
Protriptyline		Bretylium
		Reserpine
	Effector cell (alpha receptors)	
Phenylephrine		Dibenzyline
Epinephrine (high concentration)		Tolazoline
Ephedrine		Phentolamine
Norepinephrine		
	Effector cell (beta receptors)	
Isoproterenol		Propranolol
Epinephrine (low concentration)		Dichloroisoproterenol

Adrenergic blockade may be accomplished by several groups of drugs. Blockade of the alpha receptors occurs with administration of drugs such as dibenamine, phenoxybenzamine (Dibenzyline), phentolamine (Regitine), or tolazoline (Priscoline). Blockade of the beta receptors is accomplished with the administration of propranolol (Inderal) or dichloroisoproterenol. Adrenergic blockage also occurs with drugs that interfere with the synthesis, storage, and release of norepinephrine. Guanethidine appears to block the synthesis of norepinephrine or blocks granule storage. Bretylium acts by inhibiting the release of norepinephrine. Reserpine blocks vesicle storage of norepinephrine and thus causes an initial depletion from the sympathetic nerves and also prevents accumulation of effective concentrations so that stimulatory effects are not possible. The various sites of sympathetic nervous system stimulation and blockade are presented in Table 10.

APPLICATION TO OPHTHALMIC DISEASE
Cholinergic drugs

Topical administration of cholinergic drugs in the eye produces pupillary constriction, ciliary muscle contraction, dilatation of conjunctival and iris blood vessels, and increased aqueous outflow. These agents are used for their miotic effect and for the treatment of glaucoma.

Acetylcholine is unstable in solution and is not useful as an antiglaucoma drug. It is sometimes irrigated into the anterior chamber (concentrations 1:100 to 1:200) to constrict the pupil after cataract surgery.

Methacholine was formerly employed in strengths of 10% to 20% for treatment of glaucoma; at present it is seldom used for this purpose. Methacholine solutions are relatively unstable, and potency is usually lost within 2 to 3 weeks. A tonic pupil (Adie's pupil) will contract when 2.5% solution of methacholine is instilled into the eye; this response is used to establish a diagnosis of tonic pupil.

Pilocarpine is the most commonly used drug in the treatment of primary glaucoma. It may be used in strength of 0.5% to 8%, two to six times a day. Pilocarpine is also used to counteract mydriasis and to constrict the pupil after cataract surgery. It is well tolerated and may be used for years without side effects.

Carbachol (Carcholin, Doryl) is employed in strengths of 0.75% to 3% one to four times a day for the treatment of open-angle glaucoma. Since corneal penetration is poor, a wetting agent such as benzalkonium chloride is added. On a percentage basis the drug is a more powerful miotic than is pilocarpine. It is frequently employed in patients whose glaucoma is not adequately controlled with pilocarpine. An 0.01% solution of carbachol has been instilled into the anterior chamber to produce miosis after cataract surgery.

Bethanechol and furtrethonium (Furmethide) are other cholinergic drugs that are no longer used for treatment of glaucoma.

Anticholinesterase drugs

Topical administration of the anticholinesterase drugs produces contraction of the pupillary sphincter and ciliary muscle, dilatation of the blood vessels of the conjunctiva and iris, and improved aqueous outflow in most eyes. These agents are employed for the treatment of open-angle glaucoma; they are not advised for the treatment of narrow-angle glaucoma because they may produce hyperemia and edema of the iris and trabecular tissues. Since these agents act indirectly by inactivating cholinesterase and allowing prolonged effects of the natural acetylcholine, they are not effective as miotic agents when the parasympathetic fibers to the pupil are not active, as after retrobulbar injection of an anesthetic. Combinations of anticholinesterases should not be used, since they may be antagonistic to one another.

Physostigmine is employed in concentrations of 0.25% to 1% in solution or as an 0.25% ointment one to four times a day for the treatment of glaucoma. It is sometimes used in combination with pilocarpine. Systemic side reactions from topical therapy are rare, but local effects such as conjunctival folliculosis and posterior synechiae may occur after prolonged usage.

Neostigmine (Prostigmin) is occasionally used as a 5% solution two to six times a day for the treatment of open-angle glaucoma. Its use is reserved for patients who develop intolerance to other miotics. Neostigmine is also used as a diagnostic test for myasthenia gravis; an intravenous injection of 0.5 mg is used for this purpose.

Isoflurophate (DFP, Floropryl) is a powerful, long-lasting miotic. It is employed as an 0.1% solution once or twice a day in peanut oil in the treatment of glaucoma. Since severe ciliary spasm follows the application of the drug, it is usually employed only if the weaker miotics fail or in the treatment of aphakic glaucoma. This agent is also used in an 0.01% drop or ointment for the treatment of accommodative esotropia. Systemic side reactions are rare, but local side reactions include headache, and "iris cysts" are common; other ocular reactions include retinal detachment and cataracts.

Echothiophate (Phospholine) iodide is a strong, long-lasting anticholinesterase agent employed in the treatment of open-angle glaucoma and accommodative esotropia. For the treatment of glaucoma it is used in concentrations of 0.03% to 0.25% once or twice a day; solutions of 0.03% or 0.06% are advised in strabismus. Systemic side reactions of cholinergic stimulation including diarrhea, abdominal cramps, nausea, and vomiting occur in a small percentage of patients. Local reactions include iris cysts, accommodative spasm, cataracts, and retinal detachments. The incidence of iris cysts may be reduced by using 2.5% phenylephrine as the diluent.

Demecarium bromide (Humorsol) is another strong, long-lasting miotic used in the treatment of open-angle glaucoma in concentrations of 0.125% to 0.25% once or twice a day. It produces the same local and side reactions that echothiophate iodide does.

Adrenergic drugs

Adrenergic agents are employed chiefly for their mydriatic effects; in addition, levoepinephrine is used frequently as an antiglaucoma agent. These drugs are also used occasionally for their vasoconstrictive effects and for the symptomatic relief of allergic reactions and hyperemia of the conjunctiva.

Epinephrine is a poor mydriatic in the normal eye. However, instillation of 1:1,000 epinephrine in the eye of a patient with Horner's syndrome, produced by a lesion of the superior cervical sympathetic ganglion or its pupillary fibers, will dilate the pupil. Levoepinephrine preparations will reduce intraocular pressure, apparently by producing both decreased aqueous inflow and increased aqueous outflow. These agents are employed as a 1% or 2% solution and are used once or twice a day. They are usually prescribed in combination with pilocarpine in the treatment of glaucoma. Systemic side reactions may include palpitation and tachycardia. Local side reactions include rebound hyperemia, melanin deposits in the conjunctiva and cornea, and macular edema in aphakic eyes. Dipivalyl epinephrine, a congener of epinephrine, recently has been employed in concentrations of 0.025% to 0.1% in the treatment of open-angle glaucoma. In preliminary studies topical norepinephrine borate, 2% to 4%, has been shown to reduce intraocular pressure by improving aqueous humor outflow.

Phenylephrine hydrochloride as a 10% solution is an effective mydriatic agent. It is valuable in breaking posterior synechiae and is used as adjunctive treatment in iritis. Concentrations of 2.5% are used as a diluent for echothiophate iodide; this reduces the incidence of iris cysts with echothiophate treatment. Systemic side reactions to phenylephrine are uncommon but include tachycardia and palpitation; transient epithelial edema of the cornea may occur.

Hydroxyamphetamine hydrobromide is a mild mydriatic agent. It is employed as a 1% solution and is sometimes used in combination with cycloplegic agents. Hydroxyamphetamine is also used as a diagnostic agent to help localize the site of the sympathetic nerve lesion responsible for Horner's syndrome. Instillation of this agent will produce mydriasis only if the postganglionic neuron is intact.

Cocaine has been used in ophthalmology primarily for its anesthetic effect. It has been used also for its mydriatic action in eyes resistant to pupillary dilatation; most often it is combined with epinephrine or phenylephrine and a cholinergic blocking agent such as homatropine or atropine. Cocaine has been applied topically to deepen the anterior chamber in patients who have had recent cataract surgery and contact of the anterior face of the vitreous to the corneal endothelium. The mechanism of this action is not understood.

Protriptyline (a tricyclic antidepressant agent) has been applied topically for the treatment of open-angle glaucoma with limited success.

Cholinergic blocking agents

Topical application of the cholinergic blocking agents into the eye results in pupillary dilatation and paralysis of accommodation. Vascular permeability of the iris and ciliary blood vessels also occurs. The cholinergic blocking agents are used for the treatment of anterior uveitis, as an aid in refraction, and for their mydriatic effects, particularly as postoperative agents in cataract and retinal detachment surgery.

Atropine is used in strengths of 0.5% to 2% solution or as a 1% ointment administered one to three times a day. It is the strongest cycloplegic agent available. Mydriasis persists for up to 14 days, and cycloplegia lasts up to 6 days. Systemic side reactions may occur, particularly in children, and include tachycardia, dryness and flushing of the skin, and thirst. The most common local side reaction is contact dermatitis.

Scopolamine is employed topically in concentrations of 0.2% to 0.5% one to three times a day. Its cycloplegic effects last 2 to 3 days. Central nervous system excitement may follow its use. Since local sensitivity reactions are rare, it is often used in patients sensitive to atropine.

Homatropine is used in concentrations of 2% to 5%. Its cycloplegic effect lasts up to 48 hours. Side reactions are rare.

Cyclopentolate (Cyclogyl) is a short-acting cycloplegic. Duration of effect is 2 to 24 hours. It is used chiefly as an aid in refraction and may be employed along with 10% phenylephrine to dilate resistant pupils. It is used in 0.5% to 2% solutions at short intervals for two or three doses. Central nervous system toxicity, such as confusion, ataxia, dysarthria, and personality changes, may occur with cyclopentolate usage.

Tropicamide (Mydriacyl) is another short-acting cycloplegic. Its effect lasts 30 minutes to 4 hours. It is used in refraction and when a short-acting cycloplegic is desired as in retinal photography. Drops of 0.5% or 1% solution are repeated at short intervals for two or three doses.

Eucatropine (Euphthalmine) is a weak cycloplegic agent with moderate mydriatic properties. It is used as a 5% to 10% solution for mydriasis in ophthalmoscopy and as a provocative test in suspected narrow-angle glaucoma.

Adrenergic blocking agents

Adrenergic blocking agents are seldom employed by the ophthalmologist for treatment of eye disease. Their chief use is as antihypertensive agents. Some of these drugs have been used for the treatment of glaucoma, and others have been used for the treatment of retinal arterial occlusion.

Intravenous dibenamine was employed at one time as an antiglaucoma agent, but it is not used for this purpose now because of the availability of other more effective antiglaucoma drugs and because of the side reactions of this medication. Guanethidine (Ismelin) will lower intraocular pressure after systemic or topical administration, but it appears doubtful that it is particularly useful as an antiglaucoma drug. The application of 5% or 10% guanethidine, one to four times a day will often reduce lid retraction of Graves' disease. The increased sympathotonia of Müller's smooth muscle is relieved with this treatment, which also produces a miosis. Side reactions to topical guanethidine include conjunctival hyperemia and a burning sensation.

Tolazoline (Priscoline) has been used as a vasodilator in the treatment of retinal arterial disease. It may be injected retrobulbarly in a dose of 25 mg in 1 ml of solution along with a local anesthetic, or it may be given orally or parenterally in doses of 25 to 75 mg.

Recently 6-hydroxydopamine (6-HD) has been used topically to lower intraocular pressure in patients with glaucoma resistant to other medical treatment. The drug is applied by a special cornealscleral contact lens reservoir or injected subconjunctivally. A chemical sympathectomy is produced and the ocular hypotensive action of epinephrine is potentiated. The duration of the chemical sympathectomy is 2 to 6 months.

Thymoxamine, an alpha blocking agent, has been used topically as an 0.5% solution in the treatment of angle-closure glaucoma. The agent has also been used to reverse effects of phenylephrine induced angle-closure glaucoma.

Timolol, a beta adrenergic blocking agent that is more potent than propranolol, recently has been investigated in a small group of patients with open-angle glaucoma. The drug is applied topically in a 0.5% concentration. A fall in intraocular pressure occurs probably as a result of decreased aqueous humor secretion.

Ganglionic blocking agents

Ganglionic blocking agents such as hexamethonium (Bistrium) and pentolinium (Ansolysen) will lower intraocular pressure. This effect is probably secondary to a fall in systemic blood pressure, and these agents are not indicated in the therapy of glaucoma.

REFERENCES

Beasley, H.: Miotics in cataract surgery, Arch. Ophthalmol. **88**:49, 1972.
Goth, A.: Medical pharmacology; principles and concepts, ed. 8, St. Louis, 1976, The C. V. Mosby Co.
Halasa, A. H., and Rutkowski, P. C.: Thymoxamine therapy for angle-closure glaucoma, Arch. Ophthalmol. **90**:177, 1973.
Holland, M. G.: Treatment of glaucoma by chemical sympathectomy with 6-hydroxydopamine, Trans. Am. Acad. Ophthalmol. Otolaryngol. **76**:436, 1972.
Kaback, M. B., Podos, S. M., Harbin, T. S., Jr., and others: The effects of dipivalyl epinephrine on the eye, Am. J. Ophthalmol. **81**:768, 1976.
Katz, I. M., Hubbard, W. A., Getson, A. J., and Gould, A. L.: Intraocular pressure decrease in normal volunteers following timolol ophthalmic solution, Invest. Ophthalmol. **15**:489, 1976.
Koelle, G. B.: Neurohumoral transmission and the autonomic nervous system. In Goodman,

L. S., and Gilman, A., editors: The pharmacological basis of therapeutics, ed. 4, New York, 1970, Macmillan, Inc.

Langham, M. E., and Carmel, D. D.: The action of protriptyline on adrenergic mechanisms in rabbit, primate and human eyes, J. Pharmacol. Exp. Therap. **163**:368, 1968.

Leopold, I. H.: Trends in ocular therapy, twenty-third Sanford S. Gifford memorial lecture, Am. J. Ophthalmol. **65**:297, 1968.

Leopold, I. H.: Drugs for ophthalmic use. In Modell, W., editor: Drugs of choice, 1976-1977, St. Louis, 1976, The C. V. Mosby Co.

Pollack, I. P., and Rossi, H.: Norepinephrine in treatment of ocular hypertension and glaucoma, Arch. Ophthalmol. **93**:173, 1975.

Richardson, K. T.: Parasympathetic physiology and pharmacology, Surv. Ophthalmol. **14**: 461, 1970.

Richardson, K. T.: Sympathetic physiology and pharmacology, Surv. Ophthalmol. **17**:120, 1972.

Sears, M. D., McClean, E. B., and Bellows, A. R.: Drug induced retraction of the vitreous face after cataract extraction, Trans. Am. Acad. Ophthalmol. Otolaryngol. **76**:498, 1972.

CHAPTER 5

Carbonic anhydrase inhibitors and osmotherapeutic agents

CARBONIC ANHYDRASE INHIBITORS

Carbonic anhydrase is an enzyme that is widely distributed in the body, including the red blood cells, pancreas, kidney, central nervous system, and gastric mucosa. In the eye it is found in the uvea, retina, vitreous humor, and lens. Carbonic anhydrase may be regarded as an enzyme that increases the availability of the hydrogen and bicarbonate ions. The enzyme catalyzes step I in the following reaction:

$$\overset{\text{I}}{}\qquad\overset{\text{II}}{}$$
$$CO_2 + H_2O \rightleftarrows H_2CO_3 \rightleftarrows H^+ + HCO_3^-$$

Step II is an ionic dissociation reaction that proceeds very rapidly and is not under enzymatic control.

More than 90% of carbonic anhydrase inhibition must occur before clinical effects are achieved. The administration of carbonic anhydrase inhibitors results in decreased hydrogen ion available for the hydrogen and sodium ion exchange in the kidney tubules. As a consequence there is an initial diuresis, and the urine becomes alkaline. Urine sodium, potassium, and bicarbonate levels increase and the ammonia concentration decreases.

As a result of the effect on the kidney, bicarbonate in the extracellular spaces decreases, and metabolic acidosis occurs. Further acidosis does not occur with continued carbonic anhydrase inhibitor therapy, since there is compensatory increased reabsorption of bicarbonate in the proximal tubule. The diuretic effect diminishes as there is less available bicarbonate and sodium in the glomerular filtrate. Initially there is a marked increase in potassium excretion, but with continued administration of carbonic anhydrase inhibitors, the effect on potassium balance is lost. For these reasons, continuous use of carbonic anhydrase inhibitors, as in the long-term treatment of glaucoma, does not produce toxic electrolyte imbalances.

Administration of carbonic anhydrase inhibitors initially appears to increase carbon dioxide tension in tissues and to decrease carbon dioxide tension in the alveoli. The effect is usually temporary because of compensatory mechanisms. Large doses of carbonic anhydrase inhibitors can inhibit the secretion of both acidic gastric juice and alkaline pancreatic juice; with ordinary dosages this effect does not occur. Thyroid activity may be somewhat depressed with long-term therapy.

Following oral administration of acetazolamide, peak plasma levels are reached in 2 hours and are maintained for 4 to 6 hours. Complete excretion of the drug by the kidney occurs in 24 hours.

OCULAR EFFECTS

Carbonic anhydrase inhibitors generally lower the intraocular pressure (IOP) in glaucomatous eyes. The magnitude of this response depends on the type and severity of the glaucoma and other antiglaucoma agents in use. The hypotensive ocular effects appear to be independent of the diuretic effect of the drug. In the normal eye carbonic anhydrase inhibitors produce only a slight or no fall in the IOP, probably as a result of a compensatory decrease in aqueous outflow.

Most investigators believe that carbonic anhydrase inhibitors produce their effect on IOP by partial inhibition of aqueous humor. Up to 60% suppression of aqueous flow may occur with carbonic anhydrase inhibitor therapy.

The exact mechanisms of suppression of aqueous flow by carbonic anhydrase inhibitors remain unknown. Several theories exist. Becker and Shaffer divided these theories into two groups: direct actions and indirect actions. The direct effect is the decreased availability of hydrogen ion and bicarbonate ion necessary for the secretory process. During secretion these ions are either moved by carriers or exchanged for the anions or cations that are transported. The indirect effect suggests that the hydrogen and bicarbonate ions provide a buffering action. Cells secreting acid become alkaline and need hydrogen ion to maintain the pH. Cells secreting alkaline become acid and need bicarbonate ion to maintain the pH.

Other possible mechanisms of the hypotensive action of carbonic anhydrase inhibitors have been described. Suppression of the conversion of CO_2 to HCO_3, a mechanism that Friedenwald originally believed was important in aqueous humor secretion, is believed by Maren to be the route by which carbonic anhydrase inhibitors may work. Other workers have described other possible actions of carbonic anhydrase inhibitors, which include decreased venous pressure secondary to constriction of the iris artery, improved aqueous outflow, and stimulation of the beta adrenergic effector sites.

OPHTHALMIC USES

Carbonic anhydrase inhibitors are valuable agents in all forms of glaucoma. In primary glaucoma they are often employed in conjunction with miotic agents since these drugs act in a different manner than carbonic anhydrase inhibitors, namely by promoting aqueous outflow. In secondary glaucoma carbonic anhydrase inhibitors are often used with cycloplegics and topical corticosteroids, which aid in the treatment of anterior uveitis (in steroid responders the pressure may be elevated from the steroid medication). Carbonic anhydrase inhibitor therapy for glaucoma is often on a short-term basis. Long-term therapy should be used with caution to avoid serious side reactions; however, many patients have been treated with carbonic anhydrase inhibitors for more than a decade without serious side reactions. Most failures in long-term use of carbonic anhydrase inhibitors result from side effects. Other causes of failure are progressive advancement of the glaucoma, poor drug absorption, and drug tolerance.

ADVERSE EFFECTS

Undesirable side reactions are frequent but not usually serious. They are generally reversed by discontinuance of the drugs. Paresthesias occur in almost all patients taking carbonic anhydrase inhibitors; these tend to diminish with time. Gastrointestinal discomforts and anorexia occasionally become severe enough that therapy must be discontinued.

Ureteral colic and calculi formation are not uncommon with carbonic anhydrase inhibitor therapy. It has been suggested that calculi formation occurs because of lowered urinary citrate levels. Some patients who have experienced ureteral colic with acetazolamide have been free of this serious complication when maintained on methazolamide. This latter drug is a more potent carbonic anhydrase inhibitor per unit weight, and smaller therapeutic doses are required. Many methods to decrease calculus formation have been tried. Fluids can be forced to increase the 24-hour urine output; increased fluids can be spaced throughout the day to avoid exaggerated rises in IOP as in a water-drinking test. The more alkaline the urine, the more calcium is precipitated. Therefore, attempts can be made to acidify the urine with diet. John Lynn has recommended ascorbic acid in a dose of 2 to 2.5 times the dosage of carbonic anhydrase inhibitor. This lowers urine pH. However, ascorbate is converted to oxalate, which is a salt of many ureteral calculi. Oral sodium and potassium phosphate preparations (Neutra-Phos) reportedly decrease stone formation. The mechanism for this is unknown, but it has been suggested that these agents increase the amount of a naturally occurring inhibitor of calcium crystallization in the urine. Other side reactions to carbonic anhydrase inhibitors include drowsiness, myopia, headaches, altered taste and smell, skin reactions, and general malaise. Bone marrow suppression and aplastic anemia have been rare complications.

While there is an initial potassium depletion in patients receiving carbonic anhydrase inhibitor therapy, this effect does not appear to be of any clinical significance in long-term therapy if there is an adequate dietary intake of potassium. John Lynn has suggested that patients treated with acetazolamide should use Morton's Lite-Salt, half potassium chloride and half sodium chloride, as their table salt. In patients receiving digitalis the initial hypokalemia produced with carbonic anhydrase inhibitor therapy can result in bradycardia or heart block. Theoretically, patients receiving systemic steroids or thiazide diuretics that induce loss of potassium may develop symptoms of hypokalemia with carbonic anhydrase inhibitor therapy, although this is not the usual clinical situation.

Some degree of metabolic acidosis may persist with long-term carbonic anhydrase inhibitor therapy. While this decreases the diuretic effect of carbonic anhydrase inhibitors, it appears to potentiate the suppression of aqueous humor secretion. Acetazolamide appears to inhibit ciliary secretion in an acid medium. The administration of ammonium chloride in large doses potentiates the action of acetazolamide. However, since ammonium chloride produces severe acidosis, its use in conjunction with carbonic anhydrase inhibitors has been abandoned.

Long-term carbonic anhydrase inhibitor therapy has not produced cataracts and has not apparently altered lens metabolism. No retinal changes have been recognized in connection with its use.

Acetazolamide interactions with other drugs have been described. Acetazolamide inhibits methamines and nitrofurantoin and antagonizes the effects of oral hypoglycemics. It prolongs and enhances the effects of quinidine and tricyclic antidepressants. When used with other potassium-depleting diuretics, hypokalemia may occur.

PREPARATIONS AND DOSAGE

The dosage of carbonic anhydrase inhibitors should be individualized for each patient. This is especially necessary for long-term therapy.

Acetazolamide (Diamox)

>   ORAL: 125- and 250-mg tablets; usual dose is 125- to 250-mg one to four times daily; doses up to 500 mg four times per day are employed occasionally; pressure effects occur within 2 hours after ingestion, reach a maximum in 3 to 4 hours, and end in 6 to 10 hours
>
>   500-mg sequels; one to two capsules daily; maximum effects last up to 18 hours
>
>   INTRAVENOUS: 500-mg ampules; usual dose is 250 to 500 mg in 5 to 10 ml of distilled water; effect begins in a few minutes and reaches a maximum in 30 minutes to 2 hours

Dichlorphenamide (Daranide, Oratrol)

>   ORAL: 50-mg tablets; usual dose is 50 to 200 mg daily

Ethoxzolamide (Cardrase, Ethamide)

>   ORAL: 125-mg tablets; usual dose is 125 to 500 mg daily

Methazolamide (Neptazane)

>   ORAL: 50-mg tablets; usual dose is 50 to 100 mg three times per day

OSMOTIC AGENTS

Osmotic (hyperosmotic) agents produce a pharmacological effect by creating a rapid increase in extracellular fluid (primarily plasma) osmolality. A gradient is created in which the extracellular fluid is hypertonic to intracellular fluids and to other extracellular biological fluids such as intraocular fluids and cerebrospinal fluids from which they are separated by a semipermeable membrane. Following administration of osmotic agents, there is a movement of water out of the eye and cerebrospinal fluid and there is some cellular dehydration. In the eye, most of the fluid loss is from the vitreous, but there is also some loss from the aqueous humor.

The osmotic pressure of a solution is dependent on the number of particles present per unit volume. Osmotic agents with smaller molecular weights (such as urea) produce more osmotic effect per unit dose than do agents with a larger molecular weight (such as mannitol) because of the larger number of particles in solution. Agents such as mannitol that do not cross semipermeable membranes (such as the blood-brain or blood-aqueous barrier) are more effective in reduction of intraocular or intracranial pressure. Other factors important in the pharmacological effects of osmotic agents are the rate of administration and absorption and the rate of excretion or metabolism. The more rapid the administration and absorption of an agent, the more rapid and greater the osmotic gradient produced. The more rapid the excretion or metabolism of the osmotic agent, the shorter the duration of action.

OPHTHALMIC USES

Osmotic agents are employed in the management of various acute forms of glaucoma (see Chapter 13). They are also used as preoperative agents to lower IOP and reduce vitreous volume. Because of their dehydration effect on the vitreous, they have been employed to deepen the anterior chamber and to contract vitreous away from the corneal endothelium in postoperative patients.

AVAILABLE AGENTS

The commonly used osmotic agents are mannitol, urea, glycerin, and isosorbide. Other osmotic agents such as ascorbate, sucrose, and ethyl alcohol are not employed clinically. All osmotic agents may produce headaches, dizziness, and backache, presumably from cerebral dehydration and decreased cerebrospinal fluid volume.

Mannitol (Osmitrol)

Mannitol, molecular weight 182, is a 6-carbon sugar. It is the reduced form of mannose, an aldehyde sugar that resembles dextrose in its general properties. Mannitol remains in the extracellular fluid following intravenous administration. It produces less cellular dehydration than does urea, but it produces more diuresis. Problems with cardiovascular overload and pulmonary edema are more common with this agent because of the large fluid volume required. For most patients mannitol is the intravenous osmotic of choice.

Preparations. The preparations for intravenous infusion are as follows: injection (water), 5% in 1,000-ml containers, 10% in 500- and 1,000-ml containers, 15% in 150- and 500-ml containers; 5% and 10% also available in 0.3% sodium chloride in 500- and 1,000-ml containers; 15% in 0.45% sodium chloride in 500-ml containers; ampuls of 25% in 50-ml containers.

Dosage. The dosage for adults is 20% solution of mannitol in water for intravenous injection; total dose is 1.5 to 2 grams per kg of body weight given over a period of 30 to 45 minutes.

The dosage for infants is 10% solution of mannitol in water for intravenous injection; total dose is 1.5 grams per kg of body weight given over a period of 30 to 45 minutes.

NOTE: Mannitol solutions tend to crystallize at cooler temperatures. The crystals will go back into solution if the container is warmed.

Urea, intravenous (Ureaphil, Urevert)

Urea, molecular weight 60, is an inert substance with high water and low lipid solubility. After intravenous administration a maximum fall in IOP occurs within 30 to 45 minutes. IOP returns to pretreatment levels in 5 to 6 hours. Although urea slowly penetrates into the aqueous and vitreous humor, there does not appear to be any IOP rebound from this agent. It should not be used in patients with impaired renal function. Sloughing of skin and subcutaneous tissue may occur if urea extravasates outside the vein.

Preparations. Urea is prepared in packets containing either 40 grams of lyophilized urea and 93 ml of invert sugar or 90 grams of lyophilized urea and 210 ml of invert sugar; when it is prepared, a 30% solution of urea is formed. It is also available as a powder (for solution): 40 grams with 1 gram of citric acid buffer in 250-ml containers.

Dosage. Urea is given by intravenous infusion of 1 to 1.5 grams per kg of body weight at the rate of 60 drops per minute.

Glycerin, glycerol (Glyrol, Osmoglyn)

Glycerol, molecular weight 92, is a trihydric alcohol. It is a clear, colorless, syrupy liquid with a sweet taste. This agent is usually rapidly absorbed from the gastrointestinal tract after oral administration, although the uniformity of absorption may be variable. A fall in IOP develops within an hour; the pressure gradually returns to pretreatment levels by the end of the fourth or fifth hour. Unlike urea or mannitol, glycerin is only a mild diuretic. Blood glucose levels become elevated since glycerin is metabolized to carbohydrates; therefore, some caution must be exercised when glycerol is administered to diabetic patients, although difficulties are seldom encountered.

Preparations. Each milliliter of USP glycerin contains approximately 1.25

grams of glycerin. Osmoglyn is a 6-ounce preparation of flavored 50% glycerin; Glyrol is a 4-ounce preparation of 75% glycerin.

Dosage. Glycerin is administered orally, 1 to 1.5 grams per kg of body weight. The calculated volume of glycerin is mixed in an equal volume of flavored saline solution or water or in an equal volume of orange juice to provide a 50% solution of glycerin. Osmoglyn is given in a dose of 4 to 8 ounces; Glyrol is administered in a dose of 3 to 4 ounces.

Isosorbide (Hydronol, Isonol)

Isosorbide, molecular weight 146, is a dihydric alcohol. Like mannitol, it is metabolically inert and does not produce calories or elevated blood glucose levels as does glycerol. Like urea, the drug is distributed in total body water and may slowly enter the anterior chamber. Unlike glycerol, it does not usually produce nausea but may produce some diarrhea. It produces diuresis. Since 220 ml of isosorbide contains 132 mg of sodium, the repeated use of this drug should be avoided in patients on a restricted sodium intake.

Preparations. No commercial products are currently available but may be shortly.

Dosage. Isosorbide is given orally as a 50% flavored solution in a dose of 1.5 to 2 grams per kg of body weight.

REFERENCES
Carbonic anhydrase inhibitors

Becker, B.: Carbonic anhydrase and the formation of aqueous humor, Friedenwald Memorial Lecture, Am. J. Ophthalmol. 47(1, part 2):342, 1959.
Becker, B.: Use of methazolamide (Neptazane) in the therapy of glaucoma, Am. J. Ophthalmol. 49:1307, 1960.
Becker, B.: Decrease in intraocular pressure in man by a carbonic anhydrase inhibitor, Diamox, Am. J. Ophthalmol. 37:13, 1954.
Drance, S. M.: Ethoxyzolamide (Cardrase) in the management of chronic simple glaucoma, Arch. Ophthalmol. 64:433, 1960.
Ellis, P. P.: Carbonic anhydrase inhibitors: pharmacologic effects and problems of long-term therapy. In Leopold, I. H., editor: Symposium on ocular therapy, vol. 4, St. Louis, 1969, The C. V. Mosby Co.
Kolker, A. E., and Hetherington, J.: Becker and Shaffer's diagnosis and therapy of the glaucomas, ed. 4, St. Louis, 1976, The C. V. Mosby Co.
Lynn, J.: Personal communication.
Maren, T. H.: Carbonic anhydrase: chemistry, physiology, and inhibition, Physiol. Rev. 47:595, 1967.
Maren, T. H.: The rates of movement of Na^+, Cl^-, and HCO_3^- from plasma to posterior chamber: effect of acetazolamide and relation to the treatment of glaucoma, Invest. Ophthalmol. 15:356, 1976.
Spaeth, G. L.: Potassium, acetazolamide, and intraocular pressure, Arch. Ophthalmol. 78:578, 1967.

Osmotic agents

Becker, B.: Use of hyperosmotic agents in the treatment of the glaucomas, Symposium on glaucoma, Transactions of the New Orleans Academy of Ophthalmology, St. Louis, 1967, The C. V. Mosby Co.

Becker, B., Kolker, A. E., and Krupin, T.: Isosorbide, an oral hyperosmotic agent, Arch. Ophthalmol. **78:**147, 1967.

Becker, B., Kolker, A. E., and Krupin, T.: Hyperosmotic agents. In Leopold, I. H., editor: Ocular therapy, ed. 3, St. Louis, 1968, The C. V. Mosby Co.

Galin, M. A., Davidson, R., and Schacter, N.: Ophthalmological use of osmotic therapy, Am. J. Ophthalmol. **62:**629, 1966.

Harris, L. S., Cohn, K., and Galin, M. A.: Osmotic therapy in ophthalmology, Surv. Ophthalmol. **15:**237, 1971.

Jaffe, N. S., and Light, D. S.: Treatment of postoperative cataract complications by osmotic agents, Arch. Ophthalmol. **75:**370, 1966.

Krupin, T., Podos, S. M., and Becker, B.: Effect of optic nerve transection on osmotic alterations of intraocular pressure, Am. J. Ophthalmol. **70:**214, 1970.

CHAPTER 6

Local anesthetics*

Cocaine is a naturally occurring alkaloid that is used for anesthesia. The drug is derived from the leaves of *Erythroxylon coca,* found in the high altitudes of the Andes. The Indians in this region chew the leaves for their stimulating effect on the central nervous system and as part of their social and religious life. It is known that they packed ground leaves into wounds to relieve pain, and in early Indian culture cocaine might have been used as an anesthetic in some of the operations they performed. The Spaniards brought the leaves back to Europe, and a number of German chemists tried to isolate the active principle from these leaves.

In 1860 Niemann isolated cocaine and found that it had a numbing effect on the tongue. Freud and Koller tried cocaine for several purposes, one of which was to cure morphine addiction. The drug did effect a cure for morphine addiction, but it also produced cocaine addiction. In 1884 Koller tried cocaine as a local anesthetic drug in ophthalmology. He was successful in this attempt and reported his work to an international conference in Germany. Within a year the drug was in widespread use throughout the world and was quickly extended into other areas such as dentistry and urology.

Because of the addictive properties of cocaine, attempts were made to synthesize analogs that lacked addictive properties. To accomplish this it was first necessary to identify the structure of cocaine. This was achieved by Willstätter in 1895. Cocaine is quite similar in structure to atropine, but it does not have atropine's antimuscarinic properties (although atropine is a weak local anesthetic). Using the structure of cocaine as a model, Einhorn in 1904 synthesized procaine, which had the desirable local anesthetic properties without the undesirable narcotic and addictive properties and many of the systemic toxic properties of cocaine. Subsequently, many compounds were developed that were similar in structure to procaine with an ester link between the aromatic nucleus and the amine group. In 1948 Lofgren synthesized lidocaine, which has an amide rather than an ester link between the two major structural portions of the compound.

---

*A major portion of this chapter is from Ellis, P. P.: Local anesthetics. In Leopold, I. H., and Burns, P. P., editors: Symposium on ocular therapy, vol. 8, New York, copyright © 1976, John Wiley & Sons, Inc. Reprinted by permission of John Wiley & Sons, Inc.

PHARMACOLOGICAL CHARACTERISTICS

Local anesthetics produce a transient and reversible loss of sensation in the area where they are applied or injected. To understand the pharmacological action of local anesthetics it is necessary to review briefly the physiology of nerve conduction. During the resting phase, a negative potential of 50 to 70 mv exists within the nerve with respect to its external surface. With nerve excitation an initial slow phase of depolarization occurs, during which the electropotential within the nerve becomes less negative. When the potential difference between the interior and exterior surfaces of the membrane reaches a critical level (the threshold potential), rapid depolarization occurs and the electropotential is altered so that the interior of the nerve cell becomes relatively more positive. At the peak of potential the interior of the cell has an electropotential of about 40 mv compared with the outside. After the depolarization phase has ended, the inside potential again becomes negative.

In the resting state, the interior of the nerve cell has a high concentration of potassium and a low concentration of sodium, while the extracellular fluid has a high concentration of sodium and a low concentration of potassium, and the nerve cell membrane is relatively impermeable to the movement of sodium and potassium ions. However, with nerve excitation, the permeability of the nerve cell membrane increases, and there is an influx of sodium along a concentration gradient, which accounts for depolarization. At the time of maximum depolarization, the permeability of the cell membrane to sodium decreases, and the potassium ions move along a concentration gradient inside the cell, resulting in repolarization of the cell membrane. Immediately after repolarization, an excessive amount of sodium is present within the nerve cell, and an excess amount of potassium is outside the nerve. At this time sodium is actively transported from inside the nerve, with expenditure of energy derived from the metabolism of adenosine triphosphate (ATP). Potassium ions may also be transported by the same mechanism, although they may return along an electrostatic gradient.

In unmyelinated nerves, conduction occurs along the entire nerve. In myelinated nerves, breaks or pores exist within the myelin (the nodes of Ranvier), and nerve impulses are conducted from one node to the next. Propagation of the nerve impulse is much faster in myelinated nerves than in unmyelinated nerves.

It appears that local anesthetics block nerve conduction by interfering with depolarization so that the threshold potential level is not reached and nerve action potential does not occur. The apparent primary mechanism for this is a reduction of the permeability of the cell membrane to sodium ions. It has been suggested also that local anesthetics may compete with calcium for sites on the nerve membrane. Calcium may have a regulatory role in the movement of sodium across the nerve cell membrane.

The site of action of anesthetics seems to be at the nodes of Ranvier. It is thought that the pores are plugged both inside and outside by drug molecules.

However, the main effect appears to be inside the cell. In unmyelinated nerves the effect of the anesthetic is along the entire surface of drug contact. Higher concentrations of anesthetics are required to block conduction in myelinated nerves, and even higher concentrations are required to block large sheathed motor nerves.

In solution, local anesthetics exist in both charged and uncharged forms. The relative proportion of these forms depends on the pH of the solution and on the dissociation constant (pK) of the compound. With a higher pH there is a greater concentration of the free base uncharged form. Apparently the uncharged base form is important for optimal penetration of the nerve sheath. However, after diffusion through the epineurium, equilibration occurs between the charged and uncharged forms, and it is the charged form that binds the drug to the receptor site. Thus, probably both the charged and uncharged forms are important in anesthetic activity.

Local anesthetics may be divided into two structural groups: those with an ester linkage between the aromatic portion and the intermediate chain and those with an amide linkage. The ester group consists of drugs such as procaine and tetracaine and are hydrolyzed by plasma cholinesterase; the amide group such as mepivacaine and bupivacaine are metabolized in the liver. Patients with decreased amounts or abnormal plasma cholinesterase may have increased or toxic effects with the usual dosage of the ester type of anesthetic agents.

The structure of the drug molecule determines its protein-binding and lipid-solubility characteristics. The aromatic portion of the drug molecule is responsible for its lipophilic properties; the amine portion affects the lipid water distribution coefficient. Agents with high affinity for lipoproteins demonstrate prolonged activity on nerves with high lipoprotein content; on nerves without much lipoprotein these agents may not have any longer action than anesthetics without high lipoprotein affinity.

GENERAL PHARMACOLOGICAL EFFECTS

Cardiovascular. Local anesthetics such as lidocaine and procainamide are used intravenously to treat cardiac arrhythmias. These drugs decrease electrical transmission from the atrium to the ventricle and excitability of the ventricle. In the normal heart at nontoxic doses there is little or no alteration of electrical activity, hemodynamic properties of the heart, or peripheral resistance. Changes in the intra-atrial, intraventricular, and atrioventricular conduction, absolute refractive periods, and diastolic threshold are minimal. As the doses of anesthetics are increased, the conduction time in various parts of the heart is prolonged. At toxic levels, vasodilatation occurs initially, followed by decreased myocardial contractility. Systemic hypotension, depressed cardiac conduction, and ultimate cardiac arrest occur with higher doses. The often observed circulatory effects with anesthetic injections may come from epinephrine itself, which produces increased cardiac output and a decrease in peripheral resistance.

Central nervous system. Nontoxic levels of local anesthetics produce little apparent effect on the central nervous system. As doses of the drug are increased, an excitory phase may occur, which usually is manifested clinically as tremors, shivering, and ultimately convulsions. Further doses of the anesthetic produce generalized central nervous system depression leading to respiratory problems. The cause of central nervous system excitation has created much discussion. Recent studies indicate that the initial effect of anesthetics on the central nervous system is a blockade of the inhibitory cortical synapses. This permits the facilitory neurons to function unopposed, which leads to symptoms of excitation.

INJECTABLE ANESTHETICS

A list of the commonly used injectable anesthetic agents is presented in Table 11, including their maximum safe doses, delay in time of onset of action, duration of activity, and toxicity. Procaine is not often used now for intraocular procedures because of its comparatively short duration of action. Chloroprocaine is seldom used in ophthalmology for the same reason, although it is one of the least toxic agents. Lidocaine is probably the most commonly used local anesthetic in ophthalmology. The maximum safe dose of lidocaine without epinephrine is 3 to 4 mg per kg of body weight, whereas with epinephrine the maximum safe dose is 7 mg per kg of body weight.

Epinephrine frequently is added to local anesthetic solutions to prolong their duration of action. The rate of absorption is decreased by the vasoconstrictive action of epinephrine, and this prolongs the effect and decreases toxicity by permitting detoxification to proceed systematically without excess blood levels of the drug. Various concentrations of epinephrine have been recommended from 1:50,000 to 1:200,000. Concentrations greater than 1:200,000 are no more effective in producing vasoconstriction, however, and the risk of side reactions is much greater than with lower concentrations. Epinephrine is not usually added to anesthetic agents such as mepivacaine and prilocaine, which are absorbed slowly. Hyaluronidase is often added to anesthetic solutions, particularly those injected into the orbit, because it enhances the infiltration of the anesthetic. However, it does decrease the duration of the effect and may lead to increased rate of absorption, with possible increase in incidence of toxic reactions. For these reasons, epinephrine is usually combined with hyaluronidase, which generally is used in a concentration of 6 to 7 turbidity units per milliliter of anesthetic solution. Allergic reactions to hyaluronidase have been reported.

Bupivacaine hydrochloride (Marcaine) is a long-acting anilide anesthetic that was synthesized by af Ekenstam and his co-workers in 1957. It was approved for clinical use in the United States by the Food and Drug Administration in 1973. It has gained acceptance by anesthesiologists as a safe, long-acting anesthetic.

At the University of Colorado Medical Center, bupivacaine has been em-

Table 11. Local anesthetic agents*

Drug (trade name)	Supplied	Maximum permitted dose	Onset of action	Duration	Toxicity
Procaine (Novocain)	1% to 2% solution	10 to 15 mg/kg	Rapid	30 min to 1 hr	Tinnitus, nausea; convulsions rare
Chloroprocaine (Nesacaine)	1% to 2% solution	10 to 20 mg/kg	Very rapid	1 hr	Less toxic than procaine
Tetracaine (Pontocaine)	Made up from Niphinoid crystal as required to 0.05% to 0.15% solutions (10 mg crystal/vial)	1.5 mg/kg (not to exceed 150 mg)	Slow (15 to 45 min) (usually combined with faster-acting agents)	3 to 6 hrs	Drowsiness → coma; convulsions rare
Lidocaine (Xylocaine)	0.5% to 2% solution	3 to 4 mg/kg	5 to 30 min	2 hrs	Drowsiness → coma, convulsions also
Mepivacaine (Carbocaine)	1.0% to 2.0% solution	7 mg/kg (do not exceed 1,000 mg/24 hrs)	5 to 30 min	2 to 3 hrs	Drowsiness → coma, convulsions
Xylocaine with 1:200,000 epinephrine	0.5% to 2.0% solution	7 mg/kg	5 to 30 min	2 to 3 hrs	Drowsiness → coma, convulsions; do not use more than 50 ml of 1:200,000 epinephrine solution
Prilocaine (Citanest)	1.0% to 3.0% solution	Dose not to exceed 700 mg in adult	5 to 30 min	2 to 3 hrs	Drowsiness → coma, or convulsions; methemoglobinemia with overdose
Bupivacaine (Marcaine)	0.25% to 0.75% solution	Up to 300 mg in adult	7 to 30 min	4 to 6 hrs or 25% longer than tetracaine	Tremor, shivering, nausea; rare convulsions

*Adapted from Barton, D.: Anesthesia for outpatients. In Hill, G. J. II, editor: Outpatient surgery, Philadelphia, 1973, W. B. Saunders Co.

ployed as a local anesthetic in ophthalmic surgery. The drug is used in 0.75% concentration with hyaluronidase, with and without epinephrine. The duration of surgical anesthesia has been up to 4.5 hours, which is the period of the longest surgical procedure. Ocular akinesia has persisted longer than 6 hours, and patients have been free from postoperative pain for the first 12 hours after surgery. No toxic reactions have been encountered with the maximum dose of 75 mg. Many patients experience some pain when the drug is injected subcutaneously for lid anesthesia. This can be prevented by injecting lidocaine into the area of the infraorbital and supraorbital nerves before the bupivacaine injection. Anesthetic failures occur if the injection is not accurately placed, since bupivacaine diffuses rather poorly. It appears that the bupivacaine can provide excellent local anesthesia when long surgical procedures such as retinal detachment surgery, vitrectomies, and complicated keratoplasties are undertaken. Some ophthalmologists combine bupivacaine with equal amounts of another anesthetic such as mepivacaine (Carbocaine) or lidocaine (Xylocaine).

Etidocaine (Duranest) is another long-acting amide-type local anesthetic that has been recently introduced. It is available in concentrations from 0.5% to 1.5% with and without epinephrine. Its duration of action appears comparable with that of bupivacaine (Marcaine). The side reactions are similar to those encountered with other local anesthetics.

TOXICITIES AND SIDE REACTIONS

Central nervous system and cardiovascular toxicities may occur with local anesthetics. The general pharmacological effects of the anesthetic agents on the central nervous system and cardiovascular system have been described earlier. Systemic toxicity usually follows overdosage. It should be pointed out that the maximum safe dose of anesthetics is considerably reduced if the drugs are inadvertently injected intravenously.

In normal patients, central nervous system toxicity is seen first. Cardiovascular toxicity occurs with higher doses, provided the heart is normal. Central nervous system stimulation with excitement and convulsions is common and probably results from a blockage of inhibitory cortical synapses. Usually the seizures are self-limited, and drugs are not needed for control. If drugs are used to treat the seizures, the effect of the drug often lasts for many hours after the seizures have ceased. Barbiturates and diazepam (Valium) have been used to reduce the possibility of central nervous system seizures. The latter drug offers much better protection against seizures than barbiturates, which must be used in comparatively high doses.

If the central nervous system toxicity is pronounced, as manifested by severe convulsions or respiratory depression, it is important to keep the airway open and to ventilate the patient with oxygen. Experienced anesthesiologists may handle these severe reactions with succinylcholine administration, endotracheal intubation, and bag breathing. Local anesthetics should be avoided in patients who have recently eaten, since aspiration of vomitus could occur during central nervous system toxic reactions.

Cardiovascular side reactions may follow central nervous system reactions or may occur independently. Measures to improve circulation should be instituted immediately to treat cardiovascular collapse; these include administration of oxygen, intravenous fluids, vasopressor drugs, and cardiac massage if indicated.

Side reactions of confusion, a slight rise or decrease in blood pressure, and mild convulsions, particularly in elderly patients who have been overpremedicated, may be due to hypoxia. Also, it should be reemphasized that side reactions such as palpitation, tremor, tachycardia, and hypertension might be due to epinephrine. Such reactions to epinephrine usually abate within a few minutes.

Hypersensitivity reactions to local anesthetics are rare. They may take the form of urticaria, edema of the respiratory passages, and even anaphylactic shock. If there is a history of allergy to local anesthetics, the patient should be skin tested to these drugs before they are administered. However, positive skin reactions may be encountered in patients not allergic to local anesthetics. The allergic reactions may be due to the preservatives in the anesthetic solution (such as parabens, which are used in multiple dose vials) rather than to the anesthetic agent itself. Treatment of hypersensitivity reactions include the use of intravenous corticosteroids, epinephrine, antihistamines, and oxygen, depending on the seriousness of the reaction.

Local toxic reactions to local anesthetics can occur. These may be allergic or represent direct cellular toxicity. Cellular toxicity occurs only with large doses that are generally considered outside the range of clinical dosage. Ischemia and necrosis can occur from local injections of high doses of epinephrine.

TOPICAL ANESTHETICS

The pharmacological activity of topical anesthetics is similar to that of other local anesthetics. Some injectable agents such as tetracaine and lidocaine have surface anesthetic activity, whereas other drugs such as procaine have no significant topical anesthetic effects. The most common topical agents in ophthalmology are proparacaine 0.5% (Ophthaine, Ophthetic, Alcaine), benoxinate 0.4% (Dorsacaine), tetracaine 0.5% (Pontocaine), and cocaine 0.5% to 2%. The amount of the drug absorbed after topical application is so small that systemic side reactions do not occur. However, local side effects may occur and include allergic reactions of the conjunctiva and eyelid, corneal epithelial edema, and initial discomfort after instillation.

REFERENCES

Aceves, J., and Machne, X.: The action of calcium and of local anesthetics on nerve cells, and their interaction during excitation, J. Pharmacol. Exp. Ther. **140:**138, 1963.
af Ekenstam, B., Egner, B., and Pettersson, G.: N-alkyl pyrrolidine and N-alkyl piperidine carboxylic acid amides, Acta Chem. Scand. **11:**1183, 1957.

Aldrete, J. A., and Johnson, D. A.: Allergy to local anesthetics, J.A.M.A. **207**:356, 1969.

Aldrete, J. A., and Johnson, D. A.: Evaluation of intracutaneous testing for investigation of allergy to local anesthetic agents, Anesth. Analog. (Cleve.) **49**:173, 1970.

Barton, D.: Side reactions of drugs in anesthesia, Int. Ophthalmol. Clin. **11**(2):185, 1971.

Bonica, J. J., Akamatsu, T. J., Berges, P. U., Morikawa, K., and Kennedy, W. F., Jr.: Circulatory effects of peridural block. II. Effects of epinephrine, Anesthesiology **34**:514, 1971.

Blaustein, M. P., and Goldman, D. E.: Competitive action of calcium and procaine on lobster axon: a study of the mechanism of action of certain local anesthetics, J. Gen. Physiol. **49**:1043, 1966.

Carolan, J. A., Cerasoli, J. R., and Houle, T. V.: Bupivacaine in retrobulbar anesthesia, Ann. Ophthalmol. **6**:843, 1974.

Castren, J. A., and Tammisto, T.: A clinical evaluation of a new anesthetic (Marcaine-Adrenalin) in ocular surgery, Acta Ophthalmol. **44**:837, 1966.

Covino, B. J.: Local anesthesia, part I, N. Engl. J. Med. **286**:975, 1972; part II, N. Engl. J. Med. **286**:1035, 1972.

de Jong, R. H.: Physiology and pharmacology of local anesthesia, Springfield, Ill., 1970, Charles C Thomas, Publisher.

de Jong, R. H., Robles, R., and Corbin, R. W.: Central actions of lidocaine: synaptic transmission, Anesthesiology **30**:19, 1969.

Ellis, P. P., and Littlejohn, K.: Effects of topical anticholinesterases on procaine hydrolysis, Am. J. Ophthalmol. **77**:71, 1974.

Hille, B.: Common mode of action of three agents that decrease permeability in nerves, Nature (London) **210**:1220, 1966.

Laaka, V., Nikki, P., and Tarkkanen, A.: Comparison of bupivacaine with and without adrenalin and mepivacaine with adrenalin in intraocular surgery, Acta Ophthalmol. **50**:229, 1972.

Leopold, I. H.: Advances in anesthesia in ophthalmic surgery, Ophthalmic. Surg. **5**:13, 1974.

Lieberman, W. A., Harris, R. S., Katz, R. I., Lipschutz, H. M., Dolgin, M., and Fisher, V. J.: The effects of lidocaine on the electrical and mechanical activity of the heart, Am. J. Cardiol. **22**:375, 1968.

Löfström, B.: Aspects of the pharmacology of local anesthetic agents, Br. J. Anaesth. **42**:194, 1970.

Moore, D. C.: Use of hyaluronidase in local and nerve block analgesia other than spinal block: 1,520 cases, Anesthesiology **12**:611, 1951.

Narashashi, T., Frazier, D. T., and Yamada, M.: The site of action and active form of local anesthetics. I. Theory and pH experiments with tertiary compounds, J. Pharmacol. Exp. Ther. **171**:32, 1970.

Ritchie, J. M., Cohen, P. J., and Dripps, R. D.: Cocaine, procaine, and other synthetic local anesthetics. In Goodman, L. S., and Gilman, A., editors: The pharmacologic basis of therapeutics, ed. 4, New York, 1970, Macmillan, Inc.

Ritchie, J. M., Ritchie, B., and Greengard, P.: The active structure of local anesthetics, J. Pharmacol. Exp. Ther. **150**:152, 1965.

Ritchie, J. M., and Ritchie, B. R.: Local anesthetics: effect of pH on activity, Science **162**:1394, 1968.

Rosen, K. M., Lau, S. H., Weiss, M. B., and Damato, A. N.: The effect of lidocaine on atrioventricular and intraventricular conduction in man, Am. J. Cardiol. **25**:1, 1970.

Smith, R. B., and Everett, W. G.: Physiology and pharmacology of local anesthetic agents, Int. Ophthalmol. Clin. **13**(2):35, 1973.

Smith, R. B., and Linn, J. G., Jr.: Retrobulbar injection of bupivacaine (Marcaine) for anesthesia and akinesia, Invest. Ophthalmol. **13**:157, 1974.

Tanaka, K., and Yamasaki, M.: Blocking of cortical inhibitory synapses by intravenous lidocaine, Nature (London) **209**:207, 1966.

Taylor, R. E.: Effect of procaine on electrical properties of squid axon membrane, Am. J. Physiol. **196**:1071, 1959.

Wylie, W. D., and Churchill-Davidson, H. C.: A practice of anaesthesia, ed. 2, Chicago, 1966, Year Book Medical Publishers, Inc.

CHAPTER 7

Medical agents in surgical care

PREANESTHETIC MEDICATIONS

The use of preanesthetic agents is a subtle art, and the surgeon's choice of drugs is based on his familiarity with the individual patient's physical and mental status as well as on his knowledge of pharmacology. In fact, when an operation is to be performed with the patient under local anesthesia, the need for preanesthetic medication depends largely on the skill of the surgeon in handling the patient both preoperatively and during surgery.

The major considerations in the selection of preanesthetic agents are (1) the general health of the patient, (2) the type of anesthetic to be used during surgery, (3) the patient's age and weight, (4) the emotional makeup of the patient, and (5) the patient's background of any drug idiosyncrasy.

Any patient who is to undergo eye surgery should have a thorough physical examination. Some surgeons prefer that this be done before the patient enters the hospital. Others arrange for it during the preoperative hospital stay. If the patient has any systemic disease of consequence, he should be under the care of a qualified physician during his hospitalization, and preoperative orders should be modified, if necessary, to ensure the best possible treatment of the systemic disease during the patient's hospital stay for the ocular surgery. Moreover, elective surgery should not be performed until the patient's general health is satisfactory. Many patients requiring ophthalmic surgery have diabetes mellitus. These patients should be managed so that they do not become hypoglycemic during surgery, and at the same time reasonable control of hyperglycemia should be maintained. If the patient has received systemic corticosteroid therapy in the past 6 months, it may be advisable to reinstitute this medication before general anesthesia is given to prevent acute adrenal cortical insufficiency. Some anesthesiologists routinely give an intramuscular injection of 50 to 100 mg of hydrocortisone an hour before surgery and continue this medication daily for 2 to 3 days postoperatively. Others do not routinely administer corticosteroids preoperatively but are prepared to give intravenous corticosteroids if signs of acute adrenal insufficiency develop during surgery.

If general anesthesia is to be used, the anesthesiologist is responsible for writing the preoperative orders. However, the ophthalmic surgeon should consult with him concerning the types of premedication and anesthesia that would be best suited to each particular case. For example, if he is going to perform squint surgery, he may discuss the medications that might be employed in order to avoid cardiac arrest resulting from the oculocardiac reflex. If he is going to perform intraocular surgery, he should advise the anesthesiologist either to avoid using succinylcholine altogether or to administer it some time before the globe is opened, since succinylcholine causes transient contractions of the extraocular muscles and a consequent rise in intraocular pressure. These contractions may be prevented by the prior administration of nondepolarizing muscle relaxants such as curare or gallamine (Flaxedil).

If electric cautery is to be used, the anesthesiologist should be informed so that a nonexplosive anesthetic agent can be used. If the surgery is intraocular, the anesthesiologist must be warned that little or no coughing or vomiting should occur during recovery. If the patient has been receiving echothiophate iodide or demecarium bromide (Humorsol) drops, succinylcholine should not be used as a relaxant during anesthesia, since this agent is hydrolyzed by plasma cholinesterase, which is often lowered as a result of echothiophate iodide or demecarium therapy. Administration of succinylcholine to patients with decreased levels of plasma cholinesterase may result in prolonged apnea. If there is a family or patient history of malignant hyperthermia, elective survey should be postponed until adequate evaluation of the patient can be made. Appropriate modification in selection of anesthetic agents and other supportive measures can be undertaken by the anesthesiologist if surgery is necessary. If large doses of acetazolamide (Diamox) has been employed in the immediate preoperative period, carbon dioxide exchange in the alveoli from the red blood cells can be decreased. A brief conference can thus avoid possible serious consequences.

If the surgery is to be done with the patient under local anesthesia, the ophthalmic surgeon should take the responsibility of writing the preanesthetic orders, which should be individualized to the patient's needs. As a rule, patients who are 70 years old or over do not require as much premedication as do younger patients. Stoic individuals need less preoperative medication than do anxious or high-strung persons. The objective is to have the patient arrive in the operating room in a relaxed but cooperative state. Overpremedication produces as many problems as does underpremedication.

Barbiturates, opiates, and tranquilizers, either alone or in combination with one another, are the most commonly used preanesthetic agents when ocular surgery is performed with the patient under local anesthesia. The barbiturates are probably the most commonly used preanesthetic agents. They usually produce very satisfactory hypnosis and sedation. However, in a small number of people, especially the aged, they cause delirium and agitation. Pentobarbital (Nembutal) and secobarbital (Seconal) are usually prescribed. If the barbiturate is the only preanesthetic agent to be used, it is given in a single or divided dose of 100 to 200 mg 1 to 2 hours before surgery. If the patient is in his seventies or eighties, or if he is of very slight build, the dose is reduced by one third to one half. If the barbiturate is used in combination with a phenothiazine product, the dose is reduced, since the phenothiazines potentiate the action of the barbiturates. Chloral hydrate in an oral dosage of 750 to 2,000 mg is often used as a substitute for the barbiturates, since it rarely causes the agitation or delirium that may result from the barbiturates.

The drug most commonly used as a preanesthetic analgesic for ocular surgery is meperidine hydrochloride (Demerol), a synthetic opiate. It is generally given in a dose of 50 to 100 mg either orally or intramuscularly 60 to 90 minutes before surgery and is ordinarily used in combination with barbiturates and the phenothiazines, since it has little sedative or hypnotic effect.

Other agents such as morphine, methadone, anileridine, and codeine are used as preanesthetic agents by a few ophthalmic surgeons. All opiates cause some depression of respiration and may cause nausea and vomiting. The latter symptom is most often seen after the administration of morphine. Patients may be checked for their reaction to these drugs by administering a test dose 1 or 2 days before surgery.

The phenothiazine drugs have enjoyed popularity as preanesthetic agents in eye surgery during the past few years. These drugs have several actions: They are tranquilizers, they are antiemetics, and they potentiate the action of barbiturates and opiates. Chlorpromazine (Thorazine) was formerly used extensively by ophthalmologists as a preanesthetic agent, but lately it has been used less frequently because of its severe hypotensive effect. Promethazine (Phenergan) and triflupromazine (Vesprin) currently are the commonly used phenothiazines. They produce the tranquilizing and antiemetic effects of chlorpromazine, usually without its severe hypotensive effects. The dose of promethazine is 25 to 50 mg either orally or intramuscularly 60 to 90 minutes before surgery. The dose of triflupromazine is 10 to 25 mg intramuscularly 60 to 90 minutes before surgery. Perphenazine (Trilafon) is another phenothiazine without significant hypotensive effects that has been used as a preanesthetic agent. The dose is 5 to 15 mg intramuscularly 60 to 90 minutes before surgery.

Hydroxyzine pamoate (Atarax, Vistaril) is an antihistamine that is used as a preanesthetic agent for its sedative and tranquilizing effects. This drug is useful in the control of agitated patients, since it does not cause hypotension, as do the phenothiazine agents. The dose is 25 to 50 mg orally or intramuscularly 60 to 90 minutes before surgery.

Barbiturates, opiates, and phenothiazines may be usefully combined. Pentobarbital or secobarbital, 75 to 100 mg, is usually given 2 hours before surgery. Chloral hydrate, 750 to 1,000 mg, is substituted for the barbiturate in very elderly patients. Meperidine, 50 to 100 mg (or anileridine, 25 to 50 mg), and promethazine, 25 to 50 mg (or hydroxyzine, 25 to 50 mg), are usually given intramuscularly about 1 hour before surgery. I have had no serious complications with this type of premedication and have been generally quite satisfied with the results.

Diazepam (Valium), a central tranquilizing agent, recently has become popular as a preanesthetic agent. It produces retrograde amnesia and has an anticonvulsant action; it does not produce significant hypotension in the preanesthetic dosage of 5 to 10 mg intramuscularly. If used in combination with narcotics this dosage should be reduced, since the drug potentiates the action of narcotics. Innovar, a combination of the sedative droperidol and the narcotic fentanyl, is a useful adjunct when local anesthesia is planned. It is usually administered intravenously when the patient is on the operating table. Because of respiratory depression produced, the drug should be given only by an anesthesiologist.

Certain special ophthalmological situations may require additional premedication. If the intraocular tension is significantly elevated in the immediate preoperative period, intravenous or oral acetazolamide, intravenous mannitol or urea, or oral glycerol may be very helpful in lowering the pressure and thus reducing the potential hazards of operating on a "hard" eye (Chapter 13). If cataract surgery is undertaken in a patient with a smoldering uveitis, corticosteroids or ACTH should be given (Chapter 16). If the patient has had an old dacryocystitis, prophylactic antibiotics should be employed if intraocular surgery is to be performed, even though the inflammation appears to have subsided, unless the puncta are sealed.

The question of whether preoperative antibiotics should be given routinely prophylactically before intraocular surgery is controversial. Certainly, any infection about the eyes should be cleared first with antibiotics, and antibiotics should be used before emergency surgery. Topical antibiotics are more commonly employed than are systemic antibiotics for prophylaxis. Subconjunctival antibiotics at the end of surgery also are advocated by some ophthalmic surgeons.

The problems of drug sensitivity and drug toxicity, alteration of conjunctival flora, development of antibiotic-resistant strains of bacteria, and formation of mycotic organisms are all arguments against the routine use of preoperative antibiotics. On the other hand, some institutions report a significant decrease in postoperative infections with preoperative antibiotic therapy.

ANESTHETIC AGENTS (see also Chapter 6)
Topical anesthetics

The most commonly used topical anesthetics in ocular surgery are tetracaine (Pontocaine), cocaine, proparacaine (Ophthaine, Ophthetic, and Alcaine), and benoxinate (Dorsacaine). Only surface anesthesia is accomplished by these agents, and additional anesthesia must be provided for any procedure that involves deeper structures. The amount of drug absorbed after topical administration is so slight that there are no systemic reactions, but there may be some local side effects. Allergic reactions of the conjunctiva and eyelid are seen most often after the administration of tetracaine. Initially, slight pain follows the instillation of cocaine, tetracaine, and benoxinate. Corneal edema may appear with the use of topical anesthetic agents. Therefore these agents should be avoided when detachment surgery is to be performed, since they may interfere with visualization of the retina. Cocaine produces mydriasis. It should be avoided if miosis is desired during operation, as in glaucoma surgery.

Any topical anesthetic instilled into a "surgical" eye must be sterile. The use of single-dose dispensers is strongly advocated.

Local anesthetics

Procaine and lidocaine (Xylocaine) are the two most commonly used local anesthetic agents in ocular surgery. To these are frequently added epinephrine (1:50,000 to 1:200,000) and hyaluronidase (5 to 10 turbidity units per milliliter). The epinephrine is used to decrease absorption of the anesthetic, and the hyaluronidase is used to increase the diffusion of the drug. Lidocaine has better diffusion capacities than does procaine. Lidocaine has approximately 2 hours of effect, whereas procaine has a duration of action of about 1 hour. Mepivacaine (Carbocaine), an analog of lidocaine, has a duration of action and toxicity similar to lidocaine; it also has a vasoconstrictive action. Prilocaine (Citanest) is another recently introduced local anesthetic similar to lidocaine in its effects. Lower toxicity is reported with this agent, but it diffuses less than lidocaine. Bupivacaine (Marcaine) is a long-acting local anesthetic that has proved useful when prolonged ophthalmic surgical procedures are undertaken (Chapter 6).

Toxic reactions to these local anesthetics are very infrequent unless an excessive amount is given or the drug is accidentally injected intravenously. For the average adult the maximum safe dosage of procaine is 1 gram (100 ml of 1% solution or 50 ml of 2% solution). Lidocaine toxicity occurs with doses of 500 to 750 mg (75 ml of 1% solution or 25 ml of 2% solution). Maximum safe dosage is 7 mg per kg of body weight when used with epinephrine; without epinephrine the maximum safe dosage of lidocaine is 4 to 5 mg per kg of body weight. If the drug is injected intravenously, toxic reactions occur with about one tenth of the minimal safe local dosage.

Toxic reactions may be manifested as central nervous system stimulation (tremors, convulsions) or as cardiovascular collapse. Procaine may cause grand mal convulsions, whereas lidocaine occasionally causes minor central nervous system toxic reactions in the form of slight tremors. The treatment for central nervous system toxic reactions consists of giving an intravenous barbiturate, either thiopental or secobarbital; 1 ml is given and then repeated after a minute if the central nervous system irritation persists. Intravenous administration of diazepam (Valium) is a very useful drug for control of central nervous system toxicity and is preferred by many physicians. The dosage is titrated to control reactions and should be given slowly—no more than 5 mg (1 ml) in a minute. An airway must be secured and the patient ventilated with oxygen. Intravenous succinylcholine may be given instead of barbituates to control convulsive movements.

Cardiovascular collapse may follow the central nervous system symptoms or may develop independently of them. Measures to improve the circulation should be instituted immediately—oxygen, intravenous fluids, vasopressor drugs, and cardiac massage if indicated.

OFFICE SEDATION

Careful ophthalmoscopic examination of infants' eyes is often impossible without sedation. The use of rectal suppository barbiturates is not satisfactory because of variable drug absorption. Time of drug effect with oral barbiturates is too delayed.

For many years we have employed chloral hydrate syrup for the sedation of infants in our clinics; in most instances the results have been very satisfactory. Recovery time is short, and there is no residual dizziness such as is frequently encountered with barbiturate sedation. The dosage of chloral hydrate syrup is 30 to 40 mg per kg of body weight, administered orally. The desired effect is observed usually in 15 to 45 minutes.

Tonometry in infants may be performed with supplemental topical anesthesia. Chloral hydrate sedation is frequently inadequate for a long detailed examination that requires manipulation of the globe, as during ophthalmoscopy for the presence of recurrent retinoblastoma.

Ketamine anesthesia is particularly valuable for outpatient surgical procedures and ophthalmological examination in infants and children. This agent produces a dissociative state; the oral pharyngeal reflex is retained. The drug is administered intravenously in a dose of 2 mg per kg of body weight or intramuscularly in a dose of 10 mg per kg of body weight. Administration of the drug by an anesthesiologist is advisable. Atropine should be used as a preanesthetic agent to avoid excess upper respiratory secretions that could lead to laryngospasm. Ketamine produces micronystagmus and increased intraocular pressure; it should not be used for intraocular surgical procedures.

POSTOPERATIVE MEDICATIONS

Postoperative medical therapy should be directed toward (1) relieving severe pain; (2) reducing any undesirable reactions such as nausea and vomiting, over-anxiety, mental confusion, and disorientation; and (3) returning the patient to his preoperative physiological habits as soon as possible. If the patient has been under treatment for a systemic disease, this treatment should be reinstituted as soon as possible. The preoperative treatment of systemic disease can usually be reestablished within a short time after surgery, Again, it is usually wise to have another physician in attendance for the management of the systemic disease during the hospital stay.

Finally, it should be mentioned that the surgeon can make the postoperative management much simpler if he speaks a few words of reassurance to the patient after surgery and instructs him in the postoperative routine. Similarly, a brief conference with the relatives and instructions to them will be most helpful in simplifying postoperative care.

Relief of pain

Most adult patients experience a moderate amount of pain during the first few hours after major ocular surgery. This can usually be controlled with meperidine, 50 to 100 mg every 5 to 6 hours as necessary, or codeine, 60 mg, with 600 mg of aspirin. For many years it was my practice to wait until the patient developed moderately severe pain before giving analgesics, but I have found that giving 50 to 100 mg of meperidine during the early period of pain will abort the restlessness, irritability, nausea, and vomiting that seem to follow discomfort and anxiety. I prefer meperidine during the first 24 hours after surgery because codeine and aspirin lead to nausea in a high percentage of patients. Dextropropoxyphene (Darvon), in a dose of 62 mg, may be substituted for codeine. Less nausea occurs with this drug than codeine, but some authorities believe the potency is also much less. After 24 to 48 hours most patients need only APC tablets, aspirin, or equivalent drugs for pain.

Postoperative analgesics are not usually necessary for infants and young children after ocular surgery. They usually sleep most of the first 24 hours after operation, which is done with the patient under general anesthesia, and by the following day the pain has greatly diminished. In older children, analgesics are sometimes indicated for one or two doses. (See pediatrics dosage schedule in section on therapeutic agents.)

Relief of nausea and vomiting

It is much better to prevent nausea and vomiting than to treat it. Reassurance and relief of pain go a long way in the prevention of postoperative nausea and vomiting after local anesthesia. The use of phenothiazines as preoperative agents is also very helpful.

If nausea and vomiting do develop, they can usually be relieved by certain phenothiazines and antihistamines. Among those most commonly used are prochlorperazine (Compazine), promethazine (Phenergan), trimethobenzamide (Tigan), meclizine (Bonine), chlorpromazine (Thorazine), dimenhydrinate (Dramamine), diphenhydrinate (Benadryl), promazine (Sparine), triflupromazine (Vesprin), and cyclizine (Marezine). Certain ones (chlorpromazine, promazine, and prochlorperazine) may produce a hypotensive effect. It has been my practice to employ either prochlorperazine, 5 to 10 mg, four times a day; promethazine, 12.5 to 25 mg, three to four times a day; or trimethobenzamide, 200 mg three to four times a day, to combat postoperative nausea and vomiting. Butyrophenones such as droperidol (Inapsine) are effective antiemetics in postoperative patients. The dose of droperidol is 2.5 to 5 mg intravenously or intramuscularly. Rarely is it necessary to treat this condition for longer than a day.

Relief of mental confusion and disorientation

Very elderly patients and those who are likely to suffer from cerebral ischemia may become quite confused after surgery. Part of this confusion may arise from oversedation, particularly with barbiturates. Therefore these agents should be avoided in such patients. Binocular eye dressings contribute significantly to confusion and disorientation. Monocular dressings are sufficient except in retinal detachment procedures, and their use is recommended to prevent the confusion and disorientation caused by binocular dressings. The presence of relatives or friends at the bedside is of great help in relieving the patient's confusion. Finally, the use of oxygen seems to be helpful in clearing states of mental confusion.

General medical treatment

Most older patients are more comfortable if the head of the bed is elevated. Except in certain retinal detachment procedures, this is not contraindicated. Early ambulation is desirable to decrease the likelihood of thrombophlebitis and also to facilitate reestablishment of regular bowel and bladder habits. It is our practice to ambulate our patients within the first 24 hours after surgery. If early ambulation is not advisable because of the type of surgery, the patient should be instructed to exercise the arms and particularly the legs and hips. Liquid diets are usually ordered for the first postoperative day, and soft diets are prescribed for the next several days. With such diets, mastication with secondary contraction of the orbicularis oculi is reduced. Free use of laxatives or stool softeners is suggested, since a change of bowel habits is most disturbing to many elderly patients. In patients with a history of vein thrombosis, the subcutaneous injection of low doses of heparin, 5,000 units twice a day, prevents recurrent thrombosis. This dose does not cause increased hemorrhagic tendencies.

MEDICAL MANAGEMENT OF POSTOPERATIVE COMPLICATIONS

Many postoperative complications, such as prolapsed iris and wound dehiscence, require further surgery, and no medical treatment is indicated. Other complications, such as flat anterior chambers, may be better treated with a combination of surgery and medical agents. Still others, such as infections and inflammations, are usually better managed by medical methods alone. It is our purpose here to describe briefly the medical approach to certain common complications of ocular surgery.

Infections

In any mention of treatment of postoperative intraocular infections, the question of the routine use of prophylactic antibiotics postoperatively is raised. Many ophthalmologists routinely prescribe the systemic administration of antibiotics postoperatively, most commonly either a penicillin preparation or a cephalosporin, and gentamicin less commonly. Others routinely inject antibiotics such as gentamicin, cephaloridine, or one of the other penicillins into the subconjunctival space at the end of surgery. Many more surgeons are content to instill an antibiotic ointment into the conjunctival cul-de-sac. The problem is whether the risk of infection justifies the risk of possible sensitivity and toxic reactions to antibiotic therapy and of antibiotic-resistant infections. Every ophthalmic surgeon must make this value judgment, and this is usually based on his most recent experience with postoperative infections. It is my opinion that prophylactic antibiotics should not be used routinely in patients with no complications after surgery. If there is reason to suspect that the eye has become infected immediately before or during surgery, their use is justified.

If there is evidence that an intraocular infection has developed postoperatively, antibiotics should be started immediately (Chapters 3 and 14). Unfortunately, it is sometimes difficult to differentiate a true septic intraocular infection from a sterile inflammatory reaction. If symptoms of infection develop, it is advisable to institute generous antibiotic therapy, even though the reaction may prove to be of a sterile type. Corticosteroids should also be started at the same time (Chapters 2 and 16). These drugs are not only effective in suppressing the sterile inflammatory response but are also very helpful in decreasing the intraocular cellular response to an infection. Such cellular responses are often more destructive to the eye than are the infecting organisms. Although it is true that the use of broad-spectrum antibiotics and the corticosteroids might accelerate a fungus intraocular infection, their use is still justified, since the incidence of postoperative fungus infections remains very low.

This leads to the problem of determination of the specific causative organism of the postoperative infection. Unfortunately, it is often impossible to identify the offending organism. Conjunctival cultures are usually not revealing. Cultures from the anterior chamber, particularly in aphakic eyes, are often negative for bacterial growth even in the presence of overwhelming infection. Recently cultures of the vitreous humor have been recommended; positive results are reported to be higher than those from aqueous humor cultures. Although an attempt should be made to identify the organism, treatment should not be delayed until culture results are obtained. Selection of the drug is made empirically at first because of the need for rapid control of the infection. Modifications thereafter are determined by the results of culture and by the patient's response.

The subject of infections is more thoroughly discussed in Chapters 3 and 14.

Inflammations

As mentioned previously, it is sometimes difficult to differentiate early between an intraocular infection and a severe uveitis. The systemic and local use of corticosteroids, along with antibiotics, is indicated in such cases. It is usually possible to decide within a few days whether an endophthalmitis is sterile or not, and treatment can be altered accordingly.

Some degree of iritis frequently develops after an intraocular procedure. This is usually mild and is satisfactorily treated with cycloplegics and local application of corticosteroids. In the more severe forms of postoperative uveitis, corticosteroids or ACTH should be administered systemically. Some oculists still prefer to use pyrogens for this complication, but this is not recommended therapy at present for postoperative uveitis (Chapters 2 and 16).

Papillitis is usually a late complication of ocular surgery. It is almost never caused by infection with an organism. The treatment for this complication is the use of corticosteroids.

Hyphema

There is no satisfactory medical treatment for hyphema. Many drugs have been advocated, but in my experience none has been of significant help. Cycloplegics are used in a routine fashion in postcataract hyphemas but are not recommended for traumatic hyphemas. If glaucoma develops, intravenous urea or mannitol or oral glycerol should be tried. Irrigation of hyphema in an aphakic eye is dangerous and should be avoided if possible.

Flat anterior chambers

Most flat anterior chambers after cataract surgery are caused by leaking wounds. Flat chambers also may be on the basis of a pupillary block mechanism that is produced by vitreous blockade of the pupil and iridectomy site with subsequent retention of aqueous humor in the posterior chamber or vitreous cavity and a functional iris bombé (see section on p. 82 for treatment of pupillary block glaucoma). If there is an obvious defect of the wound, as indicated by inspection or a positive Seidel fluorescein test, this should be surgically repaired at the earliest convenient time. Otherwise the patient should be treated initially with bedrest, well-fitted binocular patches or a light monocular pressure dressing, and repeated applications of cycloplegic and mydriatic agents until the pupil is well dilated.

Acetazolamide has been recommended for the treatment of flat chambers, and we have seen some chambers re-form while the patient was receiving acetazolamide, but what role the treatment played in the formation of the anterior chamber is unknown. Advocates of this treatment suggest that it acts (1) by decreasing the rate of aqueous formation and thus the rate of an aqueous leak through the wound so that the wound edges tend to seal themselves, (2) by depressing the amount of aqueous formed by secretion while not affecting that portion of the aqueous formed by diffusion so that the relative pressure of the posterior chamber to the anterior chamber is decreased, and thus the iris diaphragm is allowed to fall back, or (3) by decreasing the volume of subchoroidal fluid.

Hyperosmotic agents, either intravenous mannitol or oral glycerol, are frequently effective in the treatment of flat anterior chambers. With the use of these drugs there is shrinkage of the vitreous volume and often deepening of the anterior chamber (see Chapter 13). These agents may be repeated daily or occasionally twice a day if necessary, but their use should not be regarded as an adequate substitute for surgical correction of a leaking wound. It has been claimed that the application of topical cocaine deepens the anterior chamber in patients who have had recent cataract surgery and contact of the vitreous to the corneal endothelium.

Glaucoma

Glaucoma as a complication of ocular surgery may be the result of several mechanisms. Pupillary block glaucoma after cataract surgery occurs as a result of vitreous blockage of the pupillary space and subsequent collection of aqueous humor in the posterior chamber and vitreous cavity. It may be relieved with cycloplegic drops and hyperosmotic agents; iridectomy and partial vitrectomy may become necessary. Malignant glaucoma results from forward displacement of the lens iris diaphragm after glaucoma surgery. It usually occurs after filtering procedures but may occur after iridectomy. Initial medical treatment consists of the liberal use of cycloplegics; in addition, the use of intravenous urea or mannitol or oral glycerol is indicated. If the condition is unrelieved with this treatment, surgery in the form of lens extraction, posterior sclerotomy, or discission of the hyaloid face of the vitreous or partial vitrectomy may be necessary. Glaucoma after alpha chymotrypsin irrigation during cataract surgery is transient. If the intraocular pressure becomes markedly elevated, acetazolamide or other carbonic anhydrase inhibitors may be required for several days in the postoperative period.

FLUID AND ELECTROLYTE IMBALANCES

The problems of patients with fluid and electrolyte imbalance are complex, and it is advisable for the ophthalmologist to refer these cases to physicians trained in this area. However, the ophthalmologist should be familiar with general concepts of diagnosis and treatment of fluid and electrolyte disorders and should be able to initiate diagnostic studies and therapeutic management of these problems.

If cardiac, hepatic, endocrine, and renal functions are normal, the average adult ingests about 1,500 ml of water per day. An additional 1,000 ml is derived from oxidation of ingested carbohydrates and fat. Of this 2,500 ml total, 200 ml is excreted in the stools, 400 to 800 ml is lost insensibly through the skin and respiratory tract, and the remaining 1,500 to 1,900 ml is lost as urine.

The most important electrolyte requirements are for the cations sodium and potassium. These are related. The kidneys will normally conserve sodium by excreting potassium, so that in a patient with large unreplaced sodium losses, the urinary sodium concentration decreases to zero and urinary potassium concentration increases. The normal daily maintenance requirements are 60 to 80 mEq of sodium and 40 to 60 mEq of potassium. Losses from nasogastric suction should be replaced with approximately 80 to 100 mEq of sodium per liter of drainage. Magnesium and calcium requirements are 15 to 25 mEq per day, but these requirements can safely be ignored for a few days. Anion requirements are more flexible. Chloride should be given in an amount equivalent to at least two thirds of the cation load, or approximately 80 to 100 mEq. It is common practice to give the remainder as lactate, which is metabolized to bicarbonate, to avoid the acidosis-producing effect of large amounts of chloride. Phosphate is required at about 10 millimoles per day, but this also can safely be neglected for a few days.

Therefore, when parenteral fluids are necessary, 2,000 ml of 5% glucose in water and 500 ml of 5% glucose in 0.9% saline solution is indicated; in addition, 40 to 60 mEq of potassium should be given if renal function is normal. Alternatively one fourth normal saline (37.5 mEq/L) solutions may be given intravenously. Potassium chloride, 20 mEq, is added to each 1,000-ml container, and a total volume of 2,500 ml is administered daily. A number of premixed maintenance solutions are available from various manufacturers and are very useful.

Infants require 75 to 100 ml of fluid per kg of body weight per day. Their sodium requirement is 2 to 4 mEq per kg of body weight per day. The daily potassium requirements are more difficult to define but are about 1 to 3 mEq per kg of body weight per day. Caution must be exercised in the administration of these cations until normal urine flow and a normal BUN level can be demonstrated.

Aids to management of fluid imbalance include the usual history and physical examination, a large number of laboratory procedures, and an even larger number of "simplified" schemes for replacement therapy. A history of vomiting, diarrhea, or excessive sweating may suggest at least the direction of the imbalance. Vomiting with loss of gastric hydrochloric acid results in alkalosis; diarrhea with loss of sodium bicarbonate leads to acidosis; and excessive sweating produces a low-salt syndrome. Laboratory tests that should be obtained initially include the following: determination of hematocrit values; sodium, chloride, and potassium blood levels; BUN levels; serum bicarbonate or carbon dioxide combining power; and arterial blood gases. Intake and output records should be kept, and patients should be weighed daily if possible. Determina-

Table 12. Normal values in adult human plasma

Electrolyte	
Sodium	134 to 144 mEq/L
Potassium	3.5 to 5.3 mEq/L
Chloride	98 to 105 mEq/L
Calcium	4.5 to 5.7 mEq/L
Inorganic phosphate	2.7 to 4.4 mEq/L
Total bicarbonate	23 to 29 mEq/L
Arterial pH	7.35 to 7.45
Arterial P_{CO_2}	38 to 42 mmHg

tions of urinary electrolytes with calculation of daily sodium and potassium input and output are essential in more complicated cases.

A severe water deficit is characterized by thirst, fever, hot flushed inelastic skin, dry mucous membranes, disorientation, coma, deep respirations, and terminal shock. If water is lost more rapidly than sodium, then plethora, evidence of hypermetabolism, and convulsions may predominate. Hematocrit values and plasma sodium and chloride levels will be elevated, and urine flow will be low. Therapy consists of intravenous administration of 5% or 10% dextrose in water. The rate and volume of administration is calculated by the addition of three components: (1) estimated deficit of water and electrolytes as judged by history, physical examination, and laboratory determinations; (2) daily maintenance of water and electrolyte requirements; and (3) replacement of ongoing losses.

Water intoxication is usually iatrogenic. It is characterized by edema, nausea, vomiting, salivation, headache, irritability, hypertension, and convulsions. Both plasma sodium and chloride levels are reduced. Therapy consists of restriction of fluid intake to around 500 ml per day and diuresis. Hypertonic saline solutions, 3% sodium chloride, may be necessary for control of convulsions.

The so-called low-salt syndrome is one of the most common of fluid and electrolyte disturbances. The characteristic "dilutional hypotonicity" is the result of isotonic losses replaced by water only. It is characterized by weakness, apathy, tachycardia, orthostatic or even recumbent hypertension, muscular and abdominal cramps, hypothermia, and oliguria. Depression of plasma sodium and chloride levels and elevation of hematocrit values and BUN levels may be present. Therapy consists of fluids in amounts determined by estimation of deficit, maintenance, and ongoing losses.

Other combinations of water excesses and deficits and electrolyte abnormalities are generally detectable only by laboratory findings. Acidosis and alkalosis are subclassified into metabolic and respiratory types. The basic laboratory test is arterial blood gas determination.

Metabolic acidosis is one of the most common serious electrolyte disorders. Ingestion of ammonium or calcium chloride, ketone body excess with starvation or diabetes mellitus, diarrhea, enteric fistulas, and renal insufficiency are some of the causes of metabolic acidosis. Metabolic acidosis is characterized by low arterial pH and a low serum bicarbonate level. Compensatory hyperventilation with a low Pco_2 is often present. Treatment consists of correction of the basic disease process and of the electrolyte imbalance. Ringer's lactate, sodium bicarbonate, or sodium lactate solutions may be administered parenterally for correction of the acidosis. Intravenous sodium bicarbonate is usually given rapidly during initial treatment of acute metabolic acidosis.

Respiratory acidosis results from decreased ventilation and consequent retention of carbon dioxide. Various pulmonary and central nervous system diseases may lead to this condition. It is characterized by low pH and high Pco_2. Renal compensation may produce a high serum bicarbonate level. Treatment should be directed toward improvement of respiration.

Metabolic alkalosis occurs from loss of acid or retention of base. It characteristically follows vomiting with loss of gastric acid but may occur with ingestion of sodium bicarbonate or lactate, administration of mercurial diuretics, or extracellular fluid loss. In alkalosis following vomiting, sodium and potassium deficits are usually present as well. Metabolic alkalosis is characterized by an elevated pH and serum bicarbonate level. Respiratory compensation by hypoventilation may produce a mild elevation of Pco_2. It is nearly always seen as a concomitant of sodium and potassium deficits and is best alleviated through treatment of the underlying disorder. Parenteral use of ammonium chloride, ⅙M concentration, is occasionally necessary in severe and acute alkalosis.

Respiratory alkalosis, which results from hyperventilation, is common but seldom serious. Symptoms include tingling of fingers and toes, and light-headedness. The pH and the Pco_2 are both low. If the hyperventilation is the result of basic disease, treatment should be directed toward this underlying condition. Rebreathing into a paper bag will relieve alkalosis associated with anxiety hyperventilation.

In all cases, the milliequivalent values of various solutions and salts should be determined before they are administered for treatment of electrolyte imbalances.

REFERENCES

Allen, H. F., and Mangiaracine, A. B.: Bacterial endophthalmitis after cataract extraction. II. Incidence in 36,000 consecutive operations with special reference to preoperative topical antibiotics, Arch. Ophthalmol. **91**:3, 1974.

Beasley, H.: Hyperthermia associated with ophthalmic surgery, Am. J. Ophthalmol. **77**:76, 1974.

Cotlier, E.: Aphakic flat anterior chamber. II. Effects of spontaneous reformation and medical therapy, Arch. Ophthalmol. **87**:124, 1972.

Ellis, P. P.: Postoperative endophthalmitis. In Symposium on ocular pharmacology and therapeutics, Transactions of the New Orleans Academy of Ophthalmology, St. Louis, 1969, The C. V. Mosby Co.

Fine, L. M.: Diamox in absent anterior chamber, Arch. Ophthalmol. **73**:19, 1965.

Forster, R. K., Zachary, I. G., Cottingham, A. J., Jr., and Norton, E. W.: Further observations on the diagnosis, cause, and treatment of endophthalmitis, Am. J. Ophthalmol. **81**:52, 1976.

Frezzotti, R., and Gentili, M. C.: Medical therapy attempts in malignant glaucoma, Am. J. Ophthalmol. **57**:402, 1964.

Jaffe, N. S.: Cataract surgery and its complications, St. Louis, 1972, The C. V. Mosby Co.

Kornblueth, W., Gombos, G., and Traub, B.: The effect of osmotic agents employed before cataract extraction on the position of the vitreous following removal of the lens, Am. J. Ophthalmol. **62**:220, 1966.

Krupp, M. A.: Fluid and electrolyte disorders. In Krupp, M. A., and Chatton, M. J.: Current diagnosis and treatment, Los Altos, Calif., 1976, Lange Medical Publications.

Sears, M. L., McClean, E. B., and Bellows, A. R.: Drug induced retraction of the vitreous face after cataract extraction, Trans. Am. Acad. Ophthalmol. Otolaryngol. **76**:498, 1972.

Smith, R. B., editor: Anesthesia in ophthalmology, Int. Ophthalmol. Clin. **13**(2): entire issue, 1973.

CHAPTER 8

Therapy of diseases of the eyelids

ALLERGIC REACTIONS
Contact dermatitis

Contact dermatitis results from local contact of the eyelids with a substance to which they are sensitive, and it is usually a self-limited disease. Symptoms include redness, itching, and edema of the lids. Among the most common allergens are cosmetics, soaps, hair products, ophthalmic ointments, and medical tapes. Treatment consists of removal of the causative agent, application of mild soothing compresses saturated with solutions such as Burow's 1:40 or physiological saline solution, and the use of a corticosteroid ointment, which should be applied to the eyelids several times a day until the reaction has subsided.

Urticaria and angioneurotic edema

Urticaria and angioneurotic edema of the eyelids result from ingestion of a drug or a food to which the patient is sensitive, and they occur independently or in association with acute allergic reactions elsewhere in the body. Urticaria is limited to the dermis; angioneurotic edema can involve subcutaneous tissue and viscera, in addition. If it is known what drug or food is responsible for the urticaria, the offending substance should be eliminated. Common offenders include fruits, tomatoes, shellfish, and drugs such as aspirin, barbiturates, or antibiotics. For immediate therapy epinephrine, 0.3 to 0.5 ml of 1:1,000 dilution, may be given subcutaneously. Ephedrine sulfate, 25 mg four times per day, may then be started. For general discomfort and pruritus, corticosteroids may be used systemically or topically, but their prolonged use should be avoided. Antihistamines administered systemically are also helpful in relieving these conditions. Aspirin taken orally is a valuable antipruritic agent, but as previously noted, may be the responsible agent.

Allergic dermatoconjunctivitis

Allergic dermatoconjunctivitis is almost always caused by an ophthalmic preparation. It begins as an allergic conjunctivitis that spreads to the lids. Signs and symptoms include severe itching, papillary conjunctivitis, eczema of the skin of the eyelids, and conjunctival eosinophilia. The condition is usually secondary to topical anesthetics, antibiotics, mydriatrics, or ophthalmic vehicles. Miotic alkaloids rarely cause this problem but may produce an irritative dermatitis. Treatment includes stopping the offending drug and using topical steroids if necessary.

BACTERIAL INFECTIONS

Bacterial infections of the eyelids may be very mild or quite severe. The more common infections of the eyelids are folliculitis, impetigo, erysipelas, and infectious eczematoid dermatitis. Folliculitis is a staphylococcal infection of the hair follicles around the lids, and it presents as an itching or burning sensation in affected areas. Impetigo is a vesiculopustular eruption secondary to a combined infection of staphylococci and streptococci. The lesions must be differentiated from herpes simplex, varicella, or contact dermatitis. Erysipelas is caused by β-hemolytic streptococci. Lid involvement varies from mild edema and erythema to vesicle formation, which may suppurate. If untreated, gangrene of the eyelids may develop. Systemic manifestations include fever, headache, and malaise. Infectious eczematoid dermatitis usually occurs as a toxic and allergic reaction to staphylococcal products. The eczema subsides as the infection clears. In mild infections, satisfactory treatment consists of local antibiotic therapy such as bacitracin plus hot moist compresses saturated with solutions such as boric acid or physiological saline solution. If folliculitis and superficial staphylococcic infections recur, desensitization of the patient to staphylococcus toxoid may be carried out with benefit. Measures to improve general skin hygiene such as frequent bathing with hexachlorophene soap are often beneficial in clearing recurrent superficial staphylococcic infections.

For the more severe bacterial infections the systemic use of antibiotics (penicillin for streptococcal infections and penicillin or broad-spectrum antibiotics for other infections) is recommended. Continuous hot moist compresses are of definite benefit. In all severe infections of the eyelids an attempt should be made to identify the offending organism and to determine the sensitivity of this organism to various antibiotics.

Certain rare bacterial infections of the eyelid may occur. Anthrax is responsive to systemically administered penicillin; a daily dose of 10 million units intravenously is recommended. In mild, localized cases, tetracycline in doses of 500 mg given orally every 6 hours may be used. Glanders should be treated with the systemic administration of streptomycin or one of the broad-spectrum antibiotics. Chancroid of the eyelids is extremely rare. This disease is responsive to sulfonamides, streptomycin, and tetracyclines given systemically. Additionally, cleansing of the skin lesions with soap and water should be performed. Treatment of tularemia of the eyelids consists of the systemic administration of streptomycin. This disease is also responsive to tetracyclines and chloramphenicol.

Tetanus of the eyelids is an uncommon disorder. If available, 5,000 units of human tetanus antitoxin should be given intramuscularly. If the human antitoxin is unavailable, treatment consists of the administration of large doses of equine or bovine tetanus antitoxin after the patient has been tested for hypersensitivity. The antitoxin is administered intravenously; 50,000 to 100,000 units are added to an infusion of physiological saline solution and given slowly. Alternatively, 200,000 units of antitoxin may be given intramuscularly. Large systemic doses of penicillin (10 million units daily) should be administered intravenously, or tetracyclines may be prescribed if the patient is sensitive to penicillin. Hyperbaric oxygen has been reported to greatly reduce mortality in patients with tetanus infections. The infected area should be surgically debrided. General measures include the use of sedatives and anticonvulsant therapy; tracheostomy may be necessary. After recovery the patient should be given tetanus toxoid to ensure lasting immunity.

HORDEOLUM (STYE)

Hordeolum, a staphylococcic infection of the sebaceous glands of the eyelids, is usually self-limited and responds well to hot moist applications. Removal of the lashes in the affected area sometimes promotes external drainage. Local use of antibiotic ointments is indicated, particularly if there is a tendency to recurrence of hordeola. If there are staphylococcic infections elsewhere in the body, these should be treated, since there is an association of hordeola with systemic low-grade staphylococcic infection.

VIRAL INFECTIONS
Herpetic infections

Herpes simplex. Small vesicles with surrounding erythema, sometimes associated with similar lesions of the lip, comprise the clinical picture of herpes simplex of the eyelids. The lesions should be differentiated from those of herpes zoster and impetigo. Treatment for this condition is nonspecific. Topical applications of drying solutions (spirits of camphor or 70% alcohol) to the oozing skin lesions are commonly used. If the lesions are secondarily infected, the topical or systemic use of antibiotic ointments is advisable. Antibiotics have little effect against the infectious process but are useful in the treatment of secondary infection. Corticosteroids are contraindicated for the treatment of herpes simplex of the eyelids because they may predispose to corneal involvement.

Idoxuridine (IDU) has been employed for the treatment of cutaneous herpes simplex infections with equivocal results. IDU may be injected into the lesions, administered by a spray-gun jet, or painted directly on the lesions after their surfaces have been removed. Better results are attained if IDU is used early in the infection. During acute attacks of herpes simplex of the eyelid margin, IDU ointment may be instilled into the conjunctiva as prophylaxis against corneal involvement (Chapter 11).

Neutral red dye and proflavine are photosensitizing dyes that combine with the DNA of the herpes simplex virus to inactivate it in the presence of ultraviolet or visible light. Cutaneous herpes simplex may be treated by unroofing the vesicles, applying a solution of the dye, and shining a light (tungsten or fluorescent) on the lesions at a distance of 6 inches for 15 minutes twice a day. This therapy reduces the duration of the lesions and the frequency of recurrences. Recently, evidence has been presented to suggest that photoactive dye therapy for herpes simplex lesions may be a carcinogenic stimulus.

Herpes zoster. Vesicular lesions along the superficial branches of the ophthalmic division of the trigeminal nerve characterize herpes zoster infection of the eyelids. Periocular pain usually precedes the development of vesicles by 48 hours. No specific treatment is available for herpes zoster. The application of the new potent topical corticosteroids, fluocinolone acetonide (Synalar), betamethasone 17-valerate (Valisone), flurandrenolide (Cordran), fluocinonide (Lidex), or desonide (Tridesilon), is of value in reducing the inflammation. They are used on cutaneous surfaces, but they should not be applied inside the eyelids.

Opposing views exist regarding the advisability of treatment of herpes zoster infections with systemic corticosteroids. Morbidity is reduced if high doses of systemic steroids are employed early in the course of the disease. The occurrence of postherpetic neuralgia also may be reduced. Viremia has occurred in chronically ill patients who had received systemic steroids for herpes zoster infections. Zoster immune globulin has not been found to be beneficial in the treatment or prevention of the disease. If secondary infection is present, topical antibiotics such as bacitracin may be used, although systemic antibiotic therapy is preferred by many physicians. Boric acid and aluminum acetate, 1:40 solution (Burow's solution), or calamine lotion applied topically seems to give relief. Since many patients have rather severe pain with this condition, analgesics should be prescribed in amounts necessary to provide relief. Lubricating ointments instilled into the eye are useful to prevent the complication of exposure and trichiasis that may occur with severe lid involvement.

Vaccinia

Vaccinial lesions of the eyelids present as pustules with central indentations. There is associated preauricular adenopathy. Until recently, there was no specific treatment for these lesions, and treatment was supportive, consisting of the topical use of antibiotics for secondary infection and the application of hot moist compresses for treatment of the inflammation. Vaccinia immune globulin (VIG) has become available. This vaccine provides passive antibody against the vaccinial organisms. For eyelid lesions the dose of VIG is 0.6 ml per kg of body weight, given intramuscularly. The adult dose is 15 to 20 ml of the serum; usually two doses, given intramuscularly 2 or 3 days apart, are necessary for resolution of the lesion. Methisazone (Marboran) has also been used for the treatment of serious complications of vaccinia. The initial dose is 200 mg per kg of body weight given orally, followed by 50 mg per kg of body weight every 6 hours; treatment is continued for 3 days. IDU ointment should be instilled into the conjunctival cul-de-sac three to four times a day as prophylaxis against corneal involvement.

Molluscum contagiosum

The eyelid lesions of molluscum contagiosum are nodules with umbilicated centers usually located near the margin of the eyelid. Drainage of toxic material from the lesions into the eye may produce a chronic follicular conjunctivitis. It is important to examine the lids for molluscum in cases of conjunctivitis unresponsive to routine therapy. Treatment of this viral infection is surgical excision of the lesion and cauterization of the base, using either chemical- or electrocautery.

Verucca vulgaris

Warts are common hyperkeratotic, filiform lesions caused by viral agents. Treatment includes surgical removal with pathological examination and cautery to the base of the lesion.

Miscellaneous viral infections

Rubella, rubeola, and varicella infections of the eyelids can occur with the systemic diseases. The eyelid lesions are similar to cutaneous lesions elsewhere. There is no specific therapy for the eyelid lesions, but instillation of antibiotic ointment into the eye is advisable to prevent secondary infection.

FUNGUS INFECTIONS
Superficial infections

Most superficial fungus infections are effectively treated with griseofulvin (Grifulvin, Fulvicin, or Grisactin) or local antifungal drugs, including a variety of proprietary preparations, the active ingredients of which are combinations of fatty acids and salicylic acid. Griseofulvin is especially effective in the epidermomycoses. It is administered orally, 0.5 to 1 gram daily in a single dose or divided doses, and treatment is usually continued for 1 or 2 weeks after the fungus infection appears to have subsided. For *Candida* infections of the eyelid, the treatment of choice is the topical application of nystatin ointment, 100,000 units per gram.

Deep infections

Deep fungus infections must be treated with drugs administered systemically. *Actinomyces* and *Nocardia* infections are effectively treated with sulfonamides, penicillin, and occasionally broad-spectrum antibiotics. Histoplasmosis, North American blastomycosis, sporotrichosis, aspergillosis, torulosis, cryptococcosis, and South American blastomycosis usually respond to amphotericin B treatment. The medication is given intravenously. The initial dose is usually 0.05 to 0.1 mg per kg of body weight, given in a slow intravenous drip over a period of 6 to 8 hours. The medication is dissolved in 5% dextrose in water solution, in a concentration of approximately 1 mg/10 ml of the solution. The dosage is increased gradually until a maximum of 1 mg per kg of body weight is reached. The total dose should not exceed 2 grams. Therapy is given daily and is continued for 2 to 3 weeks after the lesions have subsided. The length of treatment may be modified if toxic reactions occur. The most serious reaction is damage to the kidneys, reflected in an elevated BUN level or the appearance of casts or red blood cells in the urine. If the BUN level goes over 50, or the creatinine level over 2, the treatment should be discontinued. Amphotericin B is a toxic drug and should not be used unless specific indications are present.

BLEPHARITIS
Staphylococcal blepharitis

Staphylococcal or ulcerative blepharitis is best treated with the frequent use of antibiotic ointments. The crust should be removed from the eyelids with a moistened cotton applicator before the antibiotic is instilled. Sulfacetamide sodium and sulfisoxazole (Gantrisin) ophthalmic ointments are quite effective in the control of staphylococcal blepharitis; general measures should be used in addition to this specific therapy. Manual expression of the meibomian glands is helpful. Application of 1% silver nitrate to the eyelid margins is useful in chronic blepharitis. Certain dyes (gentian violet and green) were formerly painted on the eyelid margins but are seldom used at the present time. Recurrent staphylococcal blepharitis is often managed successfully by desensitization of the patient to staphylococcic toxoid.

Seborrheic blepharitis

Seborrheic blepharitis is a chronic condition and is difficult to manage. Therapy consists of attempts to control seborrhea elsewhere, such as in the scalp and eyebrows. Selenium sulfide (Selsun), cadmium sulfide (Capsebon), or other antiseborrheic shampoos are helpful in the removal of scalp seborrhea, and improvement of this condition seems to exert a favorable effect on the seborrheic blepharitis. In refractory cases weak corticosteroid solutions applied to the scalp or corticosteroid ointment applied to the forehead may be helpful. Local measures in the treatment of seborrheic blepharitis consist of the mechanical removal of the oily, greasy material with a moistened, warm cotton applicator. Local application of 1% silver nitrate is also effective, as is the use of 1% salicylic acid. Careful application of 0.5% selenium sulfide cream to the eyelid margins is also helpful in the control of seborrheic blepharitis. Sulfonamide ointments are valuable in this type of disorder because of their keratolytic action.

Blepharitis is frequently a mixture of the seborrheic and the staphylococcal forms, and combinations of the therapy described should be employed. Treatment of blepharitis is often frustrating, since the disease recurs. Mild blepharitis is best managed by explaining the condition to the patient and advising good hygienic habits, which consist of daily removal of the crusts and scales from the eyelid margins and the application of sodium sulfacetamide ophthalmic ointment at bedtime. Scrubbing the lid with diluted baby shampoo is a good method for the removal of scaly material. A proprietary preparation, Blephamide, which contains sodium sulfacetamide, prednisolone, phenylephrine, and polyvinyl alcohol in a liquid film form, seems to be quite effective in the treatment of mixed blepharitis. The long-term use of any preparation that contains corticosteroids may entail certain risks, and other preparations without prednisolone are now available.

Demodex blepharitis

Demodex folliculorum is a human mite that infests hair and lash follicles and causes a chronic low-grade blepharitis. Diagnosis is made by the presence of the characteristic cuff of waxy material (mite feces) around the base of the lashes on slit-lamp examination. If the affected lashes are pulled and suspended in peanut oil on a glass slide, the mites can be seen (six or more on sixteen lashes is an infestation). Therapy includes thorough cleansing of the debris from the lid margins with cotton swabs saturated in ether, followed either by 3% ammoniated mercury, 1% yellow oxide of mercury, or 10% sodium sulfacetamide ointments twice a day for 2 weeks. Alternately, ether scrubs are performed and then repeated in 5 minutes to kill the emerging mites. Weekly scrubs for 3 weeks usually lower the infestation to asymptomatic levels.

CHALAZION

A chalazion is a sterile inflammation of the meibomian glands, and it may become secondarily infected. The treatment of acute chalazion consists of the application of hot moist compresses. Local use of antibiotic ointments is not effective against the chalazion itself but might be of value in the treatment of secondary infection. If an abscess forms and localizes, it should be opened. Most chalazions are seen after they have reached a chronic stage and are well walled off. Medical treatment is ineffective in these conditions. The lesions must be opened and curetted, and they may recur, particularly if excision has been inadequate. Recurrences should make one suspicious of an adenocarcinoma of the meibomian glands. Injections of 0.25 ml of methylprednisolone (Depo-Medrol) in the cul-de-sac adjacent to the chalazion have been described as improving the acute symptoms.

MEIBOMIANITIS

Therapy for meibomianitis, a chronic inflammation of the meibomian glands, consists of the application of hot moist compresses, repeated manual expression of the meibomian glands, and local antibiotic therapy. The application of 1% silver nitrate to the eyelid margins is sometimes effective. The use of local astringent medications such as zinc sulfate or detergent drops such as aqueous benzalkonium (Zephiran) chloride 1:5,000 may be helpful.

PEDICULOSIS

Pediculosis of the cilia is easily cured by the application of 3% ammoniated mercury ointment to the eyelid margins. Physostigmine ointment and DFP drops or ointment (Floropryl) are also effective against the lice. The patient also should bathe with gamma benzene hexachloride (Kwell) to remove body lice.

ABNORMALITIES OF EYELID MUSCLES
Quivering (myokymia)

Mild fasciculations of the orbicular muscle are usually transient and need little therapy beyond reassurance of the patient. Quinine, because of its curariform action, may abolish this symptom. Dosage is 5 grains orally, two to three times per day for 2 days. The drug should be discontinued if signs of toxicity develop.

Blepharospasm

Blepharospasm may be secondary to irritation, may be associated with emotional disorders, or may result from senile degenerative changes in the brainstem. Blepharospasm resulting from an acute irritation of the eye can be relieved with the topical use of anesthetic agents; treatment of the primary condition is then undertaken. Blepharospasm in the form of a tic generally is not treated effectively with medical agents, although a tranquilizer such as diazepam (Valium) occasionally is helpful. Carbamazepine (Tegretol) and phenytoin (Dilantin) have been used with rare success. In young persons severe blepharospasm is usually the result of an emotional disorder and requires psychotherapy. In older patients the difficulty is not usually associated with an emotional problem. Surgical evulsion of the upper divisions of the facial nerve has been used successfully in patients with severe, incapacitating blepharospasm. However, since permanent facial nerve palsy occurs, the procedure should be undertaken only if the patient understands the consequences.

Orbicularis oculi paralysis

Inability to close the eyelids may be caused by a central or peripheral nervous system lesion. It can be an early sign of cerebellar-pontine angle tumor or Guillain-Barré syndrome. Peripheral facial nerve paresis (Bell's palsy) is more common. Eighty percent of cases eventually resolve, but interim therapy is designed to prevent exposure keratitis. Lubricating drops and ointments are indicated. Surgical closure of the lids may be necessary if early spontaneous improvement does not occur.

TRAUMA

Ecchymosis and edema of the eyelids resulting from blunt trauma are self-limited. Cold compresses may reduce swelling if applied during the first 48 hours after injury; thereafter warm compresses are indicated. It is important to rule out more extensive injuries such as orbital and skull fractures and intraocular damage. Lacerations of the eyelids and canaliculi should be treated surgically in a primary fashion. The systemic use of trypsin and streptodornase-streptokinase has been of little value.

MALPOSITIONS

Most malpositions of the eyelids require surgical intervention. Temporary relief of a spastic entropion can be obtained if the eyelids are taped in a position away from the globe. If the eyelid is everted (ectropion), drops and ointments should be used to protect the globe from exposure. (See discussion on exposure keratitis.)

Ptosis of the eyelids also requires surgical correction. Crutch glasses may be used temporarily and in senile patients, although their use is not generally effective. Ptosis associated with myasthenia gravis is relieved when the generalized condition is appropriately treated with neostigmine (Prostigmin).

Medical treatment of congenital or traumatic malpositions of the eyelids consists of the temporary protection of the globe with ointments and drops. Occasionally the use of cosmetic dyes can improve the appearance of the eyelids.

EYELIDS IN GENERAL DISEASE

From a therapeutic standpoint the ophthalmologist usually should not treat eyelid involvement in generalized disease as a separate entity but should consult with an internist regarding the eyelid involvement. Therapy should be directed toward the general condition.

Collagen diseases

Lupus erythematosus. Involvement of the eyelid in lupus erythematosus may occur either in the systemic forms of the disease or in the discoid type. Erythema and edema of the eyelids may be present in conjunction with the classical "butterfly rash." Edema is most common after renal involvement has developed. Therapy for the systemic type of lupus erythematosus is the systemic use of corticoids and occasionally immunosuppressive agents. The discoid type of lupus should be treated as follows: exposure to sunlight or ultraviolet light should be avoided; antimalarial drugs such as chloroquine or hydroxychloroquine may be required. Chloroquine is given in a dose of 500 mg daily for 2 weeks, then reduced to 200 mg daily, treatment being continued for many months. Hydroxychloroquine is given in a dose of 400 to 800 mg daily for several weeks; the maintenance dose is 200 to 400 mg daily. Ophthalmic side effects, including retinopathy, are minimized if low dosages are maintained. Discoid lesions are helped in the active phase with the topical application of the potent corticosteroids fluocinolone acetonide (Synalar, Fluonid), betamethasone (Valisone), or flurandrenolide (Cordran). In the atrophic phase cosmetic coverups (Covermark) may be used.

Dermatomyositis. Involvement begins as a dusky erythema of the lids, which becomes increasingly violaceous with time, eventually being called "heliotrope" eyelids. Dermatomyositis involving the eyelid is often responsive to cortisone therapy. No other treatment is effective except symptomatic therapy and removal of any systemic neoplasm responsible for the dermatomyositis.

Scleroderma. Initially there is thickening of the connective tissue of the lids with a brawny edema. Later the skin becomes atrophied with distortion of the lid margins. Scleroderma may be treated with steroids, but the results of this type of treatment are unpredictable.

Granulomas

Syphilis. The eyelids may show primary or secondary syphilitic lesions. The drug of choice in therapy for syphilis is penicillin. The administration of 4.8 million units of penicillin is the preferred therapy. Procaine penicillin is given intramuscularly in a dosage of 600,000 units daily for 8 days. The aluminum monostearate form is given in an initial dose of 2.4 million units. Patients who are sensitive to penicillin may be treated with other antibiotics such as erythromycin or the tetracyclines. The dose of the latter drugs is 40 grams given over a period of 10 to 15 days. Tertiary syphilis is treated with 600,000 units of procaine penicillin daily to a total of 12 million units. Congenital syphilis is treated with intramuscular procaine penicillin 100,000 units per kg of body weight as a single intramuscular dose. The patient should always be examined for the possibility of neurosyphilis. It is important to obtain follow-up evaluations of patients who have received antisyphilitic therapy and to check for incomplete treatment with relapse.

Tuberculosis. Lupus vulgaris is the usual type of eyelid lesion of tuberculosis. The initial treatment of tuberculosis of all organs consists of the combined use of two or three highly effective drugs, always including isoniazid. The other highly effective drugs are rifampin, ethambutol, and streptomycin. The former standard treatment consisting of isoniazid and ρ-aminosalicylic acid plus streptomycin daily for the first 30 to 90 days is still highly effective but more toxic than the newer combinations, for example, isoniazid-ethambutol, isoniazid-rifampin, and isoniazid-ethambutol-rifampin. Isoniazid is given in a divided oral dose of 8 to 10 mg per kg of body weight every day, initially; subsequently the dose is reduced to 5 to 7 mg per kg of body weight per day. Fifty mg of pyridoxine per day is added to prevent isoniazid-induced peripheral neuritis. Ethambutol is administered in a single daily dose of 15 mg per kg of body weight, but it can cause retinal damage or optic neuritis, which may lead to loss of visual acuity, visual fields, and color vision. The patient should receive a complete ophthalmological examination before treatment is started with this drug, and repeat examinations should be made regularly. Toxicity is more common at higher dosage levels and tends to regress with cessation of therapy.

Rifampin is given in a single oral daily dose of 600 mg (10 to 20 mg per kg body weight) to the average-sized adult. Side effects are infrequent, and widespread use of rifampin is limited somewhat by its expense.

Streptomycin is given daily for 30 to 90 days in a dosage depending on the patient's age and renal function. If the patient is young and has good renal function, a dose of 1 gram daily should be used, but in older patients and in those with poor renal function, a dose of 0.25 to 0.5 gram daily should be given. Dihydrostreptomycin is no longer used because of its toxicity. p-Aminosalicylic acid is administered orally in a single daily dose of 150 mg per kg of body weight.

In patients who require retreatment or in those in whom resistance to one or more of the primary drugs develops, the secondary antituberculosis drugs are to be considered. These include kanamycin, 0.5 gram twice a day intramuscularly; pyrazinamide, 750 mg orally twice daily; cycloserine, a single oral dose of 0.5 to 1 gram daily; or ethionamide, an oral dose of 0.5 to 1 gram daily. All of these agents have considerable toxicities, and they should not be used by physicians unfamiliar with them.

Sarcoidosis. Cutaneous and subcutaneous nodules of the eyelids may occur in sarcoidosis. Subcutaneous nodules located near the lid margins, which have been mistaken for chalazia, may be an early sign of sarcoidosis. The involvement is frequently self-limited and may resolve without any therapy. However, if the disease appears to be progressing, the systemic use of corticosteroids will frequently reduce the inflammation. The topical use of steroids is also effective to relieve the symptoms.

Leprosy. The eyelid lesions of leprosy may be either tuberculoid or lepromatous in type. The eyelid disease should be treated as part of the generalized process. Modern therapy consists of the use of the sulfone drugs. Dapsone (Avlosulfon, DDS) is one of the more commonly used drugs and is usually begun in oral doses of 25 mg twice a week and then increased by 50 mg every 2 weeks until the maintenance dose of 300 mg is reached. Occasionally a dose of 600 mg is required. Sulfoxone (Diasone) sodium may be given orally in a daily dose of 0.3 gram the first week and of 0.6 gram daily thereafter. Solapsone (Sulphetrone) is administered in the dose of 0.5 gram three times a day orally. The dose is gradually increased to a total daily dose of 6 to 10 grams. Diphenylthiourea (DPT) is given orally in an initial dose of 250 mg daily. This is gradually increased to a maximum dose of 2 grams per day. Streptomycin, rifampin, and cycloserine are antibiotics that may be used in addition to the sulfone therapy. Acetylsalicylic acid, 0.6 gram every 4 hours, may be helpful during severe leprous reactions. Treatment must be continued for long periods (years) because recrudescence is possible on cessation of therapy.

Other eyelid diseases

Many other systemic diseases may have eyelid manifestations. Diabetes mellitus may cause an oculomotor palsy with an associated ptosis. The pupillomotor fibers are usually not involved, and remission occurs in several weeks to months. Thyroid disease may cause edema, swelling, and puffiness of the lids in addition to lid retraction and stare. Multiple sclerosis may produce Horner's syndrome or third nerve paresis, both of which are associated with ptosis. The phakomatoses, including neurofibromatosis and Sturge-Weber syndrome, may affect the eyelids. In neurofibromatosis, subcutaneous masses and café-au-lait spots can occur on the lids. The "port wine stain" of the Sturge-Weber syndrome is often diagnostic. The fundamental treatment is proper management of the primary medical problem. In selected patients cosmetic therapy (surgery, cosmetics, and cryotreatment) may be considered.

NEOPLASMS

Neoplasms of the eyelids constitute a large group of benign and malignant lesions. These are usually treated most effectively by surgical excision, x-ray therapy, or both. Occasionally the use of chemotherapeutic drugs, alkylating agents, antimetabolites, antibiotics, or hormones might be helpful. Neonatal hemangiomas of the eyelids regress with systemic corticosteroid therapy.

XANTHELASMA

Xanthelasma, which is not a true neoplasm, is treated by surgical removal, electrocoagulation, or chemical coagulation. For the latter treatment a 50% to 75% solution of bichloroacetic or trichloroacetic acid is carefully painted on the lesion with a toothpick; this may be repeated in a few weeks. Low-fat diets may be helpful in the prevention of recurrences.

REFERENCES

Beard, C.: Diseases of the lids. In Dunlap, E. A., editor: Gordon's medical management of ocular disease, ed. 2, New York, 1976, Harper & Row, Publishers.

Boniuk, M.: Eyelids, lacrimal apparatus, and conjunctiva; annual review, Arch. Ophthalmol. **90:**239, 1973.

Brunell, P. A., and Gershon, A. A.: Passive immunization against varicella-zoster infections and other modes of therapy, J. Infect. Dis. **127:**415, 1973.

Coston, T. O.: Demodex folliculorum blepharitis, Trans. Am. Acad. Ophthalmol. Soc. **65:** 361, 1967.

Fedukowicz, H. B.: External infections of the eye; bacterial, viral and mycotic, New York, 1963, Appleton-Century-Crofts.

Fox, S. A., editor: Affections of the lids, Int. Ophthalmol. Clin. 4:1, 1964.

Hiles, D., and Pilchard, W. A.: Corticosteroid control of neonatal hemangiomas of the orbit and ocular adnexa, Am. J. Ophthalmol. 71:1003, 1971.

Locatcher-Khorazo, D., and Seegal, B.: Microbiology of the eye, St. Louis, 1972, The C. V. Mosby Co.

The Medical Drug Letter, vol. 16, No. 26, Dec. 20, 1974.

Reeh, M. J.: Treatment of lid and epibulbar tumors, Springfield, Ill., 1963, Charles C Thomas, Publisher.

Schroeter, A. L., and others: Treatment for early syphilis and reactivity of serologic tests, J.A.M.A. **221:**471, 1972.

CHAPTER 9

Therapy of diseases of the conjunctiva

ALLERGIC REACTIONS
Acute allergic reactions

Although acute allergic reactions of the conjunctiva are frequently self-limited, they may produce enough symptoms to require active therapy. Treatment should include instillation of corticosteroid drops or ointment into the conjunctival cul-de-sac at frequent intervals and the application of cold compresses to relieve the edema. Systemic antihistamines and corticosteroids may be used additionally in severe cases. Identification and removal of the allergen will facilitate management and decrease the likelihood of recurrence.

Chronic allergic conjunctivitis

In the therapy of chronic allergic conjunctivitis, a very definite effort should be made to determine the cause of the allergy. Once determined, contact with the allergen should be eliminated if possible; otherwise the severity of the symptoms may require desensitization of the antigen. Dilute epinephrine solution (25 minims of 1:1,000 epinephrine, 1 ounce of diluent) or phenylephrine, 0.125%, is frequently valuable for temporary symptomatic relief. Systemic antihistamines may be used. Antihistamines act by blocking the target cells against the effect of histamine. They are more effective in the immediate type of allergic reaction than in the delayed type. Probably most allergic conjunctivitis is of the delayed variety. Although advocated in the past, the use of topical antihistamines has proved generally inadvisable, since they may be quite sensitizing in themselves. Antazoline in an 0.5% ophthalmic solution appears to be less sensitizing than most topical antihistamines, and occasionally may be beneficial. Steroids administered systemically and locally are also helpful in giving relief, but usually the reaction is not severe enough to warrant their use for long periods of time.

Vernal conjunctivitis

Vernal conjunctivitis may present as a large "cobblestone" papillary hypertrophy in the tarsal conjunctiva or as grayish, elevated areas at the limbus. The condition is usually recurrent in the spring of the year, and intensive therapy should be used only when symptoms are active. The use of antihistamines and desensitization of the patient to allergens seem to have very little effect on the disease, but symptoms of most forms of vernal conjunctivitis are relieved with the topical use of corticosteroid drops or ointment. In severe cases it may be necessary to use them every 1 to 2 hours initially. As improvement occurs, the dosage is reduced. If there is a heavy mucus discharge, 10% acetylcysteine drops may be added. Beta-radiation, cryotherapy, or surgical excision of the papillae with grafting of mucous membranes has been advocated, but in general such treatment is unnecessary.

Recently disodium cromoglycate has been recommended in this disorder. This agent appears to stabilize mast cells and prevents histamine release. It is applied topically as a 2% solution and may be used in conjunction with topical corticosteroids.

Phlyctenular conjunctivitis

Phlyctenular conjunctivitis appears near the limbus as white-capped elevated nodules with surrounding hyperemia. There are three general causes: (1) allergy to *Staphylococcus, Pneumococcus,* and so forth; (2) allergy to tuberculoprotein; and (3) allergy to the fungus *Coccidioides immitis.* Careful examination of the lids and conjunctiva should be followed by conjunctival smears and culture. A general physical examination is recommended, including chest x-ray films, PPD skin test, and, if indicated, sputum smears and culture. Appropriate topical antibiotics can then be started, followed in 1 to 2 days by topical steroids three to four times per day. The disease tends to occur in malnourished persons who require vitamin and nutritional supplements.

Bacterial allergies

Bacterial allergies of the conjunctiva are usually secondary to chronic staphylococcic infections of the eyelids. Acute symptoms will disappear with local corticosteroid therapy but will recur unless the bacterial infection is eliminated with the local use of appropriate antibiotics. Desensitization of the patient to staphylococcal phage lysate (Delmont Laboratories) may offer some help in established chronic cases.

Reactions secondary to systemic allergies

When the conjunctiva becomes involved in systemic allergic disease such as in hay fever, relief of symptoms may be obtained by the local use of epinephrine or, occasionally, antihistamine solutions. The systemic use of antihistamines is also effective in the relief of ocular symptoms; the systemic administration of antihistamines is preferable to topical therapy, since the latter may produce local reactions. Overall therapy should be directed toward the cause of the systemic allergy. When the general condition improves, the conjunctival reaction will also subside.

BACTERIAL INFECTIONS

Most bacterial conjunctival infections are caused by staphylococcus, strepto-coccus, pneumococcus, Morax-Axenfeld bacilli, or hemophilus organisms. Smears of conjunctiva and secretions help to determine the causative organism and hence the initial selection of topical antibiotics. After the results of conjunctival cultures and sensitivity testing have been obtained, antibiotic therapy may be changed. Relief of major symptoms usually occurs in 24 to 48 hours. Hot com-presses may provide desirable symptomatic comfort in the early stages of the disease. Antibiotics should be continued 4 or 5 days after all symptoms and findings have subsided.

Topical preparations of neomycin, bacitracin, and polymyxin B are generally good combinations because of their broad antibacterial spectrum and because they are seldom used systemically. Neomycin occasionally produces allergic reac-tions and punctate epithelial erosions. Ophthalmic sulfonamide or sulfisoxazole (Gantrisin) preparations cause fewer side effects but are less effective. Erythro-mycin as an 0.5% ointment is also a useful ophthalmic preparation against gram-positive cocci, but staphylococci rapidly develop resistance to this antibiotic. Chloramphenicol ophthalmic drops (0.5% solution) are nonirritating, do not produce corneal epithelial erosions, and penetrate the cornea and conjunctiva well but lack the wide antibacterial spectrum of the combination of neomycin, polymyxin B, and bacitracin. Topical gentamicin should be reserved for very resistant cases of conjunctivitis produced by an organism sensitive to this anti-biotic. If used in this way, gentamicin will remain effective for the treatment of more serious bacterial infections of the cornea as well as intraocular and systemic infections. The classical treatment for Morax-Axenfeld conjunctivitis (that is, usually angular blepharitis) is topical zinc sulfate, 0.25% to 0.5% drops; tetra-cycline ointment is equally effective.

Systemic antibiotics are required for the treatment of diphtheric, gonococcal, tularemic, and granulomatous conjunctivitis. Diphtheric conjunctivitis may be treated by daily intramuscular injections of procaine penicillin, 300,000 to 1 mil-lion units. Erythromycin in a dosage of 1 to 2 grams per day is also effective against the diphtheria organism in adults. Diphtheria antitoxin should also be employed. The adult dose ranges from 20,000 to 100,000 units, depending on the severity of the disease. The dosage for children under 2 years of age is 5,000 to 6,000 units, and 7,000 to 8,000 units for those over 2 years of age. Early ad-ministration is important.

Gonorrheal conjunctivitis

Gonorrheal conjunctivitis should be treated vigorously in order to prevent serious involvement of the cornea. Therapy consists of the systemic administra-tion of penicillin, 300,000 to 600,000 units a day intramuscularly. Tetracycline may be substituted if the patient is sensitive to penicillin. In addition to the systemic antibiotic therapy, ocular instillation of 1% silver nitrate is advisable, followed after 30 seconds by irrigation with saline or boric acid solution. During the early stages of the disease, the eye should be irrigated several times a day to remove the purulent material. In uniocular disease care must be taken to avoid infection of the second eye. Supplemental topical penicillin (100,000 units per ml) or tetracycline (5 mg per ml) should be employed at intervals of 1 to 2 hours. Cold compresses may be useful in relieving the swelling.

In recent years gonorrhea has become a major public health problem. It is held by some authorities that treatment of acute gonorrhea in men and women should be sufficiently adequate to abort any incubating attack of syphilis. Recent recommended therapy is 4.8 million units of procaine penicillin G divided into two doses, given as two intramuscular injections at one visit, together with 1 gram of probenecid given orally at least 30 minutes before the injections, or 3.5 grams of ampicillin and 1 gram of probenecid administered orally at the same time. Alternate therapy could consist of 2 to 4 grams of spectinomycin dihydrochloride pentahydrate in one intramuscular injection, or tetracycline orally in an initial dose of 1.5 grams followed by 0.5 gram four times a day until a total dose of 9 grams is reached. The above recommendations are particularly applicable for treatment of promiscuous, vagrant young adults where follow-up examination for syphilis is impossible, and are not applicable to treatment of gonococcal conjunctivitis in the newborn.

Tularemic conjunctivitis

Tularemic conjunctivitis is characterized by the appearance of small necrotic conjunctival lesions, preauricular adenopathy, and systemic symptoms of infection. Treatment consists of giving streptomycin intramuscularly, 0.5 gram every 12 hours for 72 hours, or until the lesions subside. Chloramphenicol or tetracycline may be substituted for streptomycin. Local use of antibiotics (streptomycin, chloramphenicol, or tetracycline) hourly should be combined with the systemic treatment.

Granulomatous conjunctivitis caused by syphilis, tuberculosis, or leprosy

Granulomatous conjunctivitis resulting from syphilis, tuberculosis, or leprosy is treated in essentially the same way as diseases involving the eyelids (Chapter 8), since there is usually overlapping infection of the eyelids and conjunctiva. Treatment for these conditions should always be directed toward the generalized systemic disease. When conjunctival involvement occurs, corneal infection may be avoided with the use of topical antibiotic therapy in addition to the systemic antibiotic therapy.

VIRAL INFECTIONS

Except for infections by some of the larger viruses, the *Bedsonia-Chlamydia,* there is no specific treatment for viral conjunctivitis. Therapy should be directed toward prevention of complications, reduction of secondary bacterial infection, and relief of symptoms. The local use of broad-spectrum antibiotics and the application of hot compresses are the usual forms of treatment. Topical therapy with either autologous serum or homologous convalescent serum has been reported to be effective against certain viral infections. Its actual value, however, is doubtful. Among the viral diseases of the conjunctiva for which there is no specific treatment are Newcastle virus disease, adenovirus infections, ECHO virus disease, epidemic keratoconjunctivitis, and rubeola.

Herpes zoster

Simple herpes zoster conjunctivitis may be left untreated or treated with bland drops. More severe forms, especially when keratitis and iridocyclitis occur, are best treated with topical steroids. The use of systemic steroids has been shown to reduce the duration of acute trigeminal pain as well as the incidence of postinfection trigeminal neuralgia. When a coexistent malignant disease such as lymphoma is present, systemic steroids are contraindicated because a significant increase in mortality may occur with their use. Herpes zoster must not be confused with herpes simplex in which topical steroids aggravate an existing keratitis.

Vaccinial lesions

Vaccinial lesions of the conjunctiva should be treated with IDU. The drug is administered as an 0.1% solution every hour during the day and every 2 hours at night, or as an 0.5% ointment every 6 hours. In addition, VIG may be administered, particularly if there is considerable involvement of the eyelids. This agent is given intramuscularly in a dose of 0.6 ml per kg of body weight.

Trachoma

All three stages of active conjunctival involvement (acute catarrhal, follicular and papillary hypertrophy, and cicatricial) are treated effectively by oral and local use of sulfonamides and antibiotics, including tetracyclines, erythromycin, rifampin, penicillin, spiramycin, novobiocin, and chloramphenicol. The current recommended treatment is a 21-day course of oral tetracyclines. Topical therapy may be added. Doxycycline (Doxy-II, Vibramycin) is preferred since administration only once a day is required. In children below the age of 9 years and in pregnant women, oral sulfonamides should be given instead of tetracyclines because of the side effects of tetracyclines on developing teeth. Probably trachoma can be cured with local therapy alone. However, successful local treatment requires a much longer time than when antibiotics are also administered systemically. One percent tetracycline ointment twice a day, 6 days a week, for 10 weeks is recommended. This therapy decreases the intensity of the conjunctival disease and eliminates bacterial pathogens, which may be important in scar formation. However, because of problems of reinfection and sanitation, good follow-up therapy is necessary.

Because of many problems involved with the use of systemic sulfonamides and antibiotics, the World Health Organization has recommended topical therapy alone for communitywide trachoma control programs. In such control programs tetracycline ointment or oil suspension is applied topically twice daily for 5 days each month; this is repeated for 6 months.

Inclusion conjunctivitis

Inclusion conjunctivitis also responds well to sulfonamide and tetracycline antibiotic therapy. In children, topical tetracycline antibiotic therapy satisfactorily controls the conditions. Conjunctival scarring and corneal neovascularization can only be prevented in neonatal conjunctivitis if treatment with topical tetracycline or chlortetracycline is initiated before the twelfth day of life. In adults it is advisable to supplement the local therapy with systemic sulfonamide or tetracycline antibiotic therapy. Treatment should continue for 2 to 3 weeks.

Lymphogranuloma venereum

Conjunctivitis associated with lymphogranuloma venereum also is treated effectively with sulfonamides and broad-spectrum antibiotics, the antibiotics being given both topically and systemically. It may be necessary to use a combination of both types of drugs to effect a cure in resistant cases.

MYCOTIC INFECTIONS

The therapy of fungus infections of the conjunctiva is somewhat variable. Included in this section are infections produced by *Actinomyces* and *Leptothrix* organisms, formerly classified as fungi but having growth and inhibition characteristics of bacteria. Actinomycosis is treated effectively with penicillin, sulfonamide drugs, or any of several broad-spectrum antibiotics. If the infection exists alone in the conjunctiva, local therapy is sufficient. However, if there is other involvement of the eyelids, this local therapy should be supplemented with systemic treatment. The conjunctival infection with *Actinomyces* organisms is often secondary to canalicular disease. If so, the canaliculitis must be treated by curettage and irrigation with antibiotic solutions. Conjunctival infection with *Leptothrix* organisms is characterized by small gray necrotic lesions. The source of the organisms is usually a cat. Treatment consists of surgical excision of the involved area and/or the use of systemic sulfonamide or broad-spectrum antibiotics.

Amphotericin B, in the form of local drops in the concentration of 1.5 to 5 mg per ml, is effective against many fungus infections of the conjunctiva. Nystatin (Mycostatin) drops, in a concentration of 50,000 to 100,000 units per milliliter, are also effective as a fungicide against certain mycotic infections of the conjunctiva, particularly *Candida*.

PARASITIC INFECTIONS

Rarely, the conjunctiva may become involved with parasitic infections. Most of these, however, are not seen in the United States. Therapy should be directed toward the systemic disease. Symptoms of trichinosis involving the conjunctiva may be relieved by the systemic use of corticosteroids or corticotropin, although these drugs do not destroy the *Trichinella* organisms. Discomfort may also be relieved with the use of acetylsalicylic acid, 0.6 gram every 4 hours. Thiabendazole, an anthelmintic, has been reported to be effective in the treatment of trichinosis. The drug is administered orally in a daily dose of 50 to 60 mg per kg of body weight.

MYIASIS

Myiasis of the conjunctiva, an infection with ova of nematodes, is removed effectively by irrigation and the instillation of antiseptic solutions such as benzalkonium (Zephiran) chloride, zinc sulfate, or mercurial solutions.

NONSPECIFIC HYPEREMIA

Conjunctival hyperemia without a specific etiology such as true infection or allergy should be treated symptomatically. Any irritative cause such as exposure to smoke or fumes should be eliminated. Adequate rest and proper refraction aid in relief of this annoying symptom. The use of mild astringent drops, with or without mild vasoconstrictors, is also helpful.

BURNS
Chemical burns

Chemical burns of the eye seldom involve only the conjunctiva; frequently the cornea is involved. Immediate copious irrigation is important, but irrigation after 2 or 3 hours is probably not helpful. Topical antibiotics such as Neosporin or chloramphenicol reduce the chance of secondary infection. Topical steroids help to reduce the inflammatory response, but treatment with topical steroids must be carefully monitored, especially after 7 to 10 days, since existing corneal ulcerations may progress rapidly. Early fibrinous conjunctival adhesions may be lysed with the smooth tip of a medicine dropper or glass rod and may be discouraged from reforming with ointments. Symblepharons restricting ocular or lid motility must be reduced surgically after active inflammation subsides.

Thermal burns

Thermal burns of the conjunctiva should be treated initially the same way as chemical burns. As in the case of chemical burns it is important to prevent the formation of symblepharons. The systemic administration of analgesics is advisable for the patient with either type of burn.

Ultraviolet burns

Ultraviolet burns of the conjunctiva usually subside in a very short time without serious consequences and heal within 1 or 2 days. Treatment consists of the use of a corticosteroid and antibiotic drops or ointment instilled into the eye several times a day for 48 to 72 hours. If associated with an ultraviolet burn of the cornea, systemic analgesics and ocular patching may be necessary.

X-ray burns

X-ray burns of the conjunctiva are permanent and in the more severe cases result in extreme dryness of the eye due to mucous or aqueous tear film deficiencies or both. Conjunctival goblet cell atrophy and scarring may lead to a rapid corneal tear film breakup time and extensive symblepharons. Most cases of dryness may be improved to some extent with instillation of polymeric wetting solutions such as hydroxypropyl methylcellulose, polyvinyl alcohol, or Adsorbotear as frequently as required. In the severe cases a thin, therapeutic soft contact lens used with 0.5N saline drops every few hours provides a constant fluid layer to the corneal surface.

EXPOSURE CONJUNCTIVITIS

Lagophthalmos may develop after facial nerve palsies or periods of unconsciousness. The early stages of exposure keratitis may be treated with 1% methylcellulose or bland ophthalmic ointments. More severe transitory forms, especially with keratitis, are best treated topically by antibiotics and the lid closed by transpore tape applied directly to the lids. Permanent lagophthalmos is treated by tarsorrhaphy with or without additional lubricants. Sling operations are employed occasionally.

XEROSIS (BITOT'S SPOTS)

Bitot's spots are small, white, foamy-appearing elevations of the conjunctiva or cornea. In infants and children vitamin A deficiency is the principal cause and is readily corrected with 10,000 to 20,000 units of vitamin A daily. In older children, 25,000 to 50,000 units per day are needed. If the vitamin A deficiency is secondary to other disease such as diarrhea, the primary condition should be corrected. In adults, Bitot's spots are not always associated with vitamin A deficiency, and so administration of 50,000 to 100,000 units of vitamin A daily relieves this condition in only a minority of adults. Improvement after prolonged vitamin A treatment may only represent the natural course and healing of the disease.

MUCOCUTANEOUS DISEASES

The mucocutaneous diseases include erythema multiforme, Stevens-Johnson syndrome, and Behcet's syndrome. Erythema multiforme and Stevens-Johnson syndrome may be precipitated by treatment with hydralazine, sulfonamide, antibiotics, and other nonspecific medications. The acute mucous membrane necrotizing component in each disease may be managed by topical steroids applied three or four times a day with topical antibiotics to prevent secondary infection. A chronic phase develops in some of the more severe cases with conjunctival scarring, symblepharons and atrophy of conjunctival and goblet cells; this phase leads to a mucus-deficient or mucus and aqueous–deficient eye. If the conjunctiva fails to secrete sufficient glycoprotein for corneal epithelial adsorption, a very rapid tear film breakup time and ultimate vascularization and scarring of the cornea result. In this phase of the disease, weak concentrations of steroids two or three times a day may help to quiet the inflammatory process. Frequent applications of more concentrated steroids appreciably increase the risk of ulceration and perforation. The moderately dry eye may be treated topically with hydroxypropyl methylcellulose, 1%, Adsorbotear, or 3% polyvinyl alcohol (Liquifilm Forte). These conditions may respond favorably to surgical lysis of symblepharon, excision of corneal pannus, and fitting with a thin, therapeutic soft contact lens. To maintain hydration of the lens, 0.5N saline solution is used topically every 30 minutes to 2 hours.

Acute pemphigus is a widespread disease rarely affecting conjunctiva. Treatment of the generalized condition consists of systemic steroids; supplemental topical steroids three or four times a day should be used for conjunctival involvement. The more common chronic mucosal pemphigoid manifests itself in extensive subconjunctival scarring and shrinkage, resulting in symblepharon and even ankyloblepharon. Loss of goblet cells and scarring of the ducts from the lacrimal gland result in a very dry, keratinized epithelium on the conjunctiva and cornea. Although pemphigoid is generally a progressive subconjunctival cicatrizing process, temporary remissions may be induced or prolonged by weak topical steroids three or four times a day. Attempts should be made to reduce secondary infection, which results in further shrinkage of the conjunctiva; eyelashes that turn inward should be removed. Treatment of mucosal pemphigoid generally parallels the therapy of Stevens-Johnson syndrome.

DEGENERATIVE DISEASES

This heterogeneous group of diseases of the conjunctiva includes amyloidosis, pterygium, and pinguecula. There is no effective medical therapy for these conditions, but local instillation of mild soothing drops affords some relief. Treatment is surgical or radiological.

Triethylenethiophosphoramide (Thio-TEPA), a radiomimetic agent, has been reported to be of aid in the prevention of recurrence of pterygium after surgical removal. The drug has been employed in concentrations from 1:500 to 1:2,000 in human eyes without complications. Treatment with the 1:2,000 dilution is started 2 days after surgery and continued for 6 weeks; the medication is instilled every 3 hours during the day.

REFERENCES

Bettman, J. W., Jr.: Eye disease among American Indians of the Southwest. II. Trachoma, Arch. Ophthalmol. **90**:440, 1973.
Dawson, C. R., and others: Topical tetracycline and rifampicin therapy of endemic trachoma in Tunisia, Am. J. Ophthalmol. **79**:803, 1975.

Fedukowicz, H. B.: External infections of the eye; bacterial, viral, and mycotic, New York, 1963, Appleton-Century-Crofts.

Gasset, A. R., and Kaufman, H. E., editors: Soft contact lens, St. Louis, 1972, The C. V. Mosby Co.

Lemp, M., and Holly, F.: Ophthalmic polymers as ocular wetting agents, Ann. Ophthalmol. 4:15, 1972.

Locatcher-Khorazo, D., and Seegal, B. C.: Microbiology of the eye, St. Louis, 1972, The C. V. Mosby Co.

Meacham, C. T.: Triethylene thiophosphoramide in the prevention of pterygium recurrence, Am. J. Ophthalmol. **54**:751, 1962.

Mordhorst, C. H., and Dawson, C.: Sequelae of neonatal inclusion conjunctivitis and associated disease in parents, Am. J. Ophthalmol. **71**:861, 1971.

Rudolph, A.: Control of gonorrhea; guidelines for antibiotic therapy, J.A.M.A. **220**:1587, 1972.

Symposium on infectious diseases of the conjunctiva and cornea, Transactions of the New Orleans Academy of Ophthalmology, St. Louis, 1963, The C. V. Mosby Co.

Theodore, F. H., and Schlossman, A.: Ocular allergy, Baltimore, 1958, The Williams & Wilkins Co.

Thompson, T. R., Swanson, R. E., and Wiesner, P. J.: Gonococcal ophthalmia neonatorium, J.A.M.A. **228**:186, 1974.

Thygeson, P.: Etiology and treatment of blepharitis, Arch. Ophthalmol. **36**:445, 1946.

Thygeson, P.: The etiology and treatment of phylctenular keratoconjunctivitis, Am. J. Ophthalmol. **34**:357, 1951.

Thygeson, P., and Kimura, S. J.: Chronic conjunctivitis, Trans. Am. Acad. Ophthalmol. Otolaryngol. **67**:494, 1963.

CHAPTER 10

Therapy of diseases of the lacrimal apparatus

LACRIMAL GLAND
Inflammations

The therapy of dacryoadenitis is determined by the etiology. For dacryo-adenitis that is a complication of systemic disease, therapy should be directed toward the overall treatment of the generalized disorder. Dacryoadenitis as a complication of viral disease (most commonly, mumps) should be treated symptomatically. Local application of heat or cold over the lacrimal gland area offers relief, and bed rest and the use of salicylates are suggested. The systemic use of cortisone may reduce inflammation, but the use of corticosteroids in any viral infection entails a calculated risk.

Dacryoadenitis secondary to sarcoidosis should be treated by similar symptomatic measures. The systemic use of corticosteroids is usually quite effective in reducing the inflammation and swelling of the lacrimal gland. Infections of the lacrimal gland secondary to tuberculosis and syphilis are rare. Treatment should be directed toward the general therapy of the tuberculosis or syphilis, as mentioned elsewhere in this text.

Bacterial infections of the lacrimal gland are also rare. If the causative organism can be identified, appropriate antibiotic therapy should be given. Hot packs and other symptomatic therapy may give relief.

Insufficiency

Hyposecretion of the lacrimal gland cannot be cured. Therapy is directed toward replacement of the tear deficiency. Many commercial tear replacement agents are available. In mild cases the use of 0.5% or 1% methylcellulose solution or 1.4% polyvinyl alcohol offers sufficient protection. Symptoms of burning and irritation persist in certain patients despite the use of these solutions at frequent intervals. Hydroxypropyl methylcellulose, 1% (Ultra tears), and Adsorbotear may provide relief to some patients who do not respond to other tear replacement therapy. In patients troubled with considerable mucus, the topical application of 10% to 20% acetylcysteine, a mucolytic agent, may be of value. Hyposecretion associated with partial denervation of the lacrimal gland, as in the Riley-Day syndrome, may be helped with the topical instillation of cholinergic agents, methacholine or pilocarpine. For treatment of keratitis sicca associated with lacrimal gland insufficiency, see Chapter 11.

Hypersecretion

Hypersecretion of the lacrimal gland in the absence of any disease is seldom satisfactorily treated by medical means. The use of tranquilizers has been suggested to reduce hypersecretion, but no personal experience is available for comment. Surgical procedures to extirpate a portion of the lacrimal gland or to sever the lacrimal ducts are seldom indicated.

Tumors

Tumors of the lacrimal gland are treated surgically or with irradiation. For certain tumors, alkylating agents (such as thio-TEPA, cyclophosphamide, triethylenemelamine, uracil mustard, or chlorambucil), antimetabolites (such as methotrexate or fluorouracil), or antibiotics (such as actinomycin D) may be employed. In such cases it is wise to consult with the internist and the radiotherapist.

LACRIMAL CANALICULI AND SAC
Infections

Bacterial infections. Bacterial infections of the lacrimal canaliculi and sac should be treated according to the offending organism. If possible, cultures should be obtained before therapy is instituted. Treatment consists of the use of local and systemic antibiotics. Hot packs are valuable in speeding the recovery process. If there is obstruction to the nasal lacrimal duct, so that the tear flow is impeded, the lacrimal sac should be expressed manually at intervals, so that the topically applied antibiotic may get down into the sac. Irrigations of the canaliculi and sac with antibiotic solutions should be employed (Chapter 3). To prevent recurrence, attempts should be made to reestablish the lacrimal passage after the active inflammation has subsided. Occasionally it is necessary to drain an abscess of the lacrimal sac from the skin side. However, this should be avoided if possible to obviate the danger of a permanent fistula.

Viral infections. Viral infections of the canaliculi should be treated symptomatically. The use of hot compresses and salicylates is advised. If there is secondary bacterial infection, antibiotics should be employed.

Actinomyces **infections.** *Actinomyces* infections of the canaliculi and lacrimal sac are quite common. These organisms are not true fungi but are usually included in the discussion of mycotic infections. These infections can usually be cleared by dilatation and curettage of the canaliculi. Instillation of penicillin solutions is also helpful. Other antibiotics, including almost all the broad-spectrum antibiotics, lincomycin, and sulfonamides, are also effective against the *Actinomyces* organisms.

Mycotic infections. Mycotic infections of the canaliculi and lacrimal sac can usually be satisfactorily treated by topical administration and local syringing of the canaliculi and sac with amphotericin B and nystatin solutions. Dilutions are given in the discussion of mycotic infections in Chapter 9.

Granulomatous infections. Granulomatous infections of the canaliculi and lacrimal sac, such as tuberculosis, syphilis, and sarcoid, should be managed by the direction of therapy to the overall treatment of the patient. The specific therapy for systemic treatment of these infections should be employed.

Tumors

The treatment of tumors of the canaliculi and sac should be surgical or radiological.

Obstructions

Obstructions in the absence of infections or neoplasms are diseases requiring surgery, and medical therapy is ineffective. Most congenital blockage of the inferior portion of the nasolacrimal duct disappears without treatment. Syringing, probing, and dacryocystorhinostomy may be necessary in persistent cases of congenital and acquired obstruction.

Melanin casts within the lacrimal excretory passages may result from topical epinephrine therapy. Irrigation of these passages usually eliminates the casts. Subsequently epinephrine therapy should be discontinued if possible.

REFERENCES

Boniuk, M.: Eyelids, lacrimal apparatus, and conjunctiva; annual review, Arch. Ophthalmol. **90**:239, 1973.

Ellis, P. P., Bausor, S. C., and Fulmer, J. M.: Streptothrix canaliculitis, Am. J. Ophthalmol. **52**:36, 1961.

Jones, L. T.: Treatment of lacrimal duct obstructions in infants, J. Pediatr. Ophthalmol. 3:42, 1966.

Kohler, U., and Muller, W.: The treatment of stenosis of the lacrimal passages in infants and children, Ophthalmologica **159**:136, 1969.

Lemoine, A. N., Jr.: The lacrimal system, Surv. Ophthalmol. 7:325, 1962.

Lemp, M., and Holly, F.: Ophthalmic polymers as ocular wetting agents, Ann. Ophthalmol. 4:15, 1972.

Reese, A. B.: Tumors of the eye, ed. 3, New York, 1976, Harper & Row, Publishers.

Spaeth, G. L.: Nasolacrimal duct obstruction caused by topical epinephrine, Arch. Ophthalmol. **77**:355, 1967.

Viers, E. R., editor: The lacrimal system. Proceedings of the first international symposium,
Viers, E. R.: The lacrimal system, clinical application, New York, 1955, Grune & Stratton, Inc. St. Louis, 1971, The C. V. Mosby Co.

CHAPTER 11

Therapy of diseases of the cornea

ABRASIONS AND LACERATIONS

Simple corneal abrasions consist of epithelial loss with or without injury to the basement membrane. Because of intense blepharospasm, instillation of a topical anesthetic may be necessary immediately to relieve pain so that vision may be determined and the examination performed. Foreign bodies may be irrigated out of the eye or mechanically removed. The eyelids should be everted and inspected for foreign bodies. Loose or folded epithelium around the abrasion should be removed with a No. 15 Bard-Parker blade held perpendicular to the globe. Embedded foreign bodies may be removed with a 25-gauge needle, foreign body spud, or rust ring remover. Neosporin, chloramphenicol, or sulfacetamide drops provide good prophylactic antibiotic coverage against most bacterial pathogens. Ciliary spasm may be relieved by topical short-acting cycloplegics. Patients are more comfortable with a tight eye patch. They should be seen daily until complete epithelial regrowth has occurred. Small abrasions usually heal in 24 to 48 hours and larger abrasions in 48 to 72 hours.

Partial-thickness penetrating lacerations of the cornea should be treated in essentially the same fashion as corneal abrasions, but the time required for complete healing is longer. When the laceration is deep, it is wise to have the patient wear a shield in addition to the patch. Restriction of activity may be advisable. Full-thickness penetrating wounds of the cornea 5 mm or larger should be sutured. Recently hydrophilic contact lenses have been used to tamponade small leaking corneal lacerations. Cyanoacrylate adhesives also have been advocated to seal selected corneal lacerations.

RECURRENT EROSIONS

Recurrent epithelial erosions are usually initiated by trauma (that is, from fingernails), or infection (that is, metaherpetic ulcer). In both cases loss or injury to basement membrane interferes with the formation of tight adhesions (hemidesmosomes) between basal regenerating epithelial cells and the basement membrane. When corneal trauma does not injure the basement membrane, tight adherence of regenerated epithelium occurs in less than 5 days. If the basement membrane is destroyed, a new membrane takes about 6 weeks to form in the presence of an intact overlying epithelial layer. Fresh epithelium covering such a defect is easily stripped from the cornea during awakening when the dry lid margin scrapes over it. The use of 5% sodium chloride ointment (Mucosal No. 128) at bedtime provides lubrication for the movement of the dry lid over the corneal epithelium as well as dehydration of the new corneal epithelial layer.

BURNS
Chemical burns

The chemically burned eye should be irrigated immediately with copious amounts of any innocuous solution that is immediately available, such as tap water, saline solution, or boric acid solution. When available, weak neutralizing solutions may be used for irrigation; however, irrigation should not be delayed. For acid burns, 3% sodium bicarbonate solution is advised. For alkali burns, boric acid solution, 0.5% acetic acid solution, or acetate buffer with a pH of 4.5 is recommended. For lime burns (Ca_2OH_3), calcium may be chelated by an 0.37% solution of ethylenediamine tetra-acetate sodium (EDTA) or a 5% solution of ammonium tartrate may also be used. Treatment of tear gas burns (including Mace burns) is the same as treatment of other chemical burns.

It may be necessary to instill a topical anesthetic before irrigation if the blepharospasm is so severe that satisfactory lid manipulation cannot be accomplished. After the eye has been thoroughly irrigated, vision should be obtained and the eye inspected for possible retained chemical substances. Small pieces of lime found stuck to the cornea or in the conjunctival cul-de-sac should be mechanically removed. These pieces may be satisfactorily loosened with EDTA irrigation. Sometimes it is advisable to debride portions of the corneal epithelium to ensure removal of retained alkali particles. Antibiotic solutions should be instilled.

The follow-up treatment and end result of chemical burns of the eye depend on the nature and severity of the burn. Epithelial regrowth after mild acid and alkali corneal burns is sluggish, but regrowth is usually complete in 3 to 7 days. It is wise to continue the use of topical antibiotics, cycloplegics, and patching during the healing period. In mild cases topical steroids three or four times a day reduce the inflammatory response of the cornea, iris, and ciliary body. Corneal ulcerations rarely develop in the mild chemical injuries.

With moderately severe alkali burns, epithelial defects heal more slowly with variable scarring and vascularization. Alternately epithelial regrowth may be prolonged, allowing ulcerations to develop in the bare, vulnerable stroma 10 days to 2 weeks after injury. Severe alkali burns produce "marbleized" corneas denuded of epithelium and the whitening of the perilimbal conjunctiva. Recently it has been learned that ulcers develop in alkali-burned corneas as a result of collagenase produced by regenerating corneal epithelium and polymorphonuclear neutrophils. When epithelial defects persist for longer than a week, collagenase inhibitors must be used topically. Either EDTA (0.2M), L-cysteine (0.1 or 0.2M), or N-acetylcysteine (0.6M or 1.2M) drops in a phosphate buffer should be applied five times a day. EDTA may be quite irritating; the disodium EDTA is more effective than the calcium EDTA. Both EDTA and acetylcysteine are relatively stable at room temperatures over a 1-month period; cysteine is quite unstable and remains active for only 2 to 3 days with refrigeration. Acetylcysteine is commercially available as a 10% (0.6M) or a 20% (1.2M) solution (Mucomyst). The 20% solution can be diluted to a 10% solution with diluents such as artificial tears, saline, or Neosporin for instillation into the eye. In eyes with significant scar tissue, penetrating keratoplasty may be successful when collagenase inhibitors are used in the postoperative period.

Ether burns

Ether burns of the cornea are not serious, because involvement does not extend beneath the epithelium. Treatment consists of the instillation of a topical antibiotic and the application of an eye patch. Healing occurs rapidly, within 48 to 72 hours.

Ultraviolet burns

Ultraviolet burns of the cornea respond to medical therapy within 48 hours. Treatment consists of the instillation of topical anesthetic solutions until the pain is relieved. A drop of a mild cycloplegic is then instilled, followed by the topical application of an antibiotic ointment, with or without steroids, and a patch is placed over the eye. It is well to give the patient sedatives and analgesics systemically.

X-ray burns

X-ray burns of the cornea usually produce permanent changes that are difficult to treat. The anterior segment remains somewhat inflamed, and there is frequently a low-grade secondary iridocyclitis with persistent epithelial defects. Treatment in the early phases is topical antibiotics and steroids three or four times a day and cycloplegics one or two times a day. In moderately severe cases conjunctival scarring and goblet cell atrophy may indirectly cause corneal disease by later interference with normal globe and lid movements and by deficiencies of the aqueous and mucous components of tears. The surgical treatment of symblepharons and the use of hydroxypropyl methylcellulose, 1%, or Adsorbotear as tear replacements are of value. A therapeutic soft contact lens with added 0.5N saline drops may be necessary to maintain a tear film over the dry cornea.

ULCERS AND INFECTIONS

Successful treatment of a central corneal ulcer depends on accurate diagnosis. Predisposing factors such as anatomic irregularities, tear film disturbances, and systemic disease must be considered and treated if possible. Smears and cultures of the ulcer bed are mandatory for identification of the causative organism. A general physical examination with appropriate laboratory tests may assist in the evaluation and subsequent treatment of the corneal condition.

Bacterial ulcers

Smears made from scrapings of the ulcer base often will immediately identify the pathogen so that the proper antibiotic therapy may be started before the results of culture and sensitivity tests are available. Treatment should not be withheld pending identification of the organisms. All central corneal ulcers must be treated vigorously regardless of size.

Gram-positive cocci most likely to produce central corneal ulcers are *Staphylococcus aureus, Diplococcus pneumoniae,* and *Streptococcus pyogenes,* in that order of frequency. If the ulcer is superficial and no hypopyon is present, a combination of neomycin, polymyxin, and bacitracin (Neosporin) drops may be used every 1 to 2 hours, combined with erythromycin ointment every 8 hours. In deeply infiltrated ulcers with hypopyon, subconjunctival and systemic antibiotics should be added. Penicillin G is effective against most gram-positive organisms and is generally well tolerated. Patients allergic to penicillin may be treated with one of the cephalosporins or lincomycin. (See Chapters 3 and 14 for the antibacterial spectrum and the dosage of antibiotics.) Cycloplegics should be used in doses necessary to keep the pupil dilated. After 24 to 48 hours continued management is based on clinical response, culture identification, and sensitivity testing. If the ulcer has not improved, repeat cultures should be obtained.

Pseudomonas, Proteus, coliform, and *Klebsiella* are the most common gram-negative organisms producing corneal ulcers. Empirical treatment consists of hourly application of Neosporin, gentamicin, or tobramycin drops. Additionally subconjunctival injections of gentamicin in a dosage of 20 to 30 mg should be employed.

Of the gram-negative organisms producing corneal ulcers, *Pseudomonas* is the most common and destructive. Vigorous therapy in the form of topical and subconjunctival injections of antibiotics effective against *Pseudomonas* is required. Favorable results in the treatment of *Pseudomonas* corneal ulcers have been reported by Hessburg using an indwelling catheter through the upper lid. The irrigating solution that contains 450 mg of colistimethate sodium and 4.5 ml of 10% sodium sulfacetamide in 900 ml of physiological saline solution is given at a rate of 6 to 8 drops a minute. The lavage is continued for 14 days; thereafter polymyxin ointment is given four times a day for 4 to 6 weeks. Continuous irrigation may also be delivered through a contact lens with attached irrigating system (Medi-Flow lens). Recently topical heparin, 2,500 units per ml, applied four times a day has been recommended as adjunctive treatment for *Pseudomonas* corneal ulcers. The beneficial effects are thought to result from anticollagenase and anti-inflammatory activity.

If a corneal ulcer continues to progress despite proper antibiotic therapy, a

Gunderson-type conjunctival flap is required. It is preferable not to perform a conjunctival flap for a deep corneal ulcer with an aqueous leak, since a filtering bleb may form in the overlying conjunctiva. The resulting shallow or flat anterior chamber with loss of functional trabeculum may preclude any future rehabilitation of the eye. Closure of the leaking area by isobutyl cyanoacrylate adhesive usually effectively reestablishes anterior chamber depth and ocular integrity. If adhesive closure of the leak is unsuccessful or the perforation site and corneal ulcer are large and necrotic, a "blow out" patch corneal graft may be employed. In either case anterior chamber depth and ocular integrity are restored for future definitive optical keratoplasty.

Viral infections and ulcers

Herpes simplex ulcers. The epithelial form of herpes simplex keratitis consists of branches (dendrites) of epithelial loss in a hypoesthetic cornea. Conjunctivitis may precede the keratitis; uveitis usually occurs after keratitis has developed. Satisfactory treatment can be accomplished with either application of IDU, mechanical debridement of the corneal epithelium, or cryotherapy of the lesions.

Topical IDU therapy is employed most often. The agent acts by interfering with viral deoxribonucleic acid (DNA) synthesis. IDU may be used initially as 0.5% ointment five times a day or as 0.1% solution every hour during the day, with the ointment used at bedtime. If significant corneal improvement is not noted with IDU within 7 to 10 days, it is unlikely that additional treatment will have a favorable effect. Topical application of other antiviral agents or other modes of therapy then should be considered.

Mechanical debridement with a cotton swab or a Bard-Parker blade may be employed as initial treatment or if IDU therapy is unsuccessful. This is performed after satisfactory topical anesthesia. After debridement, pupillary dilatation and patching for 48 hours should be undertaken. Another treatment approach is the use of cryoapplications to each of the epithelial lesions at –70° to –80° C for 6 to 8 seconds.

Topical steroids are contraindicated for the epithelial form of herpes simplex. Chemicals or cautery formerly applied to herpetic corneal lesions may cause injury to underlying corneal structures and cells, especially basement membrane, giving rise to recurrent corneal ulcers. Mild to moderate uveitis is usually controlled with mydriatics and cycloplegics.

Recently two topical antiviral agents, trifluorothymidine (TFT) and vidarabine (Vira-A, adenine arabinoside, ARA-A), have been found to be effective against herpes organisms resistant to IDU. The TFT is used as a 1% solution and the vidarabine as a 3% ointment; both are applied topically several times a day. Only vidarabine is commercially available. At the present time it would not seem appropriate to initiate treatment for herpes simplex ulcers with these drugs. Instead they should be reserved for those patients who have an IDU intolerance or who fail to show a favorable response to IDU.

Stromal herpes simplex keratitis. Recurrent herpetic ulcers result from virus replication in the stroma, giving rise to uveitis and corneal infiltrates, edema, and necrosis. Overlying epithelial defects may be dendritic or patchlike. IDU ointment five times a day is indicated, but improvement is usually slow. The eye tends to remain inflamed, and stromal scarring occurs. Topical steroids used two or three times a day in addition to IDU reduces the uveitis, corneal edema, and infiltrates. If topical steroids are used extensively, progression of the ulcer with perforation of the eye may result. When steroid therapy is used, topical antibiotics should be employed to reduce the likelihood of secondary bacterial infections. IDU may not be very effective in stromal herpes due to its poor corneal penetration and failure to reach the site of viral replication. However, recent evidence suggests that vidarabine and TFT produce better results in stromal and anterior uveal herpes, probably due to better corneal permeability. Hypoxanthine arabinoside, a metabolite of vidarabine, is capable of greater penetration of the cornea than the parent compound; it has effective antiviral properties.

When medical therapy fails, a Gunderson conjunctival flap is indicated. Corneal perforations may be treated by isobutyl cyanoacrylate adhesive or a "blow out" patch corneal graft. Keratoplasty in the acute phases of the diseases should be avoided. In the quiescent phase of the disease, optical lamellar or penetrating keratoplasty may be performed with IDU coverage. A dendritic recurrent rate of 14% has been found in grafts after 2 months to 2½ years, regardless of the therapeutic regimen.

Disciform herpetic keratitis. A special form of herpetic keratitis that probably represents an immune reaction is disciform herpetic keratitis. This process is usually self-limited, but it can be prolonged and painful with temporary loss of vision. The judicious use of topical steroids usually is very effective in the reduction of the corneal edema. IDU five times a day should be given concurrently, since corticosteroids often seem to reactivate the epithelial form of the disease. Response to this treatment is usually fairly rapid and favorable.

Vaccinia infections. Vaccinia infections of the cornea should be treated with IDU therapy. The drug is administered as an 0.1% solution every hour during the day and every 2 hours at night, or as an 0.5% ointment every 6 hours. Other antiviral agents such vidarabine and TFT are probably equally effective. Cycloplegics may also be used to relieve iris spasm. Vaccinia immune globulin (VIG) was formerly advised as treatment for vaccinial keratitis, but experimental work indicates that delayed immune reactions in the cornea may be more common after use of this agent.

Herpes zoster infections. Corneal or uveal complications or both of ophthalmic herpes zoster occur in about 40% of cases. The corneal changes may be simple superficial punctate keratitis, grayish elevated subepithelial opacities, or dendritiform lesions of coarse ropy appearance without end knobs. Topical steroids three or four times a day and cycloplegics one to two times a day significantly reduce the corneal and uveal complications. If systemic prednisone in daily doses of 60 mg is given within 10 days of the development of ophthalmic zoster, the immediate severe neuralgic pain as well as postneuralgic pain can be greatly reduced. Systemic steroids should not be used in patients with associated malignant disease because of increased mortality rates. The physician must be aware that the corneal epithelial component of herpes zoster may mimic herpes simplex where topical steroids are contraindicated.

Varicella and rubeola infections. Varicella and rubeola infections of the cornea are treated symptomatically, with the use of cycloplegics to reduce any secondary iridocyclitis and the use of broad-spectrum antibiotics to prevent secondary infections. Corticosteroids should be avoided. Passive antiserum for this condition has not yet been fully evaluated. IDU therapy has been used as treatment for varicella keratitis. The varicella virus synthesizes DNA; theoretically IDU should be effective.

Trachomatous keratitis. Trachomatous keratitis is secondary to involvement of the conjunctiva. Treatment should be directed toward the primary infection in the conjunctiva. This is discussed in Chapter 9. Once scarring and vascular pannus of the cornea have occurred, little can be done for the patient medically except to give symptomatic relief. Corticosteroids may be used after the active infection has been cleared. If the disease is extensive, keratoplasty may be of benefit.

Superficial punctate keratitis. Thygeson's superficial punctate keratitis is usually a self-limited disease that has a tendency to recur at seasonal intervals for a period of a few years. The disease is thought to be viral in origin. Nonetheless, the treatment of choice appears to be the topical use of corticosteroids.

Epidemic keratoconjunctivitis. Type 8 adenovirus corneal infection produces classical epidemic keratoconjunctivitis with large, central, subepithelial, grayish macules lasting several months to years. Types 3, 4, and 7 adenoviruses generally cause pharyngoconjunctival fever with finer central subepithelial opacities lasting weeks to months. Topical steroids two or three times a day will cause both forms of subepithelial infiltrates to disappear or prevent them from appearing. However, after the steroids are stopped, infiltrates may appear. Until the effect of steroids on the natural history of the disease is known fully, topical steroids are recommended only for those cases demonstrating significant pain, irritation, or moderate visual loss.

Mycotic ulcers. A fungal etiology must be suspected in slowly progressive corneal ulcers, especially those previously treated by topical steroids or in ulcers that fail to respond to antibiotic therapy. The organism must be identified by scrapings stained with Giemsa, Gram, and potassium hydroxide as well as by culture on Sabouraud's agar. Amphotericin B is effective against a broad group of pathogenic and saprophytic fungi. It is commonly employed as a 0.15% to 5% topical solution every hour through the day and every 2 to 3 hours nightly. Nystatin (Mycostatin) in a concentration of 100,000 units per ml is effective against many fungi, particularly *Candida*. Subconjunctival injection of 0.5 ml of amphotericin B solution containing 1 to 2 mg per ml or nystatin solution containing 100,000 units per ml may be given in addition to the topical therapy. Thimerosal and potassium iodide topical solutions have also been used effectively in fungal ulcers. Recently a 5% solution of pimaricin used every 1 or 2 hours has been shown to be a very effective topical antifungal drug on the cornea. The effect of pimaricin is enhanced by simultaneous treatment with 1% or 2% potassium iodide. Other newer antifungal agents, such as clotrimazole, econazole, and thiabendazole, have been suggested. In the past, sodium iodide by mouth in doses of 15 grains three times a day and copper sulfate, 0.125 solution, applied topically or administered by iontophoresis, have also been effective against some mycotic corneal ulcers. Cycloplegics should be used to relieve the iridocyclitis that usually accompanies the mycotic corneal infection. Broad-spectrum antibiotics should also be used to combat secondary bacterial infections. If the mycotic infection persists, it may be necessary to employ surgical procedures such as conjunctival flap or keratoplasty in addition to the medical therapy.

ALLERGIC REACTIONS

Many of the corneal diseases probably represent immunological reactions. Diseases such as interstitial keratitis, phlyctenular keratitis, and sclerosing keratitis probably represent sensitivity reactions of the corneal stroma. Therapy is discussed in the chapters on specific diseases.

Allergic reactions to drugs and airborne antigens are infrequent. Therapy of these conditions begins with the determination of, if possible, the offending agent and then elimination of patient contact with it. Relief of the symptoms and of the corneal edema frequently seen in patients with these conditions is usually obtained with the topical administration of steroids. In chloroquine and indomethacin reactions with subepithelial involvement, complete clearing of the cornea will not take place until the drug has been discontinued. These latter reactions may represent drug toxicity.

Bacterial allergies of the cornea are frequently manifested by marginal corneal infiltrates or ulcerations. Although clearing of the cornea frequently follows the topical administration of steroids, a definite attempt should be made to eradicate the bacterial infection. In staphylococcic marginal ulcerations, appropriate antibiotics should be administered and desensitization of the patient to staphylococcus toxoid should be undertaken.

Limbal vernal conjunctivitis is usually satisfactorily managed with topical steroid therapy. In severe cases beta radiation has been suggested. However, this form of therapy is seldom necessary and should be avoided.

Phlyctenular keratitis

Phlyctenular keratitis may result from a sensitivity to tuberculin protein but also results from sensitivity to proteins from other bacteria such as staphylococci or fungi. The patient should be examined for systemic tuberculosis and should be referred for appropriate therapy if indicated. Steroids should be given topically to relieve symptoms and decrease the reaction. If secondary iritis is present, cycloplegic drops should be used. Desensitization of the patient to tuberculin protein was formerly recommended.

Interstitial keratitis

Interstitial keratitis is usually associated with congenital syphilis. Dramatic relief of symptoms follows the topical use of steroids. However, some workers feel steroid therapy should not be used, since it may prolong the disease. In addition, the syphilitic status of the patient should be evaluated, and active syphilis should be appropriately treated with penicillin. The topical use of atropine is recommended to relieve the iris spasm that usually develops. Interstitial keratitis from causes other than congenital syphilis is rare, although it is reported to occur as a result of tuberculosis. If there is active tuberculous infection elsewhere in the body, this should be treated. Desensitization of the patient to tuberculin protein is also still suggested, although this treatment has been largely replaced by local steroid therapy.

Parenchymatous keratitis

Parenchymatous keratitis is thought to be associated with granulomatous infections such as syphilis, tuberculosis, and sarcoidosis. Patients with parenchymatous keratitis should be examined for systemic disease, and appropriate treatment should be carried out. The topical use of steroids is of value to relieve the involvement and symptoms. Cycloplegics should also be used.

CORNEAL DRYING AND EXPOSURE
Keratitis sicca

Keratitis sicca is a condition of inadequate aqueous component of the tears resulting from a lacrimal gland deficiency. Treatment of the mild to moderate case is administration of one of a large number of commercially available artificial tears. Methylcellulose (0.5% to 1%), polyvinyl alcohol (1.4% to 3%), hydroxypropyl methylcellulose, 1% (Ultra Tears), Tears Naturale, and Adsorbotear have been used with good success in doses four times a day to every hour, depending on the severity of the disease. To conserve tears in the severe disease, cautery to the interior of the canaliculi by needle electrode offers an easy and effective method of canalicular closure. The application of a therapeutic soft contact lens, with 0.5N saline drops added intermittently, has been shown to provide a safe and effective method of maintaining a precorneal tear film in severe keratitis sicca. Acetylcysteine, as a 10% to 20% solution, has been advocated to reduce the abundant mucous and corneal filaments.

Mucus-deficient dry eyes

Stevens-Johnson syndrome and pemphigoid are examples of conjunctival goblet cell atrophy with or without aqueous tear deficiency. Tear replacements are of some use but rarely provide much improvement or reversal of symptoms.

Table 13. Artificial tear solutions

Product	Principal ingredients	Product	Principal ingredients
Adapettes	Adsorbobase* Thimerosal 0.002% Disodium edetate 0.05%	Methulose	Methylcellulose 0.25% Buffered solution Benzalkonium chloride 0.004%
Adapt	Adsorbobase Hydroxyethyl cellulose 0.55%	Pre-sert	Polyvinyl alcohol 3.0% Chlorobutanol 0.5%
Adsorbotear	Adsorbobase Hydroxyethyl cellulose Buffered isotonic solution Thimerosal 0.002% Disodium edetate 0.05%	Tearisol	Hydroxypropyl methylcellulose 0.5% Buffered isotonic solution Benzalkonium chloride 0.01%
Isopto Tears	Hydroxypropyl methylcellulose 0.5% Benzalkonium chloride 0.01%	Tears Naturale	Disodium edetate 0.01% Duasorb† Benzalkonium chloride 0.01% Disodium edetate 0.05%
Lacril	Hydroxypropyl methylcellulose Polysorbate 80, gelatin A, buffered isotonic solution, chlorobutanol 0.5%	Ultra Tears	Hydroxypropyl methylcellulose 1.0% Benzalkonium chloride 0.004%
Liquifilm Forte	Polyvinyl alcohol 3.0% Chlorobutanol 0.5%	Visculose	Methylcellulose 0.5 or 1.0% Buffered solution Benzalkonium chloride 0.004%
Liquifilm Tears	Polyvinyl alcohol 1.4% Chlorobutanol 0.5%		
Lyteers	Hydroxyethyl cellulose 0.2% Buffered isotonic solution Benzalkonium chloride 0.01% Disodium edetate 0.05%		

*Adsorbobase is polyvinyl pyrrolidine soluble polymers (PVP) 1.67% with water.
†Duasorb is manufacturer's polymetric preparation containing hydroxypropyl methylcellulose and dextran.

Newer tear substitutes such as hydroxypropyl methylcellulose, 1%, Tears Naturale, and Adsorbotear every 1 to 2 hours appear to be better tolerated. A therapeutic soft contact lens with frequent instillations of 0.5N saline drops improves vision and comfort. In some cases incision of symblepharons and closed cul-de-sacs are required before soft lens use. In selected severe cases a micropump with delivery tubes attached to spectacles may be used to deliver controlled amounts of fluid through polyethylene tubing into the eye.

Exposure keratitis

Exposure keratitis usually develops after facial nerve palsies and periods of unconsciousness or is associated with severe exophthalmos. It should be treated with lubricating and emulsifying agents. Methylcellulose, 0.5% to 1% drops, polyvinyl alcohol, 1.4% to 3%, Tears Naturale, or Adsorbotear should be used at frequent intervals. Bland ointments such as Lacri-Lube are suggested, particularly when the drops cannot be instilled at frequent intervals. If exposure keratitis is likely to become permanent, a tarsorrhaphy should be performed.

Neuroparalytic keratitis

Neuroparalytic keratitis is usually seen after the surgical treatment of trigeminal neuralgia. It is treated the same as exposure keratitis.

DEGENERATIVE CONDITIONS
Fuchs' endothelial-epithelial dystrophy

Medical management of Fuchs' dystrophy has largely been confined to dehydrating agents. Hypertonic 5% sodium chloride ointment (Mucosal No. 128) at bedtime or 40% glucose ointment and 5% sodium chloride drops (Mucosal No. 4) during the day help to maintain visual clarity, especially during the early phases of the disease. Remarkable visual improvement and loss of pain has been reported in some cases with the combined use of hypertonic sodium chloride drops and a therapeutic soft contact lens. Conjunctival flaps and cautery to Bowman's membrane offer relief of pain but no visual improvement. In the absence of other eye diseases, successful replacement of the dystrophic endothelium by penetrating keratoplasty is likely to give a good visual result.

Fatty degeneration

Fatty degeneration of the cornea cannot be treated satisfactorily. Such degenerative changes may follow any type of corneal injury or degeneration. They may also be found in patients with certain lipid metabolic disorders, and in these patients lipid-free diets might be indicated. Keratoplasty may be of value in some cases.

Band keratopathy

The calcium present in band keratopathy may be successfully removed with the use of a chelating agent—EDTA (Versenate Sodium). The epithelium is removed from the anesthetized cornea, calcium flakes are scraped off with a scalpel and an 0.01M to 0.05M solution of EDTA is applied to the cornea for 15 to 20 minutes by means of an iontophoresis cup or an inverted test tube. Alternatively the EDTA solution may be applied by continuous irrigation for 15 minutes or by placing a Weckcel sponge soaked in EDTA on the cornea. Intermittent rubbing with a cotton swab facilitates removal of calcium (see discussion of EDTA in Section 2). Cycloplegics are then instilled, and a pressure dressing is applied until the cornea has reepithelized. Dramatic improvement in vision may result after this form of therapy, but unfortunately the calcium has a tendency to recur.

VASCULARIZATION

Vascularization of the cornea may result from any condition that causes corneal edema and necrosis. Corneal vascularization may be secondary to trauma, infection, or degeneration. Once it has occurred, it is usually permanent. Thus it is better to prevent vascularization than to treat it after it has occurred. Accordingly, the best means of prevention is effective treatment of the underlying condition.

Topical thio-TEPA, a radiomimetic agent, has been used successfully to inhibit experimental corneal vacularization and to prevent regrowth of vessels after pterygium excision. The use of subconjunctival and topical corticosteroids may reduce inflammation and necrosis in some diseases, thereby decreasing corneal vascularization. After pterygium excision the application of beta radiation to the limbus is frequently successful in obliterating small vessels that enter the cornea from the limbus. Ocular irradiation to reduce corneal vascularization in other conditions is usually ineffective. Tissue injury from irradiation often makes later surgical treatment hazardous because of poor wound healing and delayed epithelial regrowth. Direct cauterization of larger vessels with an electrode is an outmoded treatment. In experimental animals argon laser photocoagulation has been used to treat corneal vascularization.

Vascularization of the cornea is frequently the body's method of healing a corneal wound or infection. Prevention of vascularization interferes with the basic healing process and thus impairs the body's ability to correct the underlying disease. The physician must make a value judgment as to whether he should allow vascularization to occur as a healing process and then, after healing has taken place, attempt to improve the condition of the cornea by means of keratoplasty.

EDEMA

Corneal edema may result from various disorders. The edema may be transitory or of an insignificant degree for which no therapy is required. In cases of moderate epithelial edema, which produces some blurriness of vision, hypertonic solutions or ointments such as 5% sodium chloride may provide some relief. Acetazolamide reduces corneal edema only when the intraocular pressure is abnormally high. Surface cautery and thin conjunctival inlay flaps may reduce pain associated with severe corneal edema, but these procedures do not improve vision. Patients with severe cases of corneal edema have shown improvement after removal of all the epithelium and application of a contact lens, which was glued in place with cyanoacrylate adhesives. Unfortunately the bond strength ultimately weakens after a variable period, and the lens falls off the cornea. A therapeutic soft contact lens, however, when used with hypertonic saline solution, 5%, often provides significant visual improvement as well as relief of pain. When other modes of therapy fail, penetrating keratoplasty is indicated.

SYSTEMIC DISEASES

The cornea is involved in a variety of systemic diseases. In such involvements it is important to recognize the underlying cause of the disease and to treat the condition appropriately.

Small calcium deposits may be formed in the corneas of patients with hyperparathyroidism. Treatment of the underlying disease will prevent progression of the calcium deposit formation. Cystine crystals are seen in patients with renal rickets (cystinosis). This condition is caused by congenital abnormalities of the renal transport system and is treated with vitamin D and sodium and potassium citrates. The fine, discrete, gray opacities seen in the central cornea of patients with myxedema disappear after proper thyroid medication.

Vitamin deficiences may cause changes in the cornea. Severe vitamin A deficiencies result in xerosis of the cornea and keratomalacia. High doses of vitamin A should be given as described under xerosis in Chapter 9. Vitamin B deficiencies are said to cause peripheral corneal vascularization. Thiamine, in a dose of 10 to 15 mg daily in divided oral doses, is recommended for this condition. Excessive intake of vitamin A may result in a form of band keratopathy. Treatment is simply elimination of the excessive amount of vitamin A intake. Peripheral corneal vascularization and infiltrates are seen in patients with acne rosacea. The eye manifestations are helped by the local use of corticosteroid preparations.

Severe marginal corneal ulceration may occur in patients with such systemic degenerative diseases as periarteritis and in those with severe debilitating diseases such as dysentery. Treatment consists of proper management of the underlying disease.

Both peripheral and central corneal ulcerations are observed in patients with arthritis. Many cases can be managed with tear replacement therapy as described in the treatment of keratitis sicca. Weak dilutions of steroids may be helpful, although in some patients the ulceration may progress more rapidly with steroid therapy. In some patients the application of a thin, therapeutic soft contact lens combined with the frequent instillation of 0.5N saline drops has been of value. Topical antibiotic drops, such as chloramphenicol, should be used concurrently to prevent a secondary infection. If perforation of the ulcer occurs, cyanoacrylate adhesive can be applied topically as a temporary seal. Keratoplasty may become necessary in some patients.

Certain corneal opacities such as occur in patients with Hurler's disease (gargoylism), a generalized disorder of connective tissue and a storage disease, are not amenable to therapy. Penetrating keratoplasty may be of value, but ultimately opacification may result from recurrence of the stored material.

REFERENCES

Allen, H. F.: Current status of prevention, diagnosis and management of bacterial corneal ulcers, Ann. Ophthalmol. 3:235, 1971.

Boruchoff, S. A., and others: Clinical applications of adhesives in corneal surgery, Trans. Am. Acad. Ophthalmol. Otolaryngol. **73**:499, 1969.

Breinin, G. M., and Devoe, A. G.: Chelation of calcium with edathamil calcium-disodium in band keratopathy and corneal calcium affections, Arch. Ophthalmol. **52**:846, 1954.

Brown, S. I., and Weller, C. A.: Collagenase inhibitors in prevention of ulcers of alkali burned cornea, Arch. Ophthalmol. **83**:352, 1970.

Dohlman, C. H., editor: Corneal edema, Int. Ophthalmol. Clin. **8**(3): entire issue, 1968.

Dohlman, C. H., and Pfister, R. R.: Management of chemical burns of the eye. In Symposium on the cornea, Transactions of the New Orleans Academy of Ophthalmology, St. Louis, 1972, The C. V. Mosby Co.

Dohlman, C. H., and others: Replacement of the corneal epithelium with a contact lens, Trans. Am. Acad. Ophthalmol. Otolaryngol. **73**:482, 1969.

Elliot, F. A.: Treatment of herpes zoster with high doses of prednisone, Lancet **2**:610, 1964.

Ellison, A. C., and Poirier, R.: Therapeutic effects of heparin on *Pseudomonas*-induced corneal ulceration, Am. J. Ophthalmol. **82**:619, 1976.

Ellison, A. C., Newmark, E., and Kaufman, H. E.: Chemotherapy of experimental keratomycosis, Am. J. Ophthalmol. **68**:812, 1969.

Fulhorst, H. W., and others: Cryotherapy of epithelial herpes simplex keratitis, Am. J. Ophthalmol. **73**:46, 1972.

Grant, W. M.: Toxicology of the eye, ed. 2, Springfield, Ill., 1974, Charles C Thomas, Publisher.

Hessburg, P. C.: *Pseudomonas* keratitis, Survey Ophthalmol. **14**:43, 1969.

Hughes, W. F.: Treatment of herpes simplex keratitis; a review, Am. J. Ophthalmol. **67**:313, 1969.

Jones, B. R.: Principles in the management of oculomycosis, Am. J. Ophthalmol. **79**:719, 1975.

Jones, D. B.: Early diagnosis and therapy of bacterial corneal ulcers, Trans. Am. Acad. Ophthalmol. Otolaryngol. **79**:95(OP), 1975.

Kaufman, H. E.: Chemotherapy of herpes simplex keratitis, Invest. Ophthalmol. **2**:504, 1963.

Kaufman, H. E., Martola, E. L., and Dohlman, C.: Use of 5-iodo-2'-deoxyuridine (IDU) in treatment of herpes simplex keratitis, Arch. Ophthalmol. **68**:235, 1962.

Langham, M. E.: The inhibition of corneal vascularization by triethylenethiophosphoramide, Am. J. Ophthalmol. **49**:1111, 1960.

Leibowitz, H. W.: Hydrophilic contact lenses in corneal disease. IV. Penetrating corneal wounds, Arch. Ophthalmol. **88**:602, 1972.

Lemp, M. A.: Tear substitutes in the treatment of dry eyes, Int. Ophthalmol. Clin. **13**:145, 1973.

Lemp, M. A.: Artificial tear solutions, Int. Ophthalmol. Clin. **13**:221, 1973.

Lemp, M. A., Dohlman, C. H., and Holly, F. J.: Corneal dessication despite normal tear volume, Ann. Ophthalmol. **1**:258, 1969.

McGill, J., Holt-Wilson, J. R., McKinnon, H. P., and others: Some aspects of the clinical use of trifluorothymidine in the treatment of herpetic ulceration of the cornea, Trans. Ophthalmol. Soc. U.K. **94**:342, 1974.

Pavan-Langston, D., Buchanan, R. A., and Alford, C. A., Jr., editors: Adenine arabinoside; an antiviral agent, New York, 1975, Raven Press.

Pavan-Langston, D., Dohlman, C. H., Geary, P., and Sulzewski, D.: Intraocular penetration of ARA-A and IDU; therapeutic implications in clinical herpetic uveitis, Trans. Am. Acad. Ophthalmol. Otolaryngol. **77**:455(OP), 1973.

Pfister, R. R., Richards, J. S., and Dohlman, C. H.: Recurrence of herpetic keratitis in corneal grafts, Am. J. Ophthalmol. **73**:192, 1972.

Scheie, H. G., and Alper, M. C.: Treatment of herpes zoster ophthalmicus with cortisone or corticotropin, Arch. Ophthalmol. **53**:38, 1955.

Slansky, H. H., Dohlman, C. H., and Berman, M. B.: Prevention of corneal ulcers, Trans. Am. Acad. Ophthalmol. Otolaryngol. **75**:2, 1971.

Wellings, P. C., Awdry, P. N., Bors, F. H., and others: Clinical evaluation of trifluorothymidine in the treatment of herpes simplex corneal ulcers, Am. J. Ophthalmol. **73**:932, 1972.

Wood, T. O., and Williford, W.: Treatment of keratomycosis with amphotericin B 0.15%, Am. J. Ophthalmol. **81**:847, 1976.

CHAPTER 12

Therapy of diseases of the sclera

EPISCLERITIS

Treatment of episcleritis should be determined by the severity of the involvement and the possible etiology or associated disease.

Mild cases of episcleritis, unassociated with any systemic disease, can be cured with minimal treatment. The local application of corticosteroid preparations, several times a day for a few days, usually resolves the lesions. In patients with a tendency to recurrence, the steroid therapy should be continued for a period of time after the recurrence is brought under control. Systemic steroids may be used concurrently in severe cases.

Episcleritis is often seen in conjunction with rheumatoid and collagen diseases. Although the therapy of the systemic manifestations of these diseases should be managed by an internist, the ophthalmologist should be aware of the coexisting disease, and his therapy of the eye condition may vary with the progress of the systemic disease. Treatment of choice is the topical use of steroids. In the very acute phases it may be necessary to use medications in the form of drops or ointments as frequently as eight or ten times a day. As the inflammation subsides, the dose may be reduced to only once or twice a day, and the medication may be discontinued as the inflammation completely recedes. In episcleritis associated with rheumatoid and collagen diseases, recurrence often occurs, and it is necessary to keep the patients on steroid therapy intermittently for several years.

The use of certain other medications, such as mild vasoconstricting agents, 0.12% phenylephrine (Neo-Synephrine) or 25 minims of 1:1,000 epinephrine (Adrenalin) in 1 ounce of mild collyria, offers symptomatic relief, but there is no pronounced suppression of the generalized inflammatory effect. Aspirin and other salicylates have been used in the past as systemic medication with some benefit. Antihistamines and histamine desensitization have been suggested, but they are not nearly so effective as local corticosteroid medication. Oxyphenbutazone, 100 mg three to four times a day, has been reported to be effective for the treatment of persistent episcleritis and scleritis.

SCLERITIS

Treatment of scleritis is determined by the severity of the involvement and the possible etiology or associated disease, as in patients with episcleritis. Associated systemic disease is present more often in patients with scleritis. Moreover, the inflammatory response is usually more severe and requires more vigorous therapy.

Scleritis is frequently associated with the arthritides, the rheumatoid group of diseases, and most of the collagen diseases. The associated scleritis usually varies with the severity of the systemic disease. Scleritis may develop while the patient is receiving active salicylate or corticosteroid therapy for the arthritis or other rheumatoid condition. In any of the forms of scleritis associated with these diseases, the treatment of choice is the topical administration of steroids in the form of ointment or drops. Systemic corticosteroids may be necessary for patients with severe involvement extending posteriorly. Subconjunctival and sub-Tenon's injections of steroids should be avoided, since the sclera is often thin and may be perforated easily. Frequency of topical administration varies with the severity of the disease, and as the disease subsides, the steroid dosage may be reduced. Despite vigorous steroid therapy, certain cases progress. If severe scleral ectasia and impending perforation of the globe occur, scleral grafting either with donor sclera or with fascia lata may become necessary.

Other forms of scleritis associated with systemic disease are sometimes encountered. In these cases, management should be directed against the systemic condition. Patients with scleritis associated with brucellosis should be treated with the tetracyclines and streptomycin. Those with scleritis associated with syphilis should be treated with penicillin in a total dose varying from 5 to 10 million units. In the treatment of scleritis associated with tuberculosis, streptomycin, rifampin, or ethambutol may be given in combination with isoniazid (Chapter 8). Patients with gouty scleritis are treated with colchicine, phenylbutazone (Butazolidin), or indomethacin (Indocin). For acute attacks of gout, colchicine, 0.6 mg, is given every 2 hours until symptoms are relieved or until gastrointestinal symptoms develop. In mild cases 0.6 mg of colchicine is given daily. Phenylbutazone is used in acute gout. The dosage is 200 to 400 mg orally initially, then 200 mg every 6 hours for four doses, followed then by doses of 100 mg three times a day until symptoms subside. Indomethacin has been found to be effective against gout. For acute attacks 50 mg three times a day is used. During the quiescent phase, the dosage is reduced to 25 mg twice a day. Uricosuric agents such as probenecid (Benemid), 500 mg twice a day; sulfinpyrazone (Anturan), 400 mg per day; or allopurinol (Zyloprim), 100 mg three times a day, are often prescribed during the quiescent phase to reduce serum levels of uric acid and prevent acute attacks of gout. Scleritis associated with leprosy should be treated with sulfone drugs in accordance with the dosage schedule given in Chapter 8.

In all of these systemic diseases with associated scleritis, the topical use of steroids in the eye affords relief and dramatic improvement of inflammation. As long as the systemic condition is being treated adequately with specific therapy, it is probably quite safe to use the corticosteroids locally at the same time.

SCLEROMALACIA PERFORANS

Scleromalacia perforans is a serious disorder that occurs in patients with rheumatoid arthritis and usually follows severe scleritis. It is characterized by extensive destruction of the sclera, exposing the underlying uvea. Perforation of the globe may occur. Various surgical procedures have been described for the treatment of scleromalacia perforans, including scleral and fascia lata grafts. Some have suggested combining antirheumatoid drugs such as penicillamine (Cuprimine) with surgery.

SCLERAL CONDITIONS ASSOCIATED WITH GENERALIZED DISEASE

Pigmentary changes in the sclera may be seen in various conditions.

The sclera may appear icteric as the result of quinacrine (Atabrine) medication or as a result of some biliary or liver disease. There is no specific treatment for this scleral condition. As the icterus subsides, the scleral pigmentation will decrease.

Ochronosis causes a grayish-brown discoloration of the sclera. This condition results from a metabolic disturbance of certain amino acids (phenylalanine and tyrosine) or as the result of a metabolic disturbance of phenols or quinones. The only effective treatment is the elimination of exposure to the phenolic substances.

There is no satisfactory medical management of osteogenesis imperfecta ("blue sclerotics").

REFERENCES

Kiss, G.: Care of scleromalacia perforans manifesting in the course of rheumatoid arthritis with D-penicillamine and facia lata autograft (English translation), Klin. Monatsbl. Augenheilkd. 167:484, 1975.

Lyne, A. J., and Pikeathley, D. A.: Episcleritis and scleritis, Arch. Ophthalmol. 80:171, 1968.

The Medical Letter on Drugs and Therapeutics, vol. 18, No. 12, June 4, 1976.

Sexton, R. R.: Diseases of the sclera. In Dunlap, E. A., editor: Gordon's medical management of ocular disease, ed. 2, New York, 1976, Harper & Row, Publishers.

Torchia, R. T., Dunn, R. E., and Pease, P. J.: Fascia lata grafting in scleromalacia perforans, Am. J. Ophthalmol. 66:705, 1968.

Watson, P. G.: Management of scleral disease, Trans. Ophthalmol. Soc. U.K. 86:151, 1966.

Watson, P. G., and Hayreh, S. S.: Scleritis and episcleritis, Br. J. Ophthalmol. 60:163, 1976.

CHAPTER 13

Therapy of glaucomas

The treatment of the glaucomas may best be considered under three general headings that correspond to the three major classifications of glaucoma:

I. Primary glaucoma
    A. Open-angle glaucoma (chronic simple)
    B. Narrow-angle or angle-closure glaucoma (acute congestive)
    C. Hypersecretion glaucoma
II. Congenital glaucoma (developmental)
    A. Infantile glaucoma
    B. Juvenile glaucoma
III. Secondary glaucoma

The treatment of open-angle glaucoma and secondary glaucoma is primarily medical, whereas the treatment of narrow-angle and congenital glaucoma is primarily surgical.

OPEN-ANGLE GLAUCOMA

The treatment of open-angle glaucoma is directed toward normalization of intraocular pressure and the prevention of deterioration of the optic nerve and the visual field. Judgment of the adequacy of therapy should be governed by the appearance of the optic nerve head, the visual fields, visual acuity, and tonometry. A fourth adjunct to this judgment is tonography, in which treatment is directed toward normalization of the coefficient of aqueous flow. Surgery should be resorted to only if vigorous medical therapy is unsuccessful in preventing progressive visual field loss.

Three groups of drugs (miotics, epinephrine derivatives, and carbonic anhydrase inhibitors) may be employed singly or in combination for the medical control of open-angle glaucoma.

Miotics

Miotics act by improving the outflow of aqueous humor from the anterior chamber. There are two general pharmacological types—the direct-acting acetylcholinelike drugs and the indirect-acting cholinesterase inhibitors. The direct-acting miotics are relatively short acting (4 to 8 hours). They may cause some irritation on instillation, transient headaches, and mild spasm of accommodation, but they seldom produce severe side reactions. The cholinesterase inhibitors have a much longer action (8 to 72 hours). They may cause severe headaches and spasm of accommodation and iris cysts at the pupillary margin. Long-term usage may produce lens opacities. This is notably true of the long-acting, water-soluble anticholinesterases—echothiophate iodide and demecarium bromide. In addition they occasionally produce systemic symptoms of acetylcholine intoxication—sweating, vomiting, diarrhea, and tachycardia. Prolonged apnea may occur after the administration of succinylcholine (Anectine) during general anesthesia as a result of depressed pseudocholinesterase levels produced by echothiophate iodide therapy. The following are the commonly used miotics:

I. Acetylcholinelike miotics
- A. Pilocarpine nitrate or hydrochloride, 0.5% to 8%
- B. Carbachol (Doryl), 0.75% to 3%

II. Cholinesterase inhibitors
- A. Eserine salicylate, 0.25% to 1%
- B. Neostigmine (Prostigmin) bromide, 2.5% to 5%
- C. Isoflurophate (DFP, Floropryl), 0.025% to 0.1%
- D. Echothiophate (Phospholine) iodide, 0.03% to 0.25%
- E. Demecarium bromide (Humorsol), 0.12% to 0.25%

The decision as to which miotic to use and in what concentration and frequency is made largely by a process of trial and error, but certain general rules may be followed. The least amount of the weakest miotic that will control the glaucoma is the treatment desired. Pilocarpine should be tried initially. In early or mild cases of open-angle glaucoma, 1% pilocarpine may be sufficient, but in well-established or chronic conditions, 2% pilocarpine or higher is usually necessary to achieve adequate results. Generally, this medication should be used at least four times a day, since the maximum drug effect lasts about 6 hours. If pilocarpine therapy proves inadequate for the control of glaucoma, epinephrine derivatives may be added or other miotics may be tried. Carbachol may be used in strengths of 0.75% to 3% four times a day. If this treatment does not achieve the desired results, stronger cholinesterase inhibitors should be tried—echothiophate iodide, demecarium bromide, or isoflurophate. These agents are generally instilled one to two times a day.

Combinations of miotics are not generally recommended. However, the combination of pilocarpine and eserine medications is sometimes advocated, either as drops only or as pilocarpine drops during the day and eserine ointment at bedtime. Combinations of cholinesterase inhibitors should not be used, since these drugs are antagonistic to one another.

Patients may become refractory to one miotic (for example, pilocarpine) after several years. However, the drug may again become effective if it is discontinued for a period of time and another miotic employed.

In recent years pilocarpine has become available for treatment of glaucoma in a continuous release device, the Ocusert. This device is a membrane-bound repository of pilocarpine, which is inserted into the conjunctival cul-de-sac.

Two pilocarpine Ocusert systems are now available. One is the Ocusert Pilo-20, which releases 20μg of pilocarpine each hour for 1 week, and the other is the Ocusert Pilo-40, which is programmed to release 40μg per hour for a week. The Pilo-20 unit has been found to provide intraocular pressure control in glaucoma patients similar to that obtained with 1% pilocarpine drops but less than that obtained with 2% drops. The Pilo-40 unit controls intraocular pressure in eyes requiring 2% and 4% pilocarpine drops, although in some eyes requiring 4% drops, the Pilo-40 unit has not completely controlled intraocular pressure.

Several advantages exist with the Ocusert system. Since there is a constant rate of drug release (zero-order kinetics), the variability of medication available to the ocular receptor sites with conventional drop technique is overcome. The total quantity of drug released is substantially reduced, which reduces the likelihood of systemic toxicity. Local side effects of miosis and accommodative spasm are reduced as well as the inconvenience of drop instillation. The disadvantages include difficulty in insertion and removal of the device for some patients and the present increased expense of these units.

Levoepinephrine derivatives

Levoepinephrine derivatives exert their favorable effect on open-angle glaucoma by increasing aqueous outflow and decreasing the secretory formation of aqueous humor. The duration of action of the medications is highly variable —from a few hours to several days. They are given once or twice a day. In the treatment of open-angle glaucoma, they are seldom employed alone but are used in addition to miotic therapy. The following are the currently available commercial products: Adrenatrate, E1, Epifrin, Epinal, Epitrate, Eppy, Glaucon, Lyophrin, and Mytrate. Among the side reactions to this type of ophthalmic medication are irritation on instillation, adenochrome deposits in the conjunctiva and cornea, chronic hyperemia of the conjunctiva, and macular edema in aphakic eyes. Often epinephrine therapy must be discontinued because of side reactions. Symptoms of epinephrine sensitivity may be overcome if the concentration of the drug is reduced, if another product is used in place of the drug, or if weak concentrations of topical corticosteroids are added. Some of the side reactions to topical epinephrine are not as pronounced with the use of dipivalyl epinephrine, a congener of epinephrine. This drug has been employed in investigational studies in a 0.2% solution; it is not yet commercially available.

A potentiated response to topical epinephrine occurs following pretreatment with 6-hydroxydopamine. Approximately 0.2 ml of this agent is injected subconjunctivally or applied by means of a corneal-scleral reservoir as a 2% solution. A localized chemical sympathectomy occurs involving the iris, ciliary body, and outflow channels and persists for 2 to 6 months. This treatment has been successful in some patients with open-angle glaucoma and in patients with various forms of secondary glaucoma whose intraocular pressures were not adequately controlled with other medical therapy.

Carbonic anhydrase inhibitors

Carbonic anhydrase inhibitors act by suppressing the secretory formation of aqueous humor (Chapter 5). The exact mechanism remains unknown. Given orally, these drugs have their maximum effect in 2 hours, and their therapeutic effectiveness is gone in 6 to 12 hours. The maximum suppression of aqueous production is achieved usually with acetazolamide (Diamox), 250 mg four times a day, or its equivalent, although in a few patients additive effects are achieved with higher doses. Open-angle glaucoma in many patients may respond well to doses of 62.5 or 125 mg three or four times a day. Carbonic anhydrase inhibitors are used only as supplementary treatment, not as substitutes for topical miotic or epinephrine therapy in the management of open-angle gluacoma. In selected patients, carbonic anhydrase inhibitors may be used in doses of 250 mg one to four times daily for prolonged periods of time. Some patients have been maintained on carbonic anhydrase inhibitor therapy for 15 years or more. However, treatment must be discontinued in many patients because of side reactions.

Undesirable side effects of carbonic anhydrase inhibitors include paresthesias, anorexia, gastrointestinal disturbances, skin eruptions, headaches, general malaise, altered taste and smell, sodium and potassium depletion, ureteral colic, and the predisposition to form renal calculi. Bone marrow suppression has been a rare complication. Generally, the different carbonic anhydrase inhibitors produce similar side reactions; however, acetazolamide appears to cause more ureteral colic than methazolamide, whereas methazolamide often produces more general malaise than other agents. Some patients who have suffered ureteral colic and calculi with acetazolamide have been free of this complication when maintained on methazolamide. Although the carbonic anhydrase enzyme is present in lens and retina, long-term use of carbonic anhydrase inhibitors has not resulted in cataract formation or retinal change.

In some patients the carbonic anhydrase inhibitors seem to lose some of their ocular hypotensive activity after producing an initial response. It has been suggested that this may be caused by potassium depletion. More recent studies indicate that the administration of potassium fails to improve the effectiveness of acetazolamide, and the use of supplemental potassium is not recommended. The administration of ammonium chloride potentiates the action of acetazolamide, but since ammonium chloride produces severe acidosis it should not be used.

Currently available carbonic anhydrase inhibitor preparations include the following: acetazolamide, 125 and 250 mg; ethoxzolamide (Cardrase, Ethamide), 125 mg; dichlorphenamide (Daranide, Oratrol), 50 mg; and methazolamide (Neptazane), 50 mg. Other preparations are found in the section on therapeutic agents.

Tranquilizers

Tranquilizers are occasionally used as supplemental therapy to local administration of miotics to control the ocular tension in patients suffering from open-angle glaucoma. The exact mechanism of action is not completely understood, but presumably the neurohumoral factors responsible for changes in ocular tension are brought under control with this treatment. Although not generally advocated, tranquilizers may be worth a trial in the emotional, very tense patient with open-angle glaucoma.

Cardiac glycosides

Preliminary studies have suggested that digoxin is an effective inhibitor of aqueous humor secretion. The mechanism of action is believed to be an inhibition of sodium-dependent and potassium-dependent adenosinetriphosphatase (Na-K-ATPase), an enzyme operative in the sodium pump. The ciliary epithelium is thought to contain a sodium pump active in the secretion of aqueous humor.

The clinical indications for the use of digoxin in the treatment of glaucoma are not yet established. It has been successfully used for short-term therapy in patients with open-angle glaucoma and a few with congenital glaucoma. However, the use of cardiac glycosides is of doubtful value as adjunctive therapy for patients already receiving other forms of maximum antiglaucoma therapy.

Phenytoin (Dilantin)

It has been suggested that phenytoin administered systemically to glaucoma patients may improve or prevent visual field loss. It was postulated that the drug may protect the optic nerve by preventing the intraneuronal buildup of sodium induced in hypoxia by potentiating the adenosine triphosphate pump mechanism. Unfortunately, the hopes held for this therapy have not been realized in studies to date.

NARROW-ANGLE GLAUCOMA

The treatment of narrow-angle glaucoma is primarily surgical. Medical therapy is usually directed toward lowering the intraocular pressure in preparation for surgery. Lowering of intraocular pressure in the presence of an acute attack is usually accomplished by the topical application of acetylcholinelike miotics at frequent intervals, combined with the oral or intravenous administration of carbonic anhydrase inhibitors or the oral administration of glycerol. If the patient is vomiting, intravenous mannitol or urea may be administered instead of oral glycerol. The cholinesterase inhibitors should be avoided because of their irritative properties and the congestion they produce in the iris and conjunctiva.

Miotics

Pilocarpine, 2% to 4%, is instilled topically into the eye every 10 to 15 minutes for 1 to 2 hours and thereafter is repeated at hourly intervals for the next

4 to 6 hours. Subsequently, it is instilled every 3 to 4 hours for the next 12 hours. After the tension is under control it may be used three times a day. It is usually wise to instill pilocarpine into the unaffected eye every 6 to 8 hours to avoid an attack in the fellow eye.

Miosis may also be produced with the topical application of thymoxamine, an alpha-adrenergic blocking agent. In preliminary studies this drug has been successfully used in a 0.5% concentration for the treatment of angle-closure glaucoma. The medication is instilled every minute for 5 doses and then every 15 minutes for 2 to 3 hours.

Carbonic anhydrase inhibitors

Acetazolamide is given as an initial dose of 500 mg orally and 250 mg every 6 hours thereafter. There is usually a delay of 2 to 3 hours before its full effect is evident; the pressure effects persist for 6 to 10 hours. If the patient is vomiting, 500 mg of acetazolamide dissolved in sterile distilled water is given intravenously as the initial dose; alternatively, 250 mg may be given intravenously and 250 mg intramuscularly. With intravenous therapy some effect is achieved in a few minutes; a maximal effect is reached in 30 to 90 minutes.

Osmotherapy

It is generally held that osmotherapeutic agents produce the ocular hypotensive effects by creating an osmotic gradient in which blood is hypertonic to the intraocular fluids. As a result, there is a movement of water out of the vitreous and aqueous humors into the bloodstream. More recent investigations indicate that in small doses osmotherapeutic agents may work through a central nervous system mechanism by stimulation of osmoreceptors with efferent transmission via the optic nerve. However, in the usual therapeutic doses they seem to act through the osmotic gradient mechanism (Chapter 5).

Oral glycerin, or glycerol, may be administered usually as a 50% solution in a dose of 1.5 grams per kg of body weight. The pure glycerin may be added to an equal volume of flavored water, or it may be mixed with an equal volume of orange or lime juice to make the 50% solution. Flavored commercial preparations of 50% glycerin (Osmoglyn) and 75% glycerin (Glyrol) are available. A fall in intraocular pressure develops within an hour, reaches a maximum in 1 to 2 hours, and lasts for 4 to 6 hours. Side effects include headaches, backache, dizziness, vomiting, and nausea; transient rises in blood glucose may occur. Glycerol is only a mild diuretic; it is metabolized. It is easily administered and should be kept in every ophthalmologist's office.

Urea (Urevert) is administered intravenously as a 30% solution. The preparation is formed when the dry powder is dissolved in a 10% solution of invert sugar. The total dose is 1 gram per kg of body weight administered at a rate of 60 drops per minute. A fall in intraocular pressure begins within 30 to 40 minutes, and the maximum effect is reached in an hour. Since this agent is a diuretic, a catheter should be introduced if the patient is to be taken to the operating room. Urea should not be used in patients with renal damage. Care must be taken to see that the drug does not extravasate outside the vein. Side effects are discussed in Chapter 5.

Mannitol is administered intravenously as a 20% solution in adults and as a 10% solution in children, over a period of 30 to 40 minutes. For adults the total dose is 1.5 to 2 grams per kg of body weight, and for children, 1.5 grams per kg of body weight. The maximum ocular hypotensive effect is reached in an hour; some effect persists for 5 to 6 hours. Unlike urea, mannitol is not contraindicated in patients with renal disease; it does not raise BUN levels. Less damage results if subcutaneous extravasation occurs. At the present time, mannitol is the intravenous osmotherapeutic agent of choice, although larger volumes of fluid must be administered. Since mannitol is a diuretic, catheterization is advisable for patients going to the operating room. Further side effects are noted in Chapter 5.

Other hyperosmotic agents effective in lowering intraocular pressure include sodium ascorbate, isosorbide, and 40% to 50% ethyl alcohol. These agents have been investigated in animals and a limited number of human subjects. Sodium ascorbate is administered as a 20% solution intravenously in doses of 0.5 to 1 gram per kg of body weight. Isosorbide (Hydronol) is given orally as a 50% solution in doses of 1 to 2 grams per kg of body weight; ethyl alcohol is given as a 40% to 50% (80 to 100 proof) oral solution in a dose of 0.8 to 1.5 grams per kg of body weight. Of these agents, isosorbide appears to be the most promising. It does not raise blood glucose levels and therefore may be of some advantage in diabetic patients. It produces less nausea and vomiting than glycerol, but diarrhea may occur.

Surgical treatment

Once the intraocular pressure has been brought under control medically, the physician must decide whether to perform a peripheral iridectomy or a filtering procedure. Peripheral iridectomy should be performed on eyes without peripheral anterior synechiae and permanent angle closure. Peripheral iridectomy with scleral cautery or iridencleisis is indicated if there is permanent angle closure. The determination of whether an angle is permanently closed is sometimes difficult. Helpful diagnostic procedures include gonioscopy, both preoperatively and at the time of surgery, and tonometry and tonography after the acute attack has subsided. Duration of the acute attack is a useful criterion—synechiae are usually permanent after 72 hours of acute unrelieved attack. When doubt remains concerning whether an iridectomy or filtering procedure is indicated, a peripheral iridectomy is performed to either side of the 12:00 meridian. Any residual glaucoma is controlled medically, or a filtering operation may be performed at a later date.

Surgical treatment of narrow-angle glaucoma is almost never contraindicated. However, should it be necessary to postpone surgical intervention, the patient should be maintained on miotics to decrease the likelihood of another acute attack.

HYPERSECRETION GLAUCOMA

Hypersecretion glaucoma, a relatively rare form, results from an overproduction of aqueous humor. It is seen in patients with vasomotor instability and hypertension. The medical treatment is directed toward reducing the secretory production of aqueous humor. Levoepinephrine ophthalmic drops may be used once or twice daily, but since they may cause elevation of systemic blood pressure they are contraindicated in patients with hypertension. The other treatment consists of the use of acetazolamide or its equivalent in the dose of 125 to 250 mg two or three times a day.

Eyes afflicted with hypersecretion glaucoma apparently withstand elevated pressures better than do eyes with other forms of glaucoma. Substantial data regarding long-term prognosis of this form of glaucoma are lacking.

CONGENITAL GLAUCOMA
Infantile glaucoma

Infantile glaucoma is a disease requiring surgery; medical therapy is ineffective. Goniotomy, either alone or in combination with goniopuncture, is the procedure of choice. Trabeculotomy has been successfully employed recently. In cases uncontrolled with these procedures, peripheral iridectomy with scleral cautery is sometimes successful. Other filtering operations are usually much less effective. Results of goniotomy are poor in newborn infants. Some surgeons prefer delaying the operation for a few months in this group of patients; pilocarpine therapy is employed in the interim.

Juvenile glaucoma

Juvenile glaucoma should be managed like open-angle glaucoma medically, with the use of miotics. However, eyes with juvenile glaucoma are much more resistant to medical therapy than eyes with presenile or senile open-angle glaucoma. Consequently, surgical treatment frequently becomes necessary. Goniopuncture, peripheral iridectomy with scleral cautery, iridencleisis, and trephination are the most commonly employed surgical procedures. Recently trabeculotomy and trabeculectomy have been advocated.

SECONDARY GLAUCOMA

The treatment of the secondary glaucomas is varied and must be directed primarily toward the cause of the elevated tension. The common causes of secondary glaucoma and their management follow.

Iris-induced secondary glaucoma

Iritis and iridocyclitis. Treatment should be directed toward the iritis. Corticosteroids systemically and topically and cycloplegics topically should be used.

If the cause of the iritis is known, specific therapy should be undertaken for this disease. The ocular tension will usually fall rapidly as the inflammation decreases. Carbonic anhydrase inhibitors should be used to control the pressure while the inflammation subsides. If an iris bombé results, an iridectomy may be necessary. If numerous peripheral anterior synechiae form, a filtering operation may become necessary after the acute inflammation has subsided.

Glaucomatocyclitic crisis. The attacks of glaucoma in glaucomatocyclitic crisis are self-limited. They are treated by topical application of steroids and cycloplegics. Carbonic anhydrase inhibitors should be used during the acute elevations of tension. Surgery is never indicated. The prolonged use of topically applied steroids between attacks may reduce recurrences. Patients should be observed in between attacks for evidence of elevated intraocular pressure in each eye.

Herpes zoster. Herpes zoster is treated as an inflammatory iridocyclitis with atropine topically and corticosteroids systemically and topically. Carbonic anhydrase inhibitors may be used if the tension becomes moderately elevated while the inflammation subsides.

Vogt-Koyanagi syndrome. Management of the Vogt-Koyanagi syndrome is the same as treatment of other glaucomas secondary to iridocyclitis.

Congenital anomalies of the iris. Posterior embryotoxon is sometimes controlled adequately with miotics. However, if medical management fails to control the glaucoma, goniopuncture, scleral cautery with iridectomy, trabeculotomy, or trabeculectomy may be employed.

Aniridia. Aniridia is an extremely difficult form of glaucoma to treat. Miotics may control the tension for many years and should be given a trial. Surgical treatment is extremely difficult. Scleral cautery with iridectomy (if residual iris is present), trabeculotomy, or trabeculectomy may be tried. It has been suggested that early goniotomy may prevent progressive contraction of the residual iris to the corneoscleral angle. Wilms' tumor is found frequently in children with aniridia. Patients should be studied for this possibility.

Degenerative diseases of the iris. Glaucoma associated with iris degeneration should be treated in the same manner as open-angle glaucoma, with miotics and epinephrine derivatives. Filtering operations such as trephination, scleral cautery with iridectomy, trabeculotomy, or trabeculectomy are probably the procedures of choice and are indicated if medical management fails.

Heterochromia. Heterochromia is usually a unilateral familial condition in which the inflammatory process results in depigmentation of the iris. The treatment is directed against the inflammatory process and consists of the topical use of atropine and corticosteroids. Carbonic anhydrase inhibitors may be indicated during acute rises of tension. No surgical treatment is indicated for the glaucoma. Surgical removal of the complicated cataract can be accomplished without undue difficulty.

Pigmentary glaucoma

Pigmentary glaucoma is seen in young adults, particularly myopic males. It is characterized by a Kruckenberg spindle, pigmentary deposits in the trabeculum, and thinning of iris pigment. It should be treated as open-angle glaucoma. Epinephrine products have been found to be particularly effective.

Essential iris atrophy. Essential iris atrophy is extremely difficult to manage. Miotics may relieve the elevated tension initially, but over a period of time they are unable to control the progressive glaucoma. Early peripheral iridectomy has been suggested. External filtering operations usually become necessary.

Glaucoma secondary to iridoschisis. Glaucoma secondary to iridoschisis should be managed in the same manner as open-angle glaucoma.

Lens-induced secondary glaucoma

Intumescent cataract. The treatment of glaucoma resulting from intumescent cataract is early surgical removal of the lens. Preoperatively an attempt should be made to normalize the intraocular pressure with the use of carbonic anhydrase inhibitors or osmotherapeutic agents.

Phacolytic glaucoma. Phacolytic glaucoma should be treated by prompt surgical removal of the lens material. The pressure should be controlled preoperatively with the use of carbonic anhydrase inhibitors or osmotherapeutic drugs. The iridocyclitis may be treated with atropine and topical application of steroids, but the physician should not delay surgical treatment while awaiting a temporary response to these agents. Oral glycerol or intravenous urea or mannitol should be given an hour before surgery if the pressure remains elevated.

Dislocated lens. Glaucoma from a dislocated lens may be secondary to a partial pupillary block and may respond to topical miotic or cycloplegic therapy. Peripheral iridectomy may relieve the glaucoma. Removal of the lens is sometimes necessary. Glaucoma associated with traumatic dislocation of the lens may in fact be due to angle recession (see p. 138).

True or pseudoexfoliation of the lens capsule. Treatment for true or pseudoexfoliation of the lens capsule is essentially the same as that for open-angle glaucoma. Removal of the lens does not improve the condition. Filtering procedures are the recommended surgery.

Secondary glaucoma from miscellaneous causes

Hyphema. Moderate hyphema may be treated conservatively by bed rest, sedation, and binocular bandages (Chapter 19). Carbonic anhydrase inhibitors may be used if there is an elevated tension. Massive hyphema with increased intraocular pressure becomes a surgical emergency. Removal of the free blood and clot from the anterior chamber of the eye should be accomplished without delay, either by wide incision and removal of the hyphema with balanced salt solution or by the use of fibrinolysin irrigation of the anterior chamber. Fibrinolysin is used in the concentration of 1,250 units per ml. It is injected and aspirated until the clot is dissolved and the chamber is free of blood, which usually requires 30 minutes.

Good results in the treatment of patients with large hyphemas and secondary glaucoma are often obtained by the intravenous administration of urea or mannitol or oral administration of glycerol. In addition to lowering the intraocular pressure by making the plasma hypertonic to the aqueous humor, these agents serve to promote aqueous circulation. I have been able to avoid surgery in many patients by employing these drugs. Several weeks after recovery from hyphema, patients should be examined by gonioscopy for evidence of angle recession.

Angle-recession glaucoma. Angle-recession glaucoma follows a contusion. Its onset may be months or years after the initial injury. Angle-recession glaucoma should be managed like open-angle glaucoma.

Ocular tumors. The most common causes of glaucoma with ocular tumors are ring melanomas of the ciliary body and retinoblastoma. In both instances enucleation is mandatory.

Sturge-Weber syndrome. Glaucoma secondary to the Sturge-Weber syndrome does not respond well to medical therapy. Nevertheless, a trial with miotics should be given. Peripheral iridectomy with scleral cautery has been successful in the control of the tension; other procedures such as trabeculectomy may be equally effective.

Endocrine exophthalmos (Graves' disease). Glaucoma is an occasional complication of endocrine exophthalmos. It should be treated similarly to open-angle glaucoma. Large doses of systemic corticosteroids or subconjunctival or retrobulbar corticosteroids may control the primary disease and thus relieve the glaucoma. Orbital decompression may be indicated if the glaucoma cannot be managed by medical means. Filtering procedures are seldom successful.

Harada's disease. Glaucoma secondary to Harada's disease is extremely difficult to treat either medically or surgically. Systemic administration of steroids, local application of atropine, and carbonic anhydrase inhibitors should be tried. Iridectomy or a filtering procedure may become necessary, despite the fact that these are seldom successful.

Neovascular (hemorrhagic) glaucoma. Hemorrhagic glaucoma may follow occlusions of either the central retinal vein or the central retinal artery. These vascular occlusions may be primary or secondary to such disorders as diabetes, carotid artery occlusion, arteriovenous fistulas, and temporal arteritis. Medical treatment is usually unsuccessful in the control of tension for any period of time. Surgical treatment is uniformly disappointing. The current most effective surgical procedure is cyclocryotherapy. Topical corticosteroids may relieve pain resulting from neovascular glaucoma, but they have little effect on the intraocular pressure. Recently panphotocoagulation of the peripheral retina and photocoagulation of the feeder vessels in the regions of the ciliary body and scleral spur utilizing a gonioscope have been reported to decrease neovascularization and improve the glaucoma.

Hemolytic glaucoma

Hemolytic glaucoma usually follows a vitreous hemorrhage of several days' to weeks' duration. Generally it has been accepted that the trabecular tissues become obstructed with macrophages laden with red blood cell debris that comes forward into the anterior chamber. More recently it has been suggested that the obstruction may occur with degenerated red blood cells (ghost cells) alone. Standard medical treatment, as used in open-angle glaucoma, should be tried first. If this is unsuccessful in the control of the intraocular pressure, irrigation of the hemolytic debris from the anterior chamber should be considered. Subtotal vitrectomy to remove the source of the blood has been suggested.

Malignant glaucoma

Malignant glaucoma is a type of glaucoma in which there is a forward displacement of the lens iris diaphragm. It is probably due to congestion of the ciliary body and occurs after glaucoma surgery, particularly after filtering operations. Initial medical treatment consists of wide dilatation of the pupil with cycloplegics and the administration of intravenous urea or mannitol or oral glycerol. If this treatment fails, surgery in the form of lens extraction with discission of the hyaloid face of the vitreous or posterior sclerotomy with aspiration of the vitreous or anterior vitrectomy may be necessary.

Pupillary block glaucoma

Pupillary block glaucoma after cataract surgery results from a vitreous blockage of the pupillary space and the subsequent collection of aqueous in the posterior and vitreous chambers. Cycloplegics may relieve the glaucoma. Osmotherapy, in the form of oral glycerol or intravenous urea or mannitol, is valuable adjunctive therapy. Iridectomy, transfixion of the iris, or other surgical procedures may become necessary. Photocoagulation iridectomy has been advocated.

Alpha-chymotrypsin glaucoma

Transient glaucoma may develop in eyes where alpha-chymotrypsin has been used for zonulysis during cataract extraction. The peak tension occurs within the first few postoperative days; thereafter the tension declines rapidly. Usually the glaucoma can be controlled with acetazolamide or similar drugs. However, the glaucoma subsides spontaneously.

REFERENCES

Armaly, M. F.: Glaucoma; annual review. Arch. Ophthalmol. 93:146, 1975.
Armaly, M. F., and Rao, K.: The effect of pilocarpine Ocusert on ocular pressure. In Leopold, I. H., editor: Symposium on ocular therapy, vol. 6, St. Louis, 1973, The C. V. Mosby Co.
Becker, B., Kolker, A. E., and Krupin, T.: Hyperosmotic agents. In Leopold, I. H., editor: Symposium on ocular therapy, vol. 3, St. Louis, 1968, The C. V. Mosby Co.
Becker, B., and others: Effects of diphenylhydantoin on glaucomatous field loss; a preliminary report, Trans. Am. Acad. Ophthalmol. Otolaryngol. 76:412, 1972.

Boniuk, M.: Cryotherapy in neovascular glaucoma, Trans. Am. Acad. Ophthalmol. Oto-laryngol. **78**:337(OP), 1974.

Campbell, D. G., Simmons, R. J., and Grant, W. M.: Ghost cells as a cause of glaucoma, Am. J. Ophthalmol. **81**: 441, 1976.

Chandler, P. A.: Choice of treatment in dislocation of the lens; the first E. B. Dunphy lecture, Arch. Ophthalmol. **71**:765, 1964.

Chandler, P. A., and Grant, W. M.: Lectures on glaucoma, Philadelphia, 1965, Lea & Febiger.

Cole, J. G., and Byron, H. M.: Evaluation of 100 eyes with traumatic hyphema; intravenous urea, Arch. Ophthalmol. **71**:35, 1964.

Drews, R. C.: Corticosteroid management of hemorrhagic glaucoma, Trans. Am. Acad. Oph-thalmol. Otolaryngol. **78**:334(OP), 1974.

Ellis, P. P.: Carbonic anhydrase inhibitors; pharmacologic effects and problems of long-term therapy. In Leopold, I. H., editor: Symposium on ocular therapy, vol. 4, St. Louis, 1969, The C. V. Mosby Co.

Grant, W. M., and Walton, D. S.: Progressive changes in the angle in congenital aniridia, with development of glaucoma, Am. J. Ophthalmol. **78**:842, 1974.

Halasa, A. H., and Rutkowski, P. C.: Thymoxamine therapy for angle-closure glaucoma, Arch. Ophthalmol. **90**:177, 1973.

Holland, M. G., Wei, C., and Gupta, S.: Review and evaluation of 6-hydroxydopamine (6-HD); clinical sympathectomy for the treatment of glaucoma, Ann. Ophthalmol. **5**:539, 1973.

Kass, M. A., Becker, B., and Kolker, A. E.: Glaucomocyclitic crisis and primary open-angle glaucoma, Am. J. Ophthalmol. **75**:668, 1973.

Kirsch, R. E.: Glaucoma following cataract extraction associated with the use of alpha-chymotrypsin, Arch Ophthalmol. **72**:612, 1964.

Kolker, A. E., and Hetherington, J., Jr.: Becker-Shaffer's diagnosis and therapy of the glaucomas, ed. 4, St. Louis, 1976, The C. V. Mosby Co.

Krupin, T., Kolker, A. E., and Becker, B.: A comparison of isosorbide and glycerol for cataract surgery, Am. J. Ophthalmol. **69**:737, 1970.

Krupin, T., Podos, S. M., and Becker, B.: Effect of optic nerve transection on osmotic alterations of intraocular pressure, Am. J. Ophthalmol. **70**:214, 1970.

Macoul, K. L., and Pavan-Langston, D.: Pilocarpine Ocusert system for sustained control of ocular hypertension, Arch. Ophthalmol. **93**:587, 1975.

Peczon, J. D.: Clinical evaluation of digitalization in glaucoma, Arch. Ophthalmol. **71**:500, 1964.

Phelps, C. D., and Watzke, R. C.: Hemolytic glaucoma, Am. J. Ophthalmol. **80**:690, 1975.

Quigley, H. A., Pollock, I. P., and Harbin, T. S., Jr.: Pilocarpine Ocuserts: long-term clinical trials and selected pharmacodynamics, Arch. Ophthalmol. **93**:771, 1975.

Scheie, H. G.: Filtering operations for glaucoma; a comparative study; the Albert C. Snell memorial lecture, Am. J. Ophthalmol. **53**:571, 1962.

Schwartz, A. L., and Anderson, D. R.: Trabecular surgery, Arch. Ophthalmol. **92**:134, 1974.

Spaeth, G. L.: Potassium acetazolamide and intraocular pressure, Arch. Ophthalmol. **78**:578, 1967.

Symposium on glaucoma, Transactions of the New Orleans Academy of Ophthalmology, St. Louis, 1975, The C. V. Mosby Co.

Symposium on microsurgery of the outflow channels, Trans. Am. Acad. Ophthalmol. Oto-laryngol. **76**:367, 1972.

CHAPTER 14

Therapy of intraocular infections

BACTERIAL INFECTIONS

Treatment of bacterial endophthalmitis or panophthalmitis is often disappointing because of the general destruction of the intraocular tissues resulting from severe bacterial infections. Early recognition and prompt vigorous treatment of the disorder is essential to maintain useful vision. Treatment should be directed toward elimination of the causative organisms and also toward reduction of the amount of damage that may result from the inflammatory process. Attempts should be made to identify the causative organisms, but this cannot be accomplished easily in many infections. Conjunctival cultures and smears are seldom revealing, unless there is actual drainage from the wound. Cultures obtained from the aqueous humor are often positive if special techniques of culture similar to techniques used for spinal fluid culture are employed. Recently, vitreous humor cultures have been recommended; positive results are reported to be higher than those from aqueous humor cultures. The initial choice of antibiotic is usually quite empirical and should be started before the results of culture and sensitivity tests are available.

Most intraocular bacterial infections, particularly postoperative infections, result from staphylococcic invasion; other offending gram-positive organisms include the pneumococci and streptococci. *Bacillus subtilis* and *Clostridium welchii* intraocular infections may follow penetrating wounds of the eye but are seldom, if ever, responsible for postoperative infections. If a staphylococcic infection was acquired in the hospital, the organisms are likely to be penicillin-resistant strains. With increasing frequency gram-negative organisms, including *Escherichia coli, Pseudomonas aeruginosa,* and various *Proteus* species, are responsible for bacterial endophthalmitis. Therefore, on an empirical basis, antibiotic therapy should be selected that will be effective against a wide range of organisms including both resistant staphylococci and gram-negative organisms. *Pseudomonas* organisms are generally affected by only a few antibiotics (Table 15).

The most effective drugs at present against resistant staphylococci include methicillin, oxacillin, nafcillin, the cephalosporins, lincomycin, and vancomycin. Of these, methicillin (Staphcillin) is the preferred agent for patients who are not sensitive to the penicillins. For patients sensitive to penicillins, the cephalosporins would appear to be the drugs of choice. Vancomycin and kanamycin are toxic drugs and have largely been replaced by the penicillinase-resistant

141

penicillins. However, they remain effective against occasional strains of staphylococci unaffected by the newer penicillins or the cephalosporins. Lincomycin is an effective agent against resistant staphylococci and is less toxic than vancomycin or kanamycin. Its bacterial spectrum is much narrower than that of cephalosporins.

Methicillin is less protein bound than oxacillin and is therefore more likely to cross the blood-aqueous barrier. This drug must be given by injection, since it is not stable in gastric acid. For intraocular infections intravenous doses of 2 to 3 grams every 6 hours are recommended. The drug is added to 25 to 100 ml of 5% glucose in water and administered over a period of 10 to 20 minutes. It may be added to a continuous intravenous infusion after it is mixed, but some antibiotic activity is lost if the intravenous solution is acidic. Therapy should be continued for several days. Intramuscular administration may be substituted for intravenous treatment as the infection subsides. Like oxacillin and nafcillin, methicillin is less effective against other gram-positive organisms such as the streptococci and pneumococci than is penicillin G, but with the recommended doses blood levels are obtained that are also effective against these organisms. Therefore it is unnecessary to use both semisynthetic penicillins and penicillin G.

Ampicillin is a semisynthetic penicillin that is effective against both gram-positive and some gram-negative organisms. However, it is not effective against resistant staphylococci. It is administered orally, intramuscularly, or intravenously, in doses of 1,000 to 2,000 mg every 6 hours. For treatment of bacterial endophthalmitis, intravenous therapy is the preferred route of drug administration. Methicillin may be given in combination with ampicillin to provide therapy against resistant staphylococci.

Cephalothin (Keflin) is a semisynthetic antibiotic that is effective against a broad spectrum of organisms including resistant staphylococci, streptococci, pneumococci, many coliform organisms, and some strains of *Proteus*. However, like other cephalosporins, it is ineffective against *Pseudomonas* organisms. It is usually given in a dose of 1 to 2 grams every 4 to 6 hours either intramuscularly or intravenously, but doses of 10 to 12 grams a day may be used. This agent would appear to be valuable for the initial treatment of bacterial endophthalmitis, particularly in patients sensitive to penicillin. Cephaloridine (Loridine) is another cephalosporin that has the same antibacterial spectrum as that of cephalothin. The dosage is 1 gram every 6 hours either intravenously or intramuscularly. Doses over 4 grams a day should not be employed because of possible renal tubular damage. The agent has low plasma protein binding and penetrates the eye in good concentrations. It is well tolerated when administered subconjunctivally. Cefazolin (Ancef, Kefzol) has to a large degree replaced cephaloridine for systemic administration because of less renal toxicity. The medication is given intravenously or intramuscularly in a dosage of 1 gram every 6 hours. Cephalexin (Keflex) is an orally administered cephalosporin. The dosage is 500 to 1,000 mg every 6 hours. Other oral cephalosporins are cephradine

Table 14. Systemic antibiotics recommended for treatment of bacterial endophthalmitis* †

Antibiotic	Adult dosage
Effective against gram-positive and some gram-negative organisms‡	
Carbenicillin (Geopen, Pyopen)	2 to 4 grams q4h
Cefazolin (Ancef, Kefzol)	1 gram IV or IM q6 to 8h
Cephalothin (Keflin)	2 grams IV or IM q6h
Cephaloridine (Loridine)	1 gram IV or IM q6h
Cephalexin (Keflex)	500 to 1,000 mg orally q6h
Cephapirin (Cefadyl)	500 to 1,000 mg orally q6h
Cephradine (Anspor, Velosef)	500 to 1,000 mg orally q6h
Chloramphenicol (Chloromycetin, Mychel, Amphicol)	1 gram IV q8h or 2 grams initial dose orally or IM; then 1,000 mg q8h
Penicillin G with streptomycin or gentamicin	Penicillin: 12 to 16 million units IV over 16- to 20-hour period
	Streptomycin: 1 gram IM q8h
	Gentamicin: 3 to 5 mg/kg/day in 3 divided doses IM or IV
Ampicillin (Polycillin, Penbritin, Amcill, Omnipen, Principen)	1 to 2 grams orally, IV, or IM q6h
Kanamycin (Kantrex)	1 gram initially IM; then 0.5 gram q 8h IM or 1 gram q12h
Tetracyclines	1 gram initial dose orally; then 500 mg q6 to 8h
Sulfadiazine, sulfamerazine, or mixed sulfonamides	2 grams initial dose orally; then 1 gram q6h
Effective against gram-positive organisms (particularly penicillin G–resistant staphylococci)	
Semisynthetic penicillins	
Methicillin (Staphcillin)	2 grams q4 to 6h IV
Nafcillin (Unipen)	1 gram q4 to 6h IV, IM, or orally
Oxacillin (Prostaphlin)	1 gram q4 to 6h IV, IM, or orally
Dicloxacillin (Dynapen, Pathocil, Veracillin)	1 gram q4 to 6h orally
Cefazolin (Ancef, Kefzol)	Same as above
Cephaloridine (Loridine)	Same as above
Cephalothin (Keflin)	Same as above
Cephalexin (Keflex)	Same as above
Cephapirin (Cefadyl)	Same as above
Cephradine (Anspor, Velosef)	Same as above
Erythromycin estolate (Ilosone)	500 mg q6h orally
Erythromycin (Erythrocin) stearate	500 mg q6h orally
Erythromycin ethyl succinate	100 mg IM qid
Erythromycin lactobionate	1 to 4 grams IV daily
Kanamycin (Kantrex)	Same as above
Lincomycin (Lincocin)	500 mg q6h
Vancomycin (Vancocin)	1 gram q6 to 8h IV for 48 hours; then 1 gram q12h
Triacetyloleandomycin (Cyclamycin, TAO)	500 mg q6h
Novobiocin (Albamycin, Cathomycin)	500 mg q6h

*Adapted from Leopold, I. H.: Problems in the use of antibiotics in ophthalmology. In Leopold, I. H., editor: Symposium on ocular therapy, vol. 5, St. Louis, 1972, The C. V. Mosby Co.
†The dosages may be reduced after several days of treatment according to the patient response.
‡Considerable variation exists in the susceptibility of gram-negative organisms to these drugs.

(Anspor, Velosef) and cephapirin (Cefadyl); the dosage for each is 500 to 1,000 mg every 6 hours.

Gentamicin is effective against most staphylococci and most gram-negative organisms, including *Pseudomonas*. It is ineffective against pneumococci and streptococci. It is frequently employed in combination with the penicillins and is administered intramuscularly or intravenously in a dose of 3 to 5 mg per kg of body weight per day in three divided doses.

Chloramphenicol (Chloromycetin) has fairly good penetration into the intraocular tissues and may be used concurrently with the penicillins. However, the use of systemic chloramphenicol has largely been abandoned because of the serious blood dyscrasias that may be associated with its use. Chloramphenicol may be given either orally or intravenously, but better concentrations can be reached by intravenous administration. Doses of 1 gram are given every 6 to 8 hours intravenously over a relatively short period of time, since better concentrations are obtained by intermittent therapy than by continuous intravenous drip. If the drug is given orally, the initial priming dose is 2 to 3 grams, followed by additional doses of 0.5 gram every 6 hours or 1 gram every 8 hours. When chloramphenicol therapy is used for an extended period of time, blood platelet and white cell counts must be followed to guard against the possibility of aplastic anemia or pancytopenia. Even so, one cannot be completely assured that these blood dyscrasias will not develop, since toxic idiosyncratic reactions to chloramphenicol occur even after one or two doses. These reactions are most common in children, and in these patients, chloramphenicol therapy should be avoided.

The author's preference for initial treatment of bacterial endophthalmitis is the use of both intravenous methicillin and gentamicin. In children, ampicillin plus gentamicin is recommended. In patients sensitive to penicillin, cephalothin is substituted for methicillin.

The response of the patient is often used as a guide to the adequacy of the therapy. If no improvement in the intraocular infection is observed within 48 to 72 hours, alterations in antibiotic therapy should be considered. A complete list of the antibiotics used in the systemic treatment of intraocular bacterial infections and adult dosage schedules are included in Table 14. Agents effective against *Pseudomonas* are shown in Table 15. The intraocular penetration of systemic antibiotics is given in Table 16. Sensitivity of common pathogens to chemotherapeutic agents is presented in Chapter 3.

In addition to the systemic antibiotic therapy, subconjunctival injection should be employed, particularly if the infection is in the anterior part of the globe. The agents used and their dosage are listed in Table 17.

Intravitreal injections of antibiotics have been advocated again recently for the treatment of bacterial endophthalmitis. The medication is injected after aspiration of 0.1 to 0.2 ml of aqueous humor and of vitreous humor if culture material is obtained from the vitreous. The medication is injected in a 0.1- to 0.2-ml volume with a 25-gauge needle (a 22-gauge needle is required for vitreous

Table 15. Antibiotics for *Pseudomonas* infections*

| Agent | Systemic | Dosage | |
		Subconjunctival	Topical
Colistin (Coly-Mycin)	1.5 to 5 mg/kg daily IM in 2 to 4 divided doses	20 mg	1.5 to 3 mg/ml
Polymyxin B (Aerosporin)	1.5 to 2.5 mg/kg daily IV as single dose or divided into 2 doses	10 mg	10,000 to 25,000 units/ml
Gentamicin (Garamycin)	3 to 5 mg/kg/day in 3 divided doses IM or IV	10 to 30 mg	3 to 10 mg/ml
Carbenicillin (Geopen, Pyopen)	25 to 35 grams daily IV	100 mg	
Tobramycin (Nebcin)	3 to 5 mg/kg/day in 3 to 4 divided doses IM or IV	2.5 mg†	1 to 10 mg/ml†

*The susceptibility of *Pseudomonas* to antibiotics is highly variable among different strains of organisms. Certain strains are susceptible to neomycin, streptomycin, or chloramphenicol. See Schneirson, S. S.: Antibiotic susceptibility of pathogenic microorganisms isolated in 1966, N.Y. J. Med. **67:**2027, 1967.
†Exact human dosage schedule is not established.

Table 16. Intraocular penetration of systemically administered antibiotics

Good	Fair*	Poor
Ampicillin	Penicillin G	Streptomycin
Chloramphenicol	Methicillin	Chlortetracycline
Cephaloridine	Kanamycin	Oxytetracycline
Dicloxacillin	Vancomycin	
	Gentamicin	
	Colistin	
	Polymyxin B	
	Amphotericin B	
	Erythromycin	
	Tetracycline	
	Lincomycin	
	Cephalothin	
	Oxacillin	

*Penetrate into inflamed eyes in therapeutic concentrations against many organisms.

aspiration) through the pars plana in phakic eyes and often through the corneal limbus and pupillary space in aphakic eyes. The medication is injected into the central portion of the vitreous. Therapeutic levels of antibiotics persist in the vitreous cavity for up to 72 to 96 hours after a single injection. The agents used and their dosages are listed in Table 18.

Intracameral (anterior chamber) injections of antibiotics do not offer significant advantages over subconjunctival injections of antibiotics. With both techniques, therapeutic levels of antibiotics are reached in the aqueous humor but persist for only a few hours. Some ophthalmologists inject antibiotics into the anterior chamber after performing aqueous humor taps for cultures. The

Table 17. Dosage of antibiotics in subconjunctival therapy

Antibiotic	Dosage
Amphotericin B	1 to 3 mg
Ampicillin	50 to 100 mg
Bacitracin	10,000 units
Carbenicillin	100 mg
Cephaloridine	50 to 100 mg
Cephalothin	50 to 100 mg
Chloramphenicol (sodium succinate)	40 to 50 mg
Colistin (Coly-Mycin)	15 to 20 mg
Erythromycin	10 to 20 mg
Gentamicin	10 to 30 mg
Kanamycin	10 to 30 mg
Lincomycin	75 mg
Methicillin	50 to 100 mg
Neomycin	100 to 500 mg
Nystatin	10,000 units
Oxacillin	50 to 100 mg
Penicillin G	500,000 units
Polymyxin B	5 to 10 mg
Streptomycin	40 to 50 mg
Tetracyclines	2.5 to 5 mg
Vancomycin	15 to 25 mg

Table 18. Dosage of antibiotics for intravitreal injections*

Antibiotic	Dosage
Ampicillin	500μg
Amphotericin B	4μg to 5μg
Cephaloridine	250μg
Gentamicin	100μg to 300μg
Lincomycin	200μg

*Administered in 0.1 to 0.2 ml volume.

Table 19. Solutions for intracameral (anterior chamber) injection or irrigation*

Antibiotic	Concentration (per ml)
Amphotericin B	500μg
Bacitracin	500 to 1,000 units
Carbomycin	1 to 2 mg
Chloramphenicol	1 to 2 mg
Erythromycin	1 to 2 mg
Methicillin	1 mg
Neomycin	2.5 mg
Penicillin	1,000 to 4,000 units
Polymyxin B	0.1 mg
Streptomycin	0.5 to 5 mg
Tetracyclines	2.5 to 5 mg

*Adapted from Leopold, I. H.: Problems in the use of antibiotics in ophthalmology. In Leopold, I. H., editor: Symposium on ocular therapy, vol. 5, St. Louis, 1972, The C. V. Mosby Co.

drugs used for anterior chamber injections and their dosages are listed in Table 19.

Steroids may be administered systemically along with antibiotics. The rationale for this approach to therapy is that the combination reduces the massive inflammatory response of the eye, which is, in itself, often as destructive as the infection. It is quite possible that there may be danger of spread if the causative organism is not susceptible to the antibiotics employed, but in such a case the eye would inevitably be lost. In my opinion the combined use of antibiotics and corticosteroids is the treatment of choice. However, a recent study has indicated that antibiotic therapy without steroids is as effective, if not more so, for the treatment of bacterial endophthalmitis.

Cycloplegics should also be employed, since synechiae are formed during the inflammatory process. If secondary glaucoma occurs, it can usually be treated satisfactorily with oral administration of acetazolamide or other carbonic anhydrase inhibitors.

Occasionally the oral application of glycerol or intravenous administration of urea or mannitol may be necessary. Before these agents were available it was the practice to perform paracentesis of the anterior chamber on these eyes, and it is still sometimes necessary to resort to this treatment. If paracentesis is performed, an attempt should be made to culture the fluid, although the cultures are often negative, as mentioned previously.

MYCOTIC INTRAOCULAR INFECTIONS

The diagnosis of postoperative or posttraumatic fungal endophthalmitis is usually made by exclusion, after an infection has failed to respond to antibiotics. The diagnosis is also made by the fact that such infections characteristically develop late, after a history of trauma or surgery. Attempts should be made to determine the exact fungus responsible for the infection. If this can be cultured, sensitivity tests to the various antifungal agents should be obtained.

Endogenous *Candida* endophthalmitis characteristically occurs in patients who are seriously ill, frequently have alimentary tract disease, are receiving large doses of antibiotics, and have a *Candida* septicemia. The vitreous contains inflammatory cells and white-gray balls of inflammatory debris. Intraretinal yellow-white exudative inflammatory lesions may be observed.

A most effective agent for the treatment of fungal endophthalmitis is amphotericin B; combined subconjunctival and systemic administration is recommended. Subconjunctival injections in doses of 1 to 2 mg may be used. For systemic administration the drug is given intravenously in an initial dose of 0.05 to 0.1 mg per kg of body weight, dissolved in 5% dextrose in water, in an intravenous drip over a period of 3 to 6 hours. Subsequently, the drug is administered on consecutive or alternate days with an increased dose of 0.1 mg per kg of body weight, and this increase is repeated each day or every other day until the dose of 1 mg per kg of body weight is reached. The medication should be continued at that level until there is a response or until there are signs of toxicity, as evidenced by a BUN level increase or other signs of renal toxicity. Alternate-day therapy is less toxic than daily therapy, but daily therapy may be necessary to control the infection. The total dosage should be kept below 2 grams, since toxic effects increase significantly after this dosage. The penetration of amphotericin B into the eye is still in some doubt. However, it is quite likely that in the inflamed eye the drug does get across the blood-aqueous barrier. Amphotericin B, $25\mu g$ to $40\mu g$, has been injected into the anterior chamber of the eye after paracentesis with beneficial effects. Intravitreal injections of $5\mu g$ of amphotericin B have been recommended for the treatment of fungal endophthalmitis.

Flucytosine (Ancobon) is a drug that is effective against some strains of *Candida* species, *Cryptococcus neoformans*, *Torulopsis glabrata*, and some *Aspergillus* species. The drug is converted by susceptible fungi to fluorouracil, which interferes with the nucleic acid synthesis. It is given orally in a daily dose of 50 to 200 mg per kg of body weight. This agent has been effective in the treatment of *Candida* endophthalmitis. Sometimes it is given following a course of intravenous amphotericin B therapy. Rifampin also has been established as effective against *Candida* and has been used in conjunction with amphotericin B. Rifampin is given orally in a dose of 15 mg per kg of body weight per day.

Nystatin (Mycostatin) is an effective antifungal drug. It is poorly absorbed after oral administration, and therefore this mode of treatment is valueless for mycotic intraocular infections. Subconjunctival injections of nystatin, 10,000 units per ml, may be given. Doses of 200 units in 0.1 ml of physiological saline solution have been injected successfully into the anterior chamber of experimental animals.

REFERENCES

Allansmith, M. R., Skaggs, C., and Kimura, S. J.: Anterior chamber paracentesis; diagnostic value in postoperative endophthalmitis, Arch. Ophthalmol. 84:745, 1970.

Allen, H. F., and Mangiaracine, A. B.: Bacterial endophthalmitis after cataract extraction. II. Incidence in 36,000 consecutive operations with special reference to preoperative topical antibiotics, Arch. Ophthalmol. 91:3, 1974.

Baum, J. L., and Rao, G.: Treatment of postcataract bacterial endophthalmitis with periocular and systemic antibiotics and corticosteroids, Trans. Am. Acad. Ophthalmol. Otolaryngol. 81:151(OP), 1976.

Ellis, P. P.: Postoperative endophthalmitis. In Symposium on ocular pharmacology and therapeutics, Transactions of the New Orleans Academy of Ophthalmology, St. Louis, 1970, The C. V. Mosby Co.

Forster, R. K., Zachary, I. G., Cottingham, A. J., and Norton, E. W. D.: Further observations on the diagnosis, cause, and treatment of endophthalmitis, Am. J. Ophthalmol. 81: 52, 1976.

Freeman, M. E., and Gay, A. J.: Systemic steroid therapy in postcataract endophthalmitis. In Becker, B., and Drews, R. C.: Current concepts in ophthalmology, vol. 1, St. Louis, 1967, The C. V. Mosby Co.

Kanski, J. J.: The treatment of late endophthalmitis associated with filtering blebs, Arch. Ophthalmol. **91**:339, 1974.

Leopold, I. H.: Problems in the use of antibiotics in ophthalmology. In Leopold, I. H., editor: Symposium on ocular therapy, vol. 5, St. Louis, 1972, The C. V. Mosby Co.

Leopold, I. H., and Apt, L.: Postoperative intraocular infections, Am. J. Ophthalmol. **50**:1225, 1960.

Lieberman, T. W.: Systemic antifungal chemotherapy in the treatment of intraocular fungal infections. In Leopold, I. H., editor: Symposium on ocular therapy, vol. 6, St. Louis, 1973, The C. V. Mosby Co.

Lou, P., Kazdan, J., Bannatyne, R. M., and Cheung, R.: Successful treatment of *Candida* endophthalmitis with a synergistic combination of amphotericin B and rifampin, Am. J. Ophthalmol. **83**:12, 1977.

Peyman, G. A., Vastine, D. W., Crouch, E. R., and Herbst, R. W.: Clinical use of intra-vitreal antibiotics to treat bacterial endophthalmitis, Trans. Am. Acad. Ophthalmol. Otolaryngol. **78**:862, 1974.

Records, R. E.: The cephalosporins in ophthalmology, Surv. Ophthalmol. **13**:345, 1969.

Records, R. E.: The penicillins in opthalmology, Surv. Ophthalmol. **13**:207, 1969.

Robertson, D. M., Riley, F. C., and Hermans, P. E.: Endogenous *Candida* oculomycosis, Arch. Ophthalmol. **91**:33, 1974.

Sonne, M., and Jawetz, E.: Combined action of carbenicillin and gentamicin on *Pseudomonas aeruginosa* in vitro, Appl. Microbiol. **17**:893, 1969.

Stern, G. A., Fetkenhour, C. L., and O'Grady, R. B.: Intravitreal amphotericin B treatment of *Candida* endophthalmitis, Arch. Ophthalmol. **95**:89, 1977.

CHAPTER 15

Therapy of diseases of the retina

VASCULAR DISEASES
Occlusion of central retinal artery

Most branch retinal artery occlusions are due to emboli. Central retinal artery obstructions are also usually due to emboli, but they may be thrombotic in nature and associated with atheroma and/or hemorrhages below the atheroma. Occlusion of the central retinal artery often occurs in patients with hypertension and arteriosclerosis. Other associated diseases include temporal arteritis, polyarteritis, orbital granuloma, hypercholesterolemia, and syphilis. The usual source of the emboli is the internal cartoid artery; occasionally the heart is the source.

The survival time of the anoxic retina is 1 to 2 hours. After total occlusion of the central retinal artery, changes in electrical activity occur within 2 to 3½ hours. By the time the diagnosis of occlusion of the retinal artery has been made, very often little can be done to restore the integrity of the retina. However, if the condition is diagnosed early, occasionally prompt treatment may restore some useful vision.

Occlusion of retinal vein

Retinal vein occlusions are often associated with retinal artery disease. Capillary obstructive disease may extend to the veins. The mechanisms and associated diseases responsible for venous obstruction include pressure on the vein by the arterial wall (in patients with hypertension, arteriosclerosis, and endarteritis), primary venous thrombosis, glaucoma, inflammatory disorders (uveitis, collagen vascular disturbance, and phlebitis), sickle cell disease, dysproteinemias, polycythemia, leukemia, trauma, and oral contraceptives.

An important factor in the development of thrombus is endothelial injury of the vascular wall. Following such injury there may be release of adenosine diphosphate (ADP), which attracts negatively charged platelets that form aggregates. There is subsequent entrapment of fibrinogen and erythrocytes and conversion of fibrinogen to fibrin. Other important factors in the development of thrombus include blood sludging, dehydration, and abnormal factors of coagulation.

Possible approaches to therapy

Measures to permit emboli to move peripherally. Tapping on the globe or massaging the globe may result in peripheral movement of an embolus. Vasodilatation may also accomplish this effect. The most effective method of producing retinal vasodilatation is the inhalation of 5% or 10% carbon dioxide with oxygen. Other smooth muscle relaxants such as the nitrites or papaverine are usually ineffective. In the past nitroglycerin tablets, 0.3 to 0.6 mg, have been given sublingually, or amyl nitrite has been administered by inhalation. Tolazoline (Priscoline) or aminophylline, 25 mg in 1 ml, has also been injected retrobulbarly.

Another method for moving emboli more peripherally is lowering intraocular pressure. The most effective method for rapidly accomplishing this is to perform a paracentesis of the anterior chamber. The use of retrobulbar anesthetic injections combined with massage also produces lowered intraocular pressure very rapidly. Intravenous administration of acetazolamide (Diamox) or osmotherapeutic agents lower intraocular pressure within 30 minutes to an hour.

Lysis of clot

Thrombolytic therapy. Lysis of clots may be accomplished with thrombolytic therapy with a plasminogen activator, such as urokinase or streptokinase. Urokinase, an enzymatic thrombolytic agent extracted from human urine and successfully used in the treatment of pulmonary embolus, has been administered for the treatment of fresh occlusions of the central retinal artery and vein. Urokinase activates the proenzyme (plasminogen) of plasma. With proper dosage the intense proteolytic activity of plasmin and subsequent degradation of proteins and clotting factors can be avoided. Urokinase is administered in a dosage of 3,300 CTA units per kg of body weight per hour. Treatment is continued over 12 to 24 hours, depending on patient response. Hemorrhages at a local level may occur. Urokinase is not presently available for treatment of ocular vascular disorders. Streptokinase is pyrogenic and highly antigenic; it is seldom used today.

Fibrinolysin therapy. Fibrinolysin therapy may be tried with the hope of dissolving the fresh intravenous clot. Treatment is more likely to be successful if started within 5 hours after a thrombotic accident since the effect of the drug is questionable once the clot is organized. Fibrinolysin is not an anticoagulant and should not be expected to prevent further thrombus formation. It becomes inactive at room temperature and therefore must be given as a freshly prepared intravenous infusion. Generally an intravenous infusion of 100,000 units of fibrinolysin dissolved in 250 ml of 5% dextrose in water is given over a 1-hour period, and this dosage is repeated for 3 to 6 hours; a freshly prepared solution is used for each infusion.

Reduction of sludging and coagulation. Low molecular weight dextran (molecular weight 40,000) reduces sludging and coagulation by several methods. It is a plasma volume expander. It appears to decrease platelet and erythrocyte adhesiveness and seems to coat the endothelial wall. Blood viscosity and platelet deposition and aggregation are decreased. The usual dose is 500 ml of a 10% solution given intravenously; it may be repeated in 12 hours. Some hemorrhagic diathesis may occur with the use of this drug. Dextran appears to have antigenic properties, and anaphylactic reactions have been reported with its use.

Anticoagulant agents

HEPARIN. Heparin may be given intravenously or by deep subcutaneous injection. Intermittent intravenous therapy is the technique usually employed; the drug is administered as a single bolus. The drug also may be injected into the tubing of an intravenous infusion or added to the intravenous solution and given in a continuous infusion. Heparinization is initiated with doses of 75 to 100 mg (7,500 to 10,000 units; 1 USP unit equals 0.01 mg of heparin). After initial intravenous injection, clotting time should be checked at the end of 1 hour to determine the extent of the anticoagulant effect and again at the end of 4 hours to determine the duration of effect and the necessary subsequent dosage. The dose is adjusted to maintain a clotting time in the range of 25 to 35 minutes when measured before the next dose (normal range, 6 to 12 minutes). The average dose for intermittent intravenous therapy is 50 mg every 4 to 6 hours. Clotting time should be checked twice daily, 3 to 4 hours after injection. For continuous intravenous therapy, 100 mg of heparin is added to 1,000 ml of physiological saline solution, and the drug is given at the rate of 25 drops per minute. The clotting time is determined after the infusion has been running for 2 hours. For deep subcutaneous use the dose is 100 to 125 mg every 12 hours, with adjustments to maintain the clotting time within the range of 20 to 30 minutes. Clotting time with this method of administration is measured immediately before the next dose.

Heparin causes a rather rapid anticoagulant effect, but the coumarin drugs do not act for 12 to 96 hours. Therefore, heparin and hypoprothrombinemic drugs are often started together, the heparin being discontinued after 24 to 48 hours and the patient maintained on the hypoprothrombinemic drugs only. The prothrombin time should not be measured when the clotting time is markedly prolonged by heparin, because the prothrombin time may be abnormally prolonged because of heparin's effect rather than the true effect of the coumarin drug.

If complications result from heparin therapy, protamine sulfate (50 mg of 1% solution) should be given slowly by the intravenous route. A second injection may be necessary if indicated by the levels of the clotting time. Blood transfusions are sometimes needed to overcome heparin toxicity. If mild bleeding occurs as a result of the hypoprothrombinemic agents, the drugs should be stopped and the prothrombin levels allowed to compensate themselves. If more severe bleeding occurs, vitamin K_1 (phytonadione), 10 to 15 mg, should be given intravenously. Subsequently, oral administration of vitamin K_1, 2.5- to 10-mg tablets, is advisable until the prothrombin levels are satisfactory.

ORAL ANTICOAGULANTS. The dosage of bishydroxycoumarin (Dicumarol) is usually 300 mg the first day, 200 mg the second day, and 50 to 75 mg daily thereafter, depending on the prothrombin activity. In older people the initial dose should be 200 mg. If warfarin sodium (Coumadin) is used instead of bishydroxycoumarin, the initial dose is 25 to 35 mg, followed by 5 to 10 mg orally for the next 2 or 3 days, adjusted to maintain the desired prothrombin levels. For older individuals the initial dose is 20 to 25 mg. Many clinicians believe it is desirable to administer oral anticoagulants by initiating therapy with maintenance doses rather than using a priming dose since antithrombotic effects are largely dependent on blood clotting factors other than prothrombin; such effects are not achieved for several days. Suppression of these factors can be accomplished by maintenance doses as readily as and more safely than with the use of priming doses. With this approach to therapy, daily doses of 50 to 75 mg of bishydroxycoumarin or 10 to 15 mg of warfarin sodium are prescribed.

Prothrombin levels should be determined before treatment with either bishydroxycoumarin or warfarin sodium is begun. (Prothrombin levels are still used to monitor dosage schedule.) It is usually desirable to change the prothrombin time to 20 to 25 seconds when the normal is about 12 seconds. If the prothrombin levels are given in terms of percentage of normal, values of 20% to 25% of normal prothrombin activity are desirable. Several other coumarin preparations available as anticoagulants are used less frequently than bishydroxycoumarin and warfarin sodium. It should be pointed out that many drugs may interact to potentiate or retard the effect of the antiprothrombin drugs such as warfarin sodium (Table 20).

Table 20. Warfarin sodium–affecting drugs*

Drugs that may potentiate the effect	Drugs that may retard the effect
Phenylbutazone	Barbiturates
Salicylates	Meprobamate
Indomethacin (Indocin)	Glutethimide (Doriden)
Acetaminophen	Ethchlorvynol (Placidyl)
Clofibrate	Griseofulvin
Bowel-sterilizing antibiotics	Estrogens
Chloramphenicol	Adrenocorticosteroids
Sulfonamides	Oral contraceptives
Quinidine sulfate	Diuretics
D-Thyroxine	Vitamin C
Anabolic steroids	
Phenytoin (Dilantin)	
Tolbutamide	
Cinchophen	
6-Mercaptopurine	
Monamine oxidase inhibitors	
Methylphenidate (Ritalin)	

*Adapted from Eipe, J.: Med. Clin. North Am. **56:**255, 1972.

Anticoagulants should not be given to patients who have evidence of other bleeding, since they may produce bleeding tendencies. If mild bleeding occurs, the drug should be stopped and the prothrombin activity allowed to compensate without specific therapy. If the bleeding is severe or if it involves a vital vascular bed, the drug should be stopped promptly, and vitamin K_1 should be administered intravenously in doses of 10 to 15 mg. With such medication, prothrombin levels can usually be improved within 4 to 12 hours. The use of vitamin K_1 orally in doses of 2.5 to 10 mg usually improves the prothrombin levels within 12 hours.

Platelet inhibitors. It is now believed that vascular retinopathies associated with some systemic diseases may be on the basis of arteriolar thrombosis in which platelets play a major role. In vivo platelet depression may occur with aspirin, clofibrate, guaifenesin, dipyridamole, and sulfinpyrazone (Anturan). The value of aspirin in preventing venous thrombosis is not established. Unfortunately there is no satisfactory laboratory method for evaluating the effectiveness of platelet inhibitors. Platelet counts themselves are unsatisfactory, and tests to measure platelet adhesiveness are not usually of any value. Furthermore, the value of therapy in clinical situations cannot be correlated with these laboratory tests to measure platelet adhesiveness. Therefore, therapy is given in an empirical manner, although patients should be observed for any tendency to develop hemorrhagic or bleeding phenomena.

Management of general medical problems and contributing ocular problems. As described earlier, many systemic disorders can be associated with retinal vascular disease. The patient should have a thorough general physical workup and appropriate laboratory tests to rule out blood dyscrasias, hypertension, and diabetes. Erythrocyte sedimentation rates should be obtained to rule out the possibility of an arteritis. It is important to determine whether the patient is taking any medication that may be contributing to alterations of the blood-clotting mechanisms. The patient should be checked for glaucoma since it is often a responsible factor in the development of retinal vascular occlusions.

Prevention of further occlusions. Treatment of any basic underlying disease should be undertaken. It should be appreciated that a sudden lowering of blood pressure in a narrowed artery may in itself precipitate a vascular occlusion. The long-term use of anticoagulants and platelet inhibitors should be discussed with the patient's internist.

Specific plan of treatment

Arterial occlusions. In acute retinal arterial occlusions it is worthwhile to admit the patient to the hospital. Before this, massage and paracentesis may be performed and osmotherapy given before the patient is sent to the hospital. Carbon dioxide, 5% or 10%, with oxygen inhalation therapy for 5 or 10 minutes every hour for 12 to 24 hours may be tried. Heparin therapy may be given unless the patient's general health contraindicates this. A careful search for systemic disease should be undertaken and appropriate therapy instituted. Particularly in older patients, tests should be obtained for evidence of temporal arteritis, and the patient should begin corticosteroid therapy if the results are positive.

In long-standing retinal arterial occlusions there is little point in admitting the patient to the hospital or in attempting vasodilatation or anticoagulant therapy. Nonetheless, the patient should receive a complete workup for evidence of systemic disease.

Vein occlusions. In fresh vein occlusions it is advisable to admit the patient to the hospital. The ophthalmologist should work closely with the internist, advising the internist of the possibilities of contributing systemic disease. A careful check should be instituted for systemic disease, and the patient should be given tests for glaucoma, including a diurnal ocular pressure check. If any disorders are found, appropriate treatment should be instituted. Anticoagulants appear to be of little value in branch occlusions but may be of some value in central vein occlusions, particularly in stagnation thrombosis and incomplete central vein occlusion. Low molecular weight dextran therapy may be worth trying, particularly if the patient's only remaining eye is involved. Platelet suppression therapy should be considered if the patient has associated capillary disease such as diabetes. Systemic administration of steroids should be instituted if the patient has some evidence of vasculitis. In younger patients a trial of corticosteroids may be employed empirically if it is thought that the thrombosis may be secondary to an acute inflammatory process. Since steroids shorten the venous clotting time, anticoagulants should be used concurrently.

Long-term therapy may require the use of photocoagulation for treatment of neovascularization with hemorrhage and for treatment of macular edema. Fluorescein angiograms should be obtained to monitor patients who have suffered retinal vascular occlusive disease.

Hayreh recently has divided central retinal vein occlusions into two categories: (1) a venous stasis type, which represents a total vein occlusion without ischemia, and (2) a hemorrhagic type, which represents total vein occlusion plus ischemia. The venous stasis type is comparatively benign and usually clears, although cystic macular edema may occur. The hemorrhagic type progresses despite any therapy, and all vision is usually lost. These observations, which need to be confirmed, suggest that anticoagulant or other medical treatment is of no real value in central retinal vein occlusions.

CENTRAL SEROUS CHOROIDOPATHY (CENTRAL SEROUS RETINOPATHY)

The etiology of central serous choroidopathy is rather obscure. Fluid accumulates beneath the retinal pigment epithelium or, as a result of breaks in the pigment epithelium, between this layer and the retinal neuroepithelium. It is frequently seen in emotionally labile, high-strung individuals, and presumably it results from vasomotor instability. Improvement usually occurs spontaneously over a period of several months, but relapses are common. Treatment is non-specific. Measures should be taken to improve the patient's mode of life, such as removal of stress situations. The use of vasodilators is not effective. During the very acute stages, the systemic administration of corticosteroids may reduce subretinal transudation, but the real value of corticosteroids is equivocal. Patients with central serous choroidopathy should have fluorescein angiograms; such studies usually show fluorescein leakage through the pigment epithelium. Most authorities now recommend argon laser photocoagulation therapy if spontaneous improvement does not occur within a few months and if the site of leakage is sufficiently far away from the fovea (outside the capillary-free zone) that treatment will not destroy central vision.

Vascular retinopathies associated with systemic diseases

In general, the improvement of the underlying disorders is the only therapy indicated for vascular retinopathies associated with systemic diseases.

Most of the changes of hypertensive retinopathy are reversible with reduction of the hypertension, and therefore the ophthalmologist should refer the patient to his attending physician for treatment of the basic disorder. The actual value of antihypertensive therapy on the basic mechanisms involved in the disease is highly questionable, and evaluation of drugs used in the treatment of hypertension is beyond the scope of this book.

Retinopathies associated with blood dyscrasias improve rapidly if and when the basic blood disorder improves. No local therapy is of value. Patients with sickling disorders, particularly sickle cell–hemoglobin C disease (SC disease) and sickle cell thalassemia (S thal), often develop retinal neovascularization, which may lead to vitreous hemorrhages and retinal detachment. Photocoagulation therapy of the retinal neovascular areas has been successfully employed.

It is now believed by some that vascular retinopathies might be on the basis of arteriolar thrombosis in which platelets play a major role. In the laboratory, many drugs, including local anesthetics, antihistamines, and analgesics have been found to affect platelet reactivity. In vivo platelet depression may occur with aspirin, clofibrate, guaifenesin, dipyridamole, and sulfinpyrazone. The value of aspirin in preventing venous thrombosis is not established.

Diabetic retinopathy appears to be related more to the duration of the disease than to its severity or control. These retinopathies are most complicated, since severe retinopathy may develop despite apparently good control of the diabetes. Optimum control of the diabetes is obviously the first consideration. Additional measures, such as the use of low-fat diets and anticholesterol agents to reduce the blood cholesterol level and alter the serum lipoprotein levels, the use of vitamin B_{12} to increase nucleotide synthesis and thus possibly local cell function, and the use of testosterone, have been tried without success. Anabolic steroids, nandrolone phenpropionate (Durabolin) and methandrostenolone (Dianabol), have been reported to be beneficial in diabetic retinopathy.

These steroids, which are androgens, induce positive nitrogen balance and are used to stimulate protein synthesis. However, it is doubtful that anabolic steroids are of any real benefit in diabetic retinopathy. Recently, clofibrate (Atromid-S), an inhibitor of cholesterol production, has been reported to be of value in the exudative form of diabetic retinopathy when employed in a dose of 250 mg three times a day. The value of this therapy, however, is equivocal.

Surgical adrenalectomy and hypophysectomy or pituitary stalk section and destruction of the pituitary gland with yttrium or betatron radiation or cryotherapy have been used in the treatment of diabetic retinopathy. Claims are made that progression of diabetic retinopathy is prevented, and in some cases retinal vasculopathy is improved with these modes of treatment. There are many problems with this type of therapy, and final evaluation of its therapeutic value is yet to be made.

In recent years photocoagulation, principally argon laser therapy, has been employed in the treatment of diabetic retinopathy. There is some disagreement regarding its value and the indications for its use. Some investigators restrict photocoagulation therapy to the treatment of macular edema and neovascular lesions, whereas others believe advanced background retinopathy should be treated. In a recent study the Diabetic Retinopathy Study Research Group reported that extensive scatter photocoagulation and focal treatment of new vessels are of benefit in the prevention of visual loss in eyes with proliferative retinopathy.

DEGENERATIVE DISEASES
Macular degenerative diseases

Degenerations of the macula are probably secondary to vascular changes. The basic process may be due to alterations in the permeability of the retinal capillaries or the choriocapillaris with resultant subretinal and intraretinal exudation, or it may result from stenosis of the fine vessels adjacent to the macula with subsequent atrophy of the retinal pigment epithelium. The treatment of these degenerations is quite unsatisfactory. Attempts have been made to show a correlation between atherosclerosis, hyperlipemia, and cholesteremia and the incidence of macular changes. Therefore attempts have been made to improve the atherosclerotic condition by the selection of diets low on saturated fatty acids, cholesterol, and the triglycerides.

Blood cholesterol–lowering agents that have been suggested as being of value in senile macular degeneration include sitosterol, clofibrate, heparin, the estrogens, and nicotinic acid. Sitosterol acts by inhibiting the absorption of exogenous cholesterol from the gastrointestinal tract and the endogenous cholesterol from the bile. The initial dose is 9 grams a day, with subsequent doses adjusted according to the patient's dietary intake and cholesterol levels. If heparin is used in the treatment of macular degeneration, it is given in doses of 50 to 75 mg per day either by intermittent intravenous injection or by intermittent deep subcutaneous injection. Clofibrate inhibits cholesterol production. The recommended dose is 500 mg four times a day. Large doses of nicotinic acid, 300 to 1,000 mg in divided doses two or three times a day, have been suggested. Periodic carbon dioxide inhalations in 5% to 10% concentration have been advocated as a means of improving the macular circulation and offering some help in treatment of macular degeneration.

Lipotropic agents, including choline, methionine, and inositol, have been used for many years by ophthalmologists in the attempt to improve choroidal circulation, but once atherosclerotic changes have occurred in the small vessels, it is doubtful that these agents are of any benefit since they are unable to mobilize these lipid deposits.

Since medical treatment is so unsatisfactory, other approaches to therapy have been sought. Fluorescein angiography studies are advisable to determine which patients may be considered for photocoagulation therapy. At the present time the value of photocoagulation therapy in patients with macular degenerative disease is still unclear.

Peripheral retinal and choroidal degenerations

In the therapeutic approach to peripheral retinal and choroidal degenerations, an attempt should be made to improve the state of atherosclerosis and the hyperlipemia or hypercholesterolemia that often accompany these conditions. Diets low in cholesterol and saturated fatty acids may be desirable. The use of cholesterol-lowering agents such as heparin, clofibrate, or nicotinic acid may be indicated. Of these agents, nicotinic acid would seem to be the most innocuous. Therefore if treatment of these conditions is indicated for long periods of time, this would seem to be the drug of choice. Evaluation of clofibrate therapy is still in progress. The results of therapy for peripheral retinal and choroidal degenerations are rather disappointing.

NEOPLASMS
Retinoblastoma

The treatment of retinoblastoma has been modified somewhat in recent years. In selected cases of uniocular involvement, or more rarely in bilateral involvement, where the lesions are small, betatron irradiation or cryotherapy or both may successfully eradicate the tumors. If there is extensive involvement in one eye, enucleation of this eye is the treatment of choice. If both eyes show considerable involvement, removal of the more involved eye is suggested, and the remaining eye treated by radiation. For advanced tumors, chemotherapy is combined with irradiation therapy.

Triethylenemelamine (TEM) is the antineoplastic agent most widely used in conjunction with x-ray therapy for the treatment of retinoblastoma. When given orally, the initial dose is 2.5 mg for children under 12 months of age, 3 mg for children from 12 to 18 months of age, and 3.5 mg for older children. The drug is administered in these doses before x-ray treatment is carried out, and a second dose is given at the conclusion of x-ray therapy. The total dose is about 15 mg in five divided doses. The interval time for the TEM therapy is determined by the white blood cell depression and the platelet depression. In general the drug is not repeated until the white blood cell count has returned to nearly normal levels.

Intramuscular use of TEM has been suggested as a replacement for oral administration, since the drug causes much nausea and vomiting when given orally. The recommended intramuscular dose of TEM is 0.082 to 0.1 mg per kg of body weight. The drug is given before x-ray therapy is started, and a second dose is given after x-ray therapy has been completed and the hemogram has returned to normal. The aim is a depression of the white blood cell count to about 3,000 and a platelet count of no less than 100,000.

In recent years, intra-arterial administration of TEM has become the preferred method. The drug may be injected into the internal carotid artery in a single dose of 0.08 mg per kg of body weight (prepared in saline solution in a concentration of 1 mg per ml). TEM is given 24 hours before radiotherapy and repeated after radiotherapy when the hemogram becomes normal. Alternatively, TEM may be administered through an indwelling catheter inserted into the superior thyroid artery of the external carotid artery. The external carotid artery is ligated distal to the superior thyroid artery so that medications injected into the catheter will go into the internal carotid artery. The catheter is kept filled with a heparin saline mixture between drug administrations. A dose of 0.03 mg per kg of body weight of TEM in 2 to 3 ml of physiological saline solution is given daily for eight to ten doses just before x-ray therapy.

Mechlorethamine hydrochloride (nitrogen mustard) is another radiomimetic agent that is similar in action to TEM. This drug has not been used widely in the treatment of retinoblastoma. The total dose of nitrogen mustard is 0.4 mg per kg of body weight for the entire course of therapy. It is given intravenously in a dose of 0.1 mg per kg of body weight on 4 successive days. Toxic reactions to this drug are the same as to TEM, including nausea and vomiting, lymphocytopenia, granulocytopenia, and occasionally skin eruptions.

Other antineoplastic agents including cyclophosphamide and vincristine have been employed.

TRAUMA
Commotio retinae

Treatment of commotio retinae should include the systemic administration of corticosteroids and bed rest. It would seem that recovery would be dependent more on the degree of involvement than on the vigorousness of the therapy. However, steroids should be of some assistance in reducing the secondary edema that may surround the initial site of trauma.

Eclipse burns

Eclipse burns of the retina should be treated by the systemic administration of corticosteroids. Long-term results depend on the severity of the burn rather than on the therapy. Rate of recovery seems faster if corticosteroids are administered systemically.

RETROLENTAL FIBROPLASIA

No satisfactory medical treatment for advanced retrolental fibroplasia has been discovered. The development of this condition seems to be associated with the administration of high levels of oxygen to premature infants. Recently, therapy employing high concentrations of oxygen to treat respiratory distress syndrome in premature infants has been used, and possibly as a result, retrolental fibroplasia is being seen again with increasing frequency. The only effective approach to this problem is one of prophylaxis, and pediatricians and obstetricians are now well informed that minimal amounts of oxygen should be given to premature infants. Monitoring of arterial oxygen is the preferred method for evaluating oxygen levels. If secondary glaucoma develops, miotics are the best treatment. Glaucoma is usually transient, and generally the eye goes on to phthisis. Many children who have had only low-grade forms of retrolental fibroplasia are myopic and should be fitted with glasses for this secondary condition. Photocoagulation or cryotherapy has been suggested to treat the proliferative stages of the disease when the condition appears to be advancing as revealed by serial examinations.

REFERENCES

Behrendt, T.: Therapeutic vascular occlusions in diabetic retinopathy; argon laser photocoagulation, Arch. Ophthalmol. **87**:629, 1972.

Coon, W. W.: Drugs affecting the coagulation of blood. In Modell, W., editor: Drugs of choice, 1976-1977, St. Louis, 1976, The C. V. Mosby Co.

The Diabetic Retinopathy Study Research Group: Preliminary report on effects of photocoagulation therapy, Am. J. Ophthalmol. **81**:383, 1976.

Duncan, L. P., and others: A three-year trial of Atromid therapy in exudative diabetic retinopathy, Diabetes **17**:458, 1968.

Gass, J. D.: Photocoagulation of macular lesions, Trans. Am. Acad. Ophthalmol. Otolaryngol. **75**:580, 1971.

Goldberg, M. F., and Acacio, I.: Argon laser photocoagulation of proliferative sickle retinopathy, Arch. Ophthalmol. **90**:35, 1973.

Hayreh, S. S.: Central retinal vein occlusion; to be published, Trans. Am. Acad. Ophthal. Otolaryngol.

Hyman, G. A., and others: Combination therapy in retinoblastoma; a 15-year summary of methods and results, Arch. Ophthalmol. **80**:744, 1968.

Nagata, M., and Tsuruoka, Y.: Treatment of acute retrolental fibroplasia with xenon arc photocoagulation, Jpn. J. Ophthalmol. **16**:131, 1972.

Newell, F. W., editor: Symposium on diabetic retinopathy, Trans. Am. Acad. Ophthamol. Otolaryngol. **72**:232, 1968.

O'Reilly, R. A., Aggeler, P. M., and Leong, L. S.: Studies on coumarin anticoagulant drugs: pharmacodynamics of warfarin in man, J. Clin. Invest. **42**:1542, 1963.

Patz, A.: Oxygen studies in retrolental fibroplasia, Am. J. Ophthalmol. **36**:1511, 1953.

Patz, A.: New role of the ophthalmologist in prevention of retrolental fibroplasia, Arch. Ophthalmol. 78:565, 1967.

Patz, A., Maumenee, A. F., and Ryan, S. J.: Argon laser photocoagulation in macular disease, Trans. Am. Ophthalmol. Soc. 69:71, 1971.

Rubin, M. L.: Cryopexy treatment for retinoblastoma, Am. J. Ophthalmol. 66:870, 1968.

Sagerman, R. H., Tretter, P., and Ellsworth, R. M.: Radiation therapy in retinoblastoma, Radiology 93:405, 1969.

Schoch, D.: Therapy of retinal vascular occlusions. In Leopold, I. H., editor: Symposium on ocular therapy, vol. 4, St. Louis, 1969, The C. V. Mosby Co.

Schoch, D.: Plasma expanders and lytic agents. In Leopold, I. H., editor: Symposium on ocular therapy, vol. 5, St. Louis, 1972, The C. V. Mosby Co.

Simmons, R. J., Dueker, D. K., and Kimbrough, R. L.: Goniophotocoagulation for neovascular glaucoma; to be published, Trans. Am. Acad. Ophthalmol. Otolaryngol.

Vannas, S., and Raitta, C.: Anticoagulant treatment of retinal venous occlusions, Am. J. Ophthalmol. 62:874, 1966.

Wessing, A.: Changing concept of central serous retinopathy and its treatment, Trans. Am. Acad. Ophthalmol. Otolaryngol. 77:275(OP), 1973.

Wetzig, P. C., and Jepson, C. N.: Further observations on the treatment of diabetic retinopathy by light coagulation, Trans. Am. Acad. Ophthalmol. Otolaryngol. 71:902, 1967.

CHAPTER 16

Therapy of uveitis

Inflammations of the uveal tract present a complex problem, and often the etiology and specific treatment are not clearly understood. Exogenous inflammatory reactions occur after accidental introduction of pathogenic organisms or foreign substances into the eye, whereas endogenous inflammations are the result of various systemic processes. Uveitis may be further classified according to the type of tissue reaction—suppurative or nonsuppurative. The first part of this chapter will deal with the management of endogenous nonsuppurative uveitis. Treatment of other types of uveal inflammation is discussed later in the chapter.

Endogenous uveitis may be classified in many ways: acute and chronic; anterior and posterior; granulomatous and nongranulomatous. The terms "granulomatous" and "nongranulomatous" are strictly speaking pathological classifications. At one time it was believed that granulomatous uveitis was usually the result of intraocular invasion of microorganisms. Today it is thought that this frequently is not the case. Nonetheless, certain clinical findings and disease entities can be associated with these terms, and they are still employed. Uveitis is considered by many workers to be entirely an immunological disorder. Much has been learned about the immunopathological mechanisms of uveitis, particularly in the pathogenesis of recurrent uveitis. It should be stressed that the etiology of endogenous uveitis is usually obscure from a pathological standpoint. Moreover, the relationship between systemic disease and uveal tract disease may be incidental. An apparently successful treatment of systemic disease does not always result in cure of the uveitis.

Woods outlined the etiology of granulomatous uveitis as follows:
  I. Nonpyogenic microorganisms pathogenic for man
     A. Syphilis
     B. Tuberculosis
     C. Brucellosis
     D. Leptospirosis
     E. Infections with other nonpyogenic organisms (leprosy, and so forth)
  II. Filterable viruses and rickettsia
     A. Behçet's syndrome (uveitis with aphthous ulcers)
     B. Vogt-Koyanagi-Harada syndrome
     C. Herpes simplex virus
     D. Herpes zoster virus

      E. Lymphogranuloma venereum
      F. Undetermined and unknown viruses
  III. Protozoan infections
      A. Trypanosomiasis
      B. Toxoplasmosis
  IV. Fungus infections
      A. Actinomycosis
      B. Blastomycosis
      C. Histoplasmosis
      D. Infection with other rare or unidentified fungi
  V. Helminth infestation
      A. Nematodes
          1. Onchocerciasis
          2. Ancylostoma larvae
      B. Cestodes
          1. *Taenia echinococcus*
          2. *Cysticercus cellulosae*
      C. Diptera larvae
  VI. Unknown agents
      A. Sympathetic ophthalmia
      B. Sarcoidosis

The more common of these infections are probably toxoplasmosis, sarcoidosis, syphilis, histoplasmosis, brucellosis, tuberculosis, sympathetic ophthalmia, and herpetic lesions.

In general, granulomatous uveitis tends to follow a chronic low-grade inflammatory course with remissions and exacerbations. When the anterior segment of the eye is involved, there is minimal to moderate external inflammatory reaction, minimal flare, large coalescent keratic precipitates, and occasionally the formation of "Koeppe nodules" on the iris at the pupillary border. Depending on the duration and intensity of the inflammatory process, the picture may be complicated by opacification of the cornea and/or lens, secondary glaucoma resulting from obstruction of the angle of the anterior chamber by inflammatory products or iris bombé, and vascular disturbance. When the posterior segment is involved, the inflammation may be discrete and focal, without involvement of the vitreous humor and lens. In other instances it may be diffuse, with profound inflammatory reaction in the vitreous humor and secondary lens involvement.

In contrast, nongranulomatous uveitis tends to be more acute in onset and follows a shorter, more intense, self-limited course. The keratic precipitates tend to be finer and more discrete and the anterior chamber flare more intense. With involvement of the posterior uveal tract, there may be a diffuse inflammatory reaction, coincident with irritation of the choroidal and retinal vascular tree. The most common etiological factors are rheumatoid arthritis, trauma, bacterial sensitivity, food and pollen allergies, heterochromic iridocyclitis, and viral diseases

Table 21. Major types of uveitis, listed according to frequency of occurrence*

Anterior only	Both segments	Posterior only
Unknown	Toxoplasmosis	Histoplasmosis†
Peripheral uveitis	Peripheral uveitis	Unknown
Ankylosing spondylitis	Unknown	Toxoplasmosis
Herpes simplex	Syphilis	Syphilis
Herpes zoster	Tuberculosis	Toxocariasis
Sarcoidosis	Sarcoidosis	Sarcoidosis
Tuberculosis	Vogt-Koyanagi-Harada syndrome	
Endophthalmitis phacoanaphylactica		
Syphilis		

*From Schlaegel, T. F., Jr.: Essentials of uveitis, Boston, 1969, Little, Brown and Co.
†Most common only in endemic areas such as Ohio-Missippi Valley.

such as mumps, measles, chickenpox, influenza, herpes simplex, and herpes zoster.

The frequency of occurrence of the major types of uveitis is presented in Table 21.

Treatment will be discussed under two headings: nonspecific treatment and therapy of specific uveal diseases.

NONSPECIFIC TREATMENT
General medical workup

Formerly, patients who developed uveitis often were subjected to needlessly extensive medical workups in the hopes of determining an etiology. It is certainly important for the ophthalmologist to inquire into the nature of the patient's general health, and a general physical examination is appropriate although usually unrevealing. A chest x-ray, lumbosacral x-rays, a complete blood count, and erythrocyte sedimentation rate are reasonable tests to obtain. In addition, blood tests for rheumatoid factor and serum protein level are good screening tests in many patients. Usually skin tests offer little helpful information. Patients with posterior uveitis or granulomatous anterior uveitis probably should be studied more extensively than patients with anterior nongranulomatous uveitis. Depending on the clinical appearance of the lesions and the course of the disease, additional tests, such as a methylene blue dye test for toxoplasmosis, may be obtained.

Cycloplegics

Cycloplegics put the iris and ciliary body at rest, allay pain from ciliary and pupillary spasm, reduce the protein content of the aqueous humor, and tend to prevent formation of posterior synechiae. The use of topically applied 1% or 2% atropine sulfate solution or ointment one to three times daily in the affected eye is essential in anterior segment involved. Scopolamine, 0.25% solution or ointment, may be used in persons sensitive to atropine. Shorter-acting cycloplegics such as 5% homatropine and 1% cyclopentolate may be used.

Mydriatics

The use of topically applied 10% phenylephrine (Neo-Synephrine) hydrochloride is often extremely helpful in producing wide pupillary dilatation and breaking up and preventing posterior synechiae. Phenylephrine hydrochloride may be applied as drops or used to saturate a cotton pledget that is placed in the inferior or superior conjunctival cul-de-sac.

Combination of mydriatic and cycloplegic agents

A combination of mydriatic and cycloplegic drugs may be injected subconjunctivally when posterior synechiae cannot be broken up with topically applied medications. One to two minims each of sterile 1% atropine sulfate solution, 4% cocaine hydrochloride solution, and 1:10,000 epinephrine or 1:1,000 norepinephrine solution are injected. Systemic side reactions may occur.

Corticosteroids

In the treatment of uveitis, corticosteroids may be used topically as drops or ointment, they may be injected subconjunctivally or retrobulbarly, or they may be administered systemically. For inflammations of the anterior uvea, topical administration is effective. The frequency of application varies with the severity of the disease—from two to three times a day to every hour. Subconjunctival injections of corticosteroids are used in the more severe forms of anterior uveitis. An injection of 0.5 to 1 ml is made beneath the bulbar conjunctiva. Any of the corticosteroid solutions or suspensions may be used, but the repository steroids are often preferred because of their delayed absorption and prolonged effectiveness. Such a technique of administration gives effective concentrations of the drug for prolonged periods, but the number of injections is limited because of the discomfort and local reaction. Frequently used corticosteroids are methylprednisolone acetate (Depo-Medrol), triamcinolone acetonide suspension (Kenalog), and triamcinolone diacetate (Aristocort Forte), which apparently give satisfactory drug levels in the anterior segment of the eye for as long as 4 to 6 weeks. Some ophthalmologists prefer to use betamethasone acetate and disodium phosphate combination (Celestone Soluspan Suspension). The phosphate solution portion of this combination provides short-term high tissue steroid levels, while the acetate suspension portion provides a prolonged effect. Retrobulbar injections of corticosteroids have been advocated in patients with posterior uveitis unresponsive to systemic therapy and in patients who develop severe side reactions to systemic therapy. To keep the medication in close apposition to the sclera, techniques of injecting the medication in the posterior sub-Tenon's space have been described, and an injection of 0.5 to 1 ml of a repository steroid preparation is made. Accidental intraocular injections have occurred, and caution is urged with this technique.

The systemic administration of corticosteroids is indicated in posterior uveitis and severe anterior uveitis. In the latter involvement, systemic therapy is used in addition to topical therapy. The dosage should be individualized to each patient. If the uveitis is acute and severe, daily administration of 40 to 60 mg of prednisone or its equivalent is suggested. If clinical improvement is not observed within 72 hours, it may be necessary to increase the dosage to 80 mg or in exceptional cases even higher. The dosage should be reduced when clinical improvement occurs, since severe complications may develop with continued high dosage. Reduction should be in gradual decrements (10 mg for large initial doses and 5 mg for smaller initial doses) over a period of days or weeks, depending on the total time of treatment. Once a dosage level of 15 to 20 mg is reached, it is sometimes better to maintain the patient at this dosage for 2 weeks, since further rapid reduction of steroids frequently results in a flare-up of the inflammation. If the uveitis is only moderately severe, a total daily dose of 30 to 40 mg of prednisone or its equivalent is advisable. Again, gradual reduction should be accomplished as soon as possible. In mild cases of uveitis a dose of 20 mg of prednisone or its equivalent is sufficient.

The alternate-day administration of corticosteroids (Chapter 2) is useful when long-term therapy is required, as in the treatment of chronic uveitis or in a case of sympathetic ophthalmia in a relatively quiescent state. It is advisable in the treatment of children with chronic uveitis. However, when it is necessary to minimize quickly the reaction of an acute severe inflammation, intermittent dosage is advisable to maintain high therapeutic drug levels.

When long-term systemic corticosteroid therapy is necessary, it is important to maintain the patient on as small a dose as possible. If the involvement is primarily anterior, the total dose of corticosteroid given systemically may be reduced if steroids applied topically are also used. Whenever prolonged therapy is required, the patient should be checked for the development of any side reactions. Repeated consultations with an internist are advisable in these cases. The side effects and contraindications to corticosteroid therapy are discussed in Chapter 2 and also in the section on therapeutic agents.

ACTH

ACTH is administered either intramuscularly or intravenously. The usual intramuscular dose is 40 to 80 USP units in four divided doses. Larger doses (up to 100 USP units) may be necessary to obtain satisfactory response. The dose of the gel form of ACTH is the same as that of regular ACTH. Injections are given at 24-hour intervals.

For intravenous use 40 USP units are dissolved in 500 to 1,000 ml of 5% dextrose in water and given over a period of 8 to 12 hours. A continuous intravenous infusion of ACTH over a 24-hour period produces a response equivalent to that resulting from 75 to 100 mg of prednisone.

Antimetabolites (immunosuppressives)

Antimetabolite immunosuppressive drugs such as mercaptopurine, cyclophosphamide, chlorambucil, azathioprine, and methotrexate have been used successfully in patients with resistant chronic uveitis. Unfortunately, flare-ups often have occurred when immunosuppressive therapy has been discontinued. These agents were developed primarily as antineoplastic drugs and are cytotoxic; however, they are effective in suppressing inflammation and antibody formation.

Since these drugs are very toxic, many serious side reactions can occur, including bone marrow depression, thrombocytopenia, leukopenia, bleeding, nausea, vomiting, and stomatitis. Their use in the treatment of uveitis is still in the experimental stage, and they should not be used by physicians unprepared to handle the toxic reactions.

Typhoid vaccine

The administration of typhoid vaccine is one of the older methods of treating uveitis. It has largely been replaced by corticosteroid therapy. The exact mechanism of action of typhoid vaccine is somewhat obscure. It probably exerts its maximum effect through stimulation of the adrenal cortex. In addition, it causes hyperpyrexia, leukocytosis, and stimulation of the reticuloendothelial system. Two forms of typhoid vaccine are available: the pure H form and the triple vaccine. The initial intravenous dose of the H antigen is usually 5 to 15 million organisms. For the triple vaccine, the initial dose is 10 to 25 million organisms. After injection the patient should be kept in bed and observed for untoward reactions. The temperature should be taken every hour for a 12-hour period. White blood cell counts should be obtained at the end of 6 hours and at the end of 12 hours. A temperature of about 103° F is desirable, with a white blood cell count response of 15,000. The intravenous typhoid therapy is repeated after a rest of 1 or 2 days. The dosage is increased by 50% to 100%. A third dose may be given after another rest period.

Typhoid vaccine should not be given to patients who have recently received corticosteroids systemically, since the adrenal cortex may not be capable of withstanding the "shock" produced by the typhoid therapy.

Salicylates

The salicylates may be given either in the form of acetylsalicylic acid or sodium salicylate. The total daily dosage for a severe uveitis is 6 to 10 grams per day, divided into doses to be given at 4-hour intervals. For less severe uveitis the initial daily dose is 4 to 6 grams. The dosage is governed by the developing signs of tinnitus. A dose just under the amount that produces this symptom is desired. Gastric irritation from salicylates may be reduced by the addition of an antacid or sodium bicarbonate. Salicylates may be used concurrently with corticosteroids.

Phenylbutazone

Phenylbutazone (Butazolidin) is occasionally used for the treatment of uveitis. This agent, closely related to aminopyrine, has anti-inflammatory, antipyretic, and analgesic actions. It is used chiefly for the treatment of arthritis and related conditions and has therefore been advocated for the treatment of uveitis associated with arthritis. In a high percentage of patients it produces undesirable side reactions and toxic effects, including edema, nausea, drug rash, stomatitis, and epigastric pains. Less common reactions are activation of peptic ulcer, agranulocytosis, hepatitis, and central nervous system stimulation. The adult dose is 300 to 600 mg, divided into four equal doses, daily for 1 week. Then, if no favorable results occur, the drug is discontinued, but if beneficial effects are observed, the drug may be continued at a maintenance dosage of 100 to 200 mg per day.

Oxyphenbutazone is an analogue of phenylbutazone. It has essentially the same pharmacological actions and side effects as phenylbutazone, although the incidence of gastric irritation is less. The dosage is 100 mg three to four times a day.

Indomethacin

Indomethacin (Indocin) is an anti-inflammatory drug with analgesic and antipyretic properties. The drug resembles aspirin in its effect, but its action is independent of the pituitary adrenal axis. It is effective in the treatment of rheumatoid arthritis, osteoarthritis, and gout. There is some evidence it may be of value in the treatment of anterior uveitis, possibly by an antiprostaglandin mechanism. A dose of 50 mg three times a day is suggested for the control of acute inflammatory states in adults. Smaller initial doses, 25 mg three times a day, are usually employed in chronic rheumatoid disorders. Topical application of indomethacin, 0.1% to 0.5%, has been found to reduce postoperative anterior chamber inflammatory reactions.

Other antiarthritic drugs

A new group of antiarthritic drugs have recently become available. These include ibuprofen (Motrin), fenoprofen (Nalfon), naproxen (Naprosyn), and tolmetin (Tolectin). The precise mechanisms of action of these drugs are unknown, but all have anti-inflammatory effects as well as analgesic and antipyretic actions. Their potential usefulness in the treatment of ocular inflammations including uveitis is not yet established.

Antilymphocyte serum

Antilymphocyte serum has been used experimentally to treat uveitis. Human antilymphocyte serum is prepared by injecting splenic tissue from human cadavers into horses. The serum has been used primarily to prevent rejection after human heart, kidney, and liver transplantation. Antilymphocyte serum reduces antibody formation; the exact mechanism is unknown. There are many side reactions to antilymphocyte serum, including anemias, thrombocytopenia, leukopenia, and serum sickness. Because of the high risks involved, antilymphocyte serum should not be used.

Other measures

It is important to monitor the intraocular pressure in patients with uveitis, particularly in those with primarily anterior segment involvement. Increased intraocular pressure can result from the disease process or from treatment (corticosteroids and cycloplegics). If secondary glaucoma occurs, it can usually be controlled with carbonic anhydrase inhibitors (Chapter 5). The patient should also be observed for possible development of cataracts and retinal detachment.

THERAPY OF UVEITIS ASSOCIATED WITH SPECIFIC DISEASES
Toxoplasmosis

Toxoplasma organisms invade the retina and cause a primary retinitis; involvement of the choroid is secondary. In the acute stages there is necrosis of the retina and inflammation of the underlying choroid; exudation into the vitreous is common. As the acute reaction subsides, there is a colobomatouslike crater lesion of the posterior segment of the globe that often involves the macular area. In the acute lesion there are both the free and the encysted parasites; in the inactive lesion encysted parasites may be present. The disease may be transmitted during fetal life or may be acquired in adulthood. Treatment of the congenital form is useless because at the time of diagnosis the disease is quiescent, and only scar formation remains. In acquired toxoplasmosis, however, there are often focal lesions, which may become active and lead to the development of daughter lesions.

Medical treatment is probably effective against the free forms of the parasite, but it is probably ineffective against the encysted parasites.

Treatment of toxoplasmosis consists of the combined use of sulfadiazine or triple sulfonamides and pyrimethamine (Daraprim) administered systemically. Corticosteroids may be administered systemically at the same time to reduce the inflammation. Pyrimethamine, 25 mg twice a day, and sulfadiazine or triple sulfonamides, 1 gram four times a day, are given for 1 to 3 weeks. Some physicians recommend that pyrimethamine be administered in priming doses of 50 mg two or four times a day for 1 to 2 days. After 1 to 3 weeks, the pyrimethamine is reduced to 25 mg daily and the sulfadiazine or triple sulfonamides to 2 grams daily, depending on the patient's response and drug toxicity. Long-term pyrimethamine therapy in a dose of 25 mg a week, without the sulfadiazine, may be continued for several months. Pyrimethamine is a folic acid antagonist, and patients may develop megaloblastic anemia or leukopenia. They should be checked twice a week with blood counts for this complication. If blood cell depression occurs, pyrimethamine should be stopped and folinic acid (Leucovorin calcium) administered in a daily dose of 5 to 15 mg until the blood cell depression has cleared. At the present time only the intramuscular form of folinic acid is available commercially. Folinic acid does not antagonize the effects of sulfadiazine or pyrimethamine and cannot be utilized by *Toxoplasma gondii*. Sulfonamides such as sulfisoxazole (Gantrisin) and sulfisomidine (Elkosin) should not be used, since these drugs are primarily distributed in the extracellular fluid.

Spiramycin (Rovamycin) has been used clinically and experimentally for the treatment of toxoplasmosis. The initial dose is 1.5 grams four times the first day and 1 gram four times a day thereafter. The effectiveness of this drug in the treatment of toxoplasmosis is still unknown. The drug is not commercially available in the United States.

Tetracyclines, lincomycin, and clindamycin also are believed somewhat effective against toxoplasma. Photocoagulation, laser therapy, and cryocautery, with or without concomitant medical therapy, have also been employed in the treatment of toxoplasmic retinochoroiditis.

Histoplasmosis

Infection with *Histoplasma*, one of the pathogenic fungi, may be acquired in childhood or in adult life. The disease is not directly transmissible from person to person but is usually acquired by inhalation of the fungi from a reservoir of the dung of pigeons or poultry. It is apparently endemic in the regions of the Ohio River Valley and the Missouri River Valley. Ocular lesions attributable to histoplasmosis have been described, although pathological examination of such lesions has failed to demonstrate the presence of *Histoplasma* organisms. The typical ocular findings of histoplasmosis are: central disciform elevations of the macula with hemorrhagic phenomena, circumpapillary choroiditis, and small peripheral punched-out depigmented lesions. There is often associated pulmonary calcification, as evidenced by x-ray films of the chest, with a negative serological test for histoplasmosis and a positive skin test for the fungi.

Patients who have the histoplasmosis syndrome should have fluorescein angiography. If discrete leaks can be identified, photocoagulation therapy may be indicated. Systemic or retrobulbar corticosteroid therapy has been recommended, but its usefulness in this disorder is controversial. In the past amphotericin B (Fungizone) was administered intravenously. At the present time this treatment is not considered to be of any value and should be avoided because of the toxicity of this drug.

Amebiasis

Amebiasis is thought to produce a picture in the choroid similar to that described for histoplasmosis. Demonstration of *Entamoeba histolytica* cyst organisms in the stool may be justification for the administration of antiamebic therapy. This therapy varies with the severity of the disease and the symptoms. Iodochlorhydroxyquin (Vioform) may be used in a dosage of 1.25 grams three times a day orally for 14 days.

Emetine hydrochloride, 60 mg daily by subcutaneous injection for 4 days, combined with carbarsone, 0.25 gram three times daily for 10 days, is also recommended for the treatment of amebiasis. All these drugs are somewhat toxic, and treatment should be supervised by a competent internist. Glycobiarsol (Milibis) is a less toxic amebicide. The dose is 500 mg three times a day for 7 days. Oxytetracyclines may be given concurrently to clear the frequently associated bacterial infections.

The stool should be reexamined after 2 weeks of therapy, and the treatment should be repeated if cysts are again formed during the cycle of the organism.

Toxocara

There is no specific treatment for *Toxocara* infections (visceral larva migrans). Thiabendazole, an antihelminthic, may be tried; the recommended dosage is 50 to 60 mg per kg of body weight daily. Corticosteroids, analgesics, and antihistamines have been used to provide relief of generalized symptoms. Some workers have recommended the administration of diethylcarbamazine or piperazine to household dogs and cats as a prophylaxis.

Syphilis

Uveal lesions may occur in congenital, late secondary, and tertiary syphilis. Either the anterior or posterior segment of the globe may be involved. The treatment of choice is penicillin. For secondary syphilis, the recommended total dose is 4.8 to 6 million units. Tertiary syphilis is treated with 600,000 units of procaine penicillin daily to a total dose of 9 to 12 million units. The dose for congenital syphilis varies with the age of the child. For a child under 2 years of age, the total dose is approximately 2 million units; for a child from 2 to 10 years old, the dose is 3 to 4 million units. If the patient has a sensitivity to penicillin, the tetracyclines or erythromycin may be substituted in a total dose of 30 to 40 grams over a period of 10 to 15 days (Chapter 8).

Tuberculosis

The uveal tract may be invaded in any stage of tuberculosis. The uveitis may be acute and fulminating, or it may follow a very chronic, prolonged course. In proved tuberculosis, treatment should be supervised by a physician familiar with the systemic disease. Treatment most commonly used at present is the combined use of isoniazid with one or two of the following drugs: streptomycin, p-aminosalicylic acid, or rifampin. Isoniazid is given in a divided oral dose of 10 mg per kg of body weight daily. Streptomycin is administered in a dose of 1 gram daily; if the patient is elderly or has poor renal function, the dose is reduced. p-Aminosalicylic acid is administered in a single oral dose of 150 mg per kg of body weight. Rifampin is given in a single daily oral dose of 600 mg. The systemic administration of steroids in combination with other antituberculosis drugs for tuberculous uveitis has not been clearly defined. However, it might be of value to use steroids in selected patients. Again, it should be stated that because tuberculous infections are so variable the management of the patients should be placed in the hands of a physician familiar with the treatment of the underlying disease.

Brucellosis

Brucellosis is sometimes a cause of posterior segment uveitis and also may involve the entire uveal tract. Specific therapy consists of the systemic administration of tetracyclines, 500 to 750 mg four times a day. Streptomycin, 1 to 2 grams a day, may be used concurrently. It is usually necessary to continue this active treatment for 3 to 4 weeks. In the chronic localized form of brucellosis, treatment may be necessary for more prolonged periods. In such cases, tetracyclines, 250 mg four times a day, are usually adequate and should be continued until all symptoms have subsided.

Sarcoidosis

Any portion of the uveal tract may become involved in sarcoidosis, although iritis is the most common inflammatory lesion. The systemic use of corticosteriods is indicated in ocular sarcoidosis. Cycloplegics and topically applied steroids should also be employed if the lesions are in the anterior portion of the uveal tract.

Rheumatoid arthritis

Anterior segment inflammation is the form of uveitis usually associated with rheumatoid arthritis. Treatment consists of the use of cycloplegics and topically applied steroids. Oral administration of salicylates may also be helpful in controlling the inflammatory reaction. The systemic use of steroids may become necessary. However, the use of these agents in patients with generalized rheumatoid arthritis should be delayed until consultation with an internist has been obtained.

Lens-induced uveitis

A severe uveitis may be induced by sensitivity to cortical material of the lens. By leading to leakage of cortical material through the capsule, a hypermature lens may induce a uveitis with secondary glaucoma. This type of uveitis is best treated by extraction of the lens together with any cortical material. Preoperative and postoperative corticosteroid therapy, both systemic and topical, is valuable in controlling the uveitis. Cycloplegics should be given, and any secondary glaucoma should be controlled with acetazolamide (Diamox) or osmotherapy.

Heterochromic iridocyclitis

Heterochromic iridocyclitis is usually unilateral and is characterized by small keratitic precipitates and minor symptoms of redness and photophobia. The disease is usually unilateral and depigmentation of the involved iris occurs. Synechiae are uncommon, but cataract formation is common. Corticosteroids do not significantly alter the course of the chronic inflammatory process.

Pars planitis (chronic cyclitis)

This form of uveitis is usually found in younger patients and, as the name implies, principally involves the region of the pars plana of the ciliary body. Bilateral involvement occurs in most patients. It often runs a chronic course with remissions and exacerbations. Clinically the disorder is characterized by cells and exudates in the anterior vitreous, mainly inferior, white "snowbank" deposits in the region of the ora serrata of the retina and pars plana, and often some sheathing of the peripheral retinal vessels. Cystoid macular edema occurs in approximately one quarter of the patients.

Management of pars planitis frequently can be quite difficult. Intensive therapy should be used only for acute flare-ups or if the posterior pole becomes involved. Low degrees of inflammation require little or no therapy. Corticosteroids are the mainstay of therapy. Probably the most effective method of administering them is with subconjunctival or periocular injections. Topical therapy does not usually achieve desired levels in the ciliary body region. Systemic administration of steroids is effective for both anterior and posterior segment involvement, but because of the age of the patients and the long-term course of the disease, the use of systemically administered steroids should be minimized. In some patients corticosteroids seem to be relatively ineffective in controlling the disease process. Immunosuppressive therapy has been used in some patients, but the risks of this treatment are so high that their use is seldom indicated. Photocoagulation and cryotherapy of the pars plana and ora serrata regions have been advocated, but the value of such therapy is not firmly established.

Sympathetic ophthalmia

No panacea has been discovered for this distressing complication of ocular injury. The disease may, of course, be averted in some cases by enucleation of a possibly exciting eye that has become hopeless visually and has received a severe injury to the ciliary body. Once sympathetic ophthalmia has been established, however, the vigorous use of corticosteroids is mandatory. Steroids should be employed systemically in sufficient concentration to control the inflammation. Daily doses up to 60 to 80 mg of prednisone or its equivalent may be necessary. As the inflammation subsides, the dosage should be decreased gradually. Supplemental topical corticosteroid therapy and cycloplegics should be employed. Long-term therapy is usually necessary, and maintenance dosages of topically and systemically administered corticosteroids may be required to prevent a flare-up of the uveitis. Alternate-day administration of systemic steroids may successfully control the disease once the acute inflammation has subsided.

Antimetabolites have been used successfully in the treatment of sympathetic ophthalmia in patients unresponsive to corticosteroid therapy.

Uveitis secondary to infections elsewhere in the body

When the cause of the uveitis is unknown, the eradication of any overt infection elsewhere in the body may well be indicated to prevent bacterial invasion into the eye or a hypersensitivity phenomenon. In my experience, frank abscesses of the teeth or the paranasal sinuses are the two most common causes as well as the two most abused so-called foci of infection. The use of antibiotic therapy, as indicated by culture and sensitivity reactions of the organisms to antibiotics, is probably indicated. In addition, general supportive therapy for the uveitis should be given.

Trauma

An iridocyclitis often accompanies contusions or other injuries of the globe and is usually well controlled by supportive therapy. Cycloplegics and topically and systemically administered corticosteroids are usually successful in controlling the inflammatory reaction.

Herpetic lesions

Herpes simplex. An anterior iridocyclitis may accompany the keratitis produced by herpes simplex. The iridocyclitis is best controlled with topically applied cycloplegics and salicylates. Phenylbutazone may be of value. Steroids should be avoided in the early stages of this disease because it is probable that they promote growth and spread of the virus. Mild uveitis usually subsides as the keratitis improves. Steroids may be used systemically or topically as treatment for severe uveitis associated with long-standing keratitis. In the event that corticosteriods are used, they should be employed in minimal doses, and IDU should be administered concurrently to reduce the likelihood of a flare-up of the superficial keratitis. It has been suggested that vidarabine may be a more valuable agent than IDU in the treatment of herpes simplex keratouveitis. A metabolite of vidarabine, hypoxanthene arabinoside, is much more soluble than the parent compound and is capable of greater penetration of the cornea. It has effective antiviral properties. Vidarabine has also been administered systemically for treatment of severe forms of herpes simplex uveitis with limited success. (See treatment of herpes simplex keratitis.)

Herpes zoster. Keratitis and iridocyclitis often accompany herpes zoster ophthalmicus. This disease is not easily cured, but it is usually improved with the topical and systemic administration of steroids concurrently with the use of cycloplegics and mydriatics.

REFERENCES

Aronson, S. B., Gamble, C. N., Goodner, E. K., and O'Connor, G. R.: Clinical methods in uveitis, St. Louis, 1968, The C. V. Mosby Co.

Coles, R. S.: Steroid therapy in uveitis, Int. Ophthalmol. Clin. 6:869, 1966.

Ellis, P. P.: Non-corticosteroid anti-inflammatory drugs. In Symposium on ocular pharmacology and therapeutics, Transactions of the New Orleans Academy of Ophthalmology, St. Louis, 1969, The C. V. Mosby Co.

Giles, C. L.: Pyrimethamine (Daraprim) and the treatment of toxoplasmic uveitis, Surv. Ophthalmol. 16:88, 1971.

Karlsberg, R. C., Gordon, D. M., and Kaufman, H. E.: Uveitis. In Dunlap, E. A., editor:

Gordon's medical management of ocular disease, New York, 1976, Harper & Row, Publishers.

Kaufman, H. E., editor: Symposium on ocular anti-inflammatory therapy, Springfield, Ill., 1970, Charles C Thomas, Publisher.

Leopold, I. H.: Drug therapy in uveitis; the XVII Francis I. Proctor lecture, Am. J. Ophthalmol. **56:**709, 1963.

O'Conner, G. R.: The uvea; annual review, Arch. Ophthalmol. **93:**675, 1975.

Pavan-Langston, D., and Dohlman, C.: A double-blind study of adenine arabinoside therapy of keratoconjunctivitis, Am. J. Ophthalmol. **74:**81, 1972.

Richardson, K. T.: Pharmacology and pathophysiology of inflammation, Arch. Ophthalmol. **86:**706, 1971.

Schlaegel, T. F., Jr.: Essentials of uveitis, Boston, 1969, Little, Brown and Co.

Smith, R. E., Godfrey, W. A., and Kimura, S. J.: Chronic cyclitis, Trans. Am. Acad. Ophthalmol. Otolaryngol. **77:**760(OP), 1973.

Tabbara, K. F., Nozik, R. A., and O'Connor, G. R.: Clindamycin effects on experimental toxoplasmosis in the rabbit, Arch. Ophthalmol. **92:**244, 1974.

Wong, V. G.: Immunosuppressive agents in ophthalmology, Surv. Ophthalmol. **13:**290, 1968.

Woods, A. C.: Endogenous inflammations of the uveal tract, Baltimore, 1961, The Williams & Wilkins Co.

CHAPTER 17

Therapy of optic neuritis

For purposes of this chapter, optic neuritis is defined as any relatively acute, presumed inflammatory insult to the optic nerve. Consideration is not given to the anatomic divisions of the optic nerve (retrobulbar, anterior, axial, peripheral, and so forth) relative to treatment. A modified etiological classification is utilized for discussing therapy: specific infection, demyelination (postviral, multiple sclerosis), ischemia, toxic, nutritional (systemic), malignant infiltration, and idiopathic.

Although the treatment for many types of optic neuritis is nonspecific, a genuine attempt should be made to determine the etiology of the disease so that treatment can be directed toward the specific cause. Even though results are often less than optimal, several diseases associated with optic neuritis can be treated specifically. These include diabetes mellitus, syphilis, orbitis, hyperthyroidism, lead and methanol intoxication, hypertension, and severe vitamin deficiency. In toxic optic neuropathy treatment primarily consists of stopping exposure to the toxic substance.

Nonspecific treatment should be directed toward reducing the inflammatory edema of the optic nerve as rapidly as possible. This can be done in several ways, the most effective treatment being the use of anti-inflammatory agents—corticosteroids or ACTH. Vasodilating agents have been used in the treatment of optic neuritis without significant success; among the agents employed were tolazoline hydrochloride (Priscoline) both orally and retrobulbarly, nicotinic acid orally, and the various nitrites. Vitamin B complex and antibiotics were once used with enthusiasm but have now been largely abandoned.

When specific infections are responsible for optic neuritis, it is frequently advisable to use corticosteroids in addition to specific anti-infective agents. Irreversible changes can occur in the optic nerve during the inflammatory response, and corticosteroid therapy is designed to reduce the likelihood that permanent damage to the axon cylinders might occur during the inflammatory or healing process.

SPECIFIC INFECTIONS

When a specific bacterial infection is responsible for the optic neuritis, it should be appropriately treated with antibiotics. The choice of antibiotic is, of course, dependent on determination of the responsible bacteria. In syphilitic infections (the most common bacterial cause of optic neuritis) the antibiotic of choice is penicillin. If the causative organism cannot be isolated in other bacterial infections, as in an orbititis, either ampicillin or other broad-spectrum antibiotics may be tried. In addition to antibiotic therapy effective against the bacteria, it is advisable to use a corticosteroid to reduce the inflammatory process. Vasodilators and vitamin B complex therapy are of no great help in most of these cases.

OPTIC NEURITIS SECONDARY TO INTOXICANTS

Optic neuritis secondary to intoxicants should be treated by elimination of the offending agent, by the use of available specific antitoxic agents, by the systemic administration of corticosteroids or corticotropic hormones, and by the administration of vitamin B complex if a vitamin deficiency is present.

At one time or another almost every therapeutic drug agent has been reported to cause optic neuritis. If the disease is secondary to drug reactions or sensitivity, the offending drug should be eliminated as rapidly as possible, and corticosteroids should be given orally or systemically to reduce the inflammation.

In my experience, tobacco-alcohol amblyopia is an uncommon and difficult diagnosis to confirm. Optic neuritis suspected to be secondary to tobacco or ethyl alcohol should be treated by the elimination of these agents. In addition, vitamin B complex should be given orally in substantial doses since many of these so-called tobacco-alcohol optic neuritides are in reality optic neuritis secondary to vitamin B complex deficiency. It has been suggested that tobacco amblyopia may result from chronic cyanide poisoning. Although agents, such as sodium thiosulfate, used in the treatment of cyanide poisoning have been reported to be of some value, basic treatment consists of good diet and elimination of tobacco. Large doses of hydroxocobalamin (a preparation for treatment of vitamin B_{12} deficiencies) may be tried.

The treatment of optic neuritis secondary to methyl alcohol intoxication is seldom satisfactory since permanent damage to the optic nerve has occurred before the ophthalmologist sees the patient. Methanol is oxidized to formaldehyde. It is unknown whether destruction of retinal ganglion cells occurring with the methanol intoxication is due to formaldehyde or to other metabolites. General measures to combat acidosis should be employed—either intravenous injection of 5% sodium bicarbonate in a dose not to exceed 6 ml per kg of body weight, given slowly over a period of at least 30 minutes, or the use of $\frac{1}{6}$M sodium lactate solution given in doses up to 25 ml per kg of body weight. The exact total dosage of the alkali should be determined by the blood pH and blood carbon dioxide content. It has been suggested by a few that visual results after methanol intoxication are better if shortly after ingestion of the methyl alcohol, the patient is given ethanol either orally or intravenously in a dosage of 0.75 gram per kg of body weight initially, followed by 0.5 gram per kg of body weight every 4 hours for a period of 56 to 64 hours. Hemodialysis has been employed for treatment of severe methanol intoxication. Methyl alcohol, formaldehyde, and formate are dialyzable products.

For optic neuritis secondary to lead poisoning, the most effective treatment consists of trying to accomplish deleading. This is best done with edathamil calcium-disodium, administered intravenously or intramuscularly. For intravenous administration the maximum dose should not exceed 1 gram per kg of body weight per hour, or 1 gram per 30 pounds of body weight in a 24-hour period. Treatment should be limited to 10 days and may be repeated after an interval of 1 week. Usually not more than two courses of therapy are given.

NUTRITIONAL (SYSTEMIC) OPTIC NEURITIS

Optic neuritis secondary to systemic diseases should be treated by measures directed against the specific underlying diseases.

Optic neuritis secondary to certain blood dyscrasias, principally pernicious anemia or iron-deficiency anemias, should be treated primarily by correction of the blood dyscrasias. Supplemental vitamin therapy is also advisable, but it would probably be well to avoid using corticosteroids in these cases since these drugs alter the blood picture and might confuse the response to the therapy. The vitamin B group probably reduces the inflammation of the nerve by improving the nutrition of the optic nerve tissue.

It has been said that optic neuritis may result from pregnancy or lactation. This is probably a nutritional problem and should be handled by standard medical methods.

DEMYELINATING OPTIC NEURITIS

Optic neuritis is frequently seen with demyelinating diseases such as multiple sclerosis, neuromyelitis optica, Schilder's disease, or disseminated encephalomyelitis following infectious diseases. The value of any therapy is highly questionable since most of the patients have spontaneous remissions of the optic neuritis. Some neurologists and ophthalmologists favor the use of corticosteroids or ACTH in this type of optic neuritis, particularly in the acute phases of the disease. It is quite possible that these are of benefit, and they are frequently employed since they may shorten the period of visual dysfunction. However, it is not known if final morbidity due to visual loss is less. I have observed several cases of optic neuritis that were improved with steroids, worsened after the discontinuance of the steroids, and improved again after steroids were reinstituted. Some ophthalmologists and neurologists believe that treatment with the corticosteroids offers no benefit. This is undoubtedly true in many instances.

If steroids are employed, moderately large doses (60 to 80 mg of prednisone or its equivalent) are advised for a period of 7 to 10 days. Some physicians state that ACTH is more valuable than corticosteroid therapy in the treatment of optic neuritis; this claim is difficult to substantiate. Retrobulbar (posterior sub-Tenon's) injections of corticosteroids also have been recommended.

ISCHEMIC OPTIC NEURITIS

Ischemic optic neuritis is very difficult to treat. Most cases show very little vision return. Temporal arteritis is usually treated with high doses of prednisone (60 mg or more per day) for days to weeks. If there is clinical systemic improvement, the dose is reduced slowly to the lowest dose that will control symptoms and/or keep the erythrocyte sedimentation rate normal or near normal. Treatment may continue for some months on an everyday or every-other-day basis. When the two parameters mentioned do not provide enough information to rationally prescribe continued steroid treatment, a repeat temporal artery biopsy may be considered. I am unaware of a double-blind study demonstrating the efficacy of steroids in reducing visual morbidity in temporal arteritis even though patients frequently report they feel better. The primary aim of treatment is to prevent involvement of the second eye.

Optic neuritis secondary to diabetes should be treated with adequate control of the primary disease. Since corticosteroids tend to exaggerate the diabetic state, they should be given cautiously.

Optic neuritis secondary to thyroid dysfunction may respond to high doses of systemically applied corticosteroids coupled with control of thyroid function.

The use of steroids in the treatment of ischemic optic neuritis secondary to collagen vascular disease, acute multifocal pigment epitheliopathy, or atherosclerosis has little support in scientific fact. The treatment of hypertension may be helpful in preventing ischemic disease of the optic nerve, but it needs to be done carefully since lowering systemic pressure in the presence of atherosclerosis may itself cause ischemia of the nerve. Dilantin probably does not help ischemic neuritis.

MALIGNANT INFILTRATION OF CELLS

Cellular infiltrates in or about the optic nerve may be controlled with chemotherapy or radiation in some cases.

IDIOPATHIC OPTIC NEURITIS

Idiopathic optic neuritis is treated with steroids by some, but good data are not available on the efficacy of such therapy.

REFERENCES

Austin, W. H., Lope, C. P., and Burnham, H. N.: Treatment of methanol intoxication by hemodialysis, N. Engl. J. Med. **265:**334, 1961.

Bowden, A. N., Bowden, P. M., Friedmann, A. I., and others: A trial of corticotrophin gelatin injection in acute optic neuritis, J. Neurol. Neurosurg. Psychiatry **37:**869, 1974.

Burde, R. M.: Ischemic optic neuropathy. In Smith, J. L., and Glaser, J. S., editors: Neuro-ophthalmology, Symposium of the University of Miami and the Bascom Palmer Eye Institute, vol. 7, St. Louis, 1973, The C. V. Mosby Co.

Carroll, F. C., and others: Symposium; diseases of the optic nerve, Trans. Am. Acad. Ophthalmol. Otolaryngol. **60:**7, 1956.

Cohen, D. N.: Temporal arteritis; improvement in visual prognosis and management with repeated biopsies, Trans. Am. Acad. Ophthalmol. Otolaryngol. **77:**74(OP), 1973.

Day, R. M., and Carroll, F. D.: Corticosteroids in the treatment of optic nerve involvement, associated with thyroid dysfunction, Arch. Ophthalmol. **79**:279, 1968.

Ellenberger, C., Keltner, J. L., and Burde, R. M.: Acute optic neuropathy in older patients, Arch. Neurol. **28**:182, 1973.

Giles, C. L., and Isaacson, J. D.: The treatment of acute optic neuritis; an analysis of eighty cases, Arch. Ophthalmol. **66**:176, 1961.

Gilger, A. P., Farkas, I. S., and Potts, A. M.: Studies on the visual toxicity of methanol X; further observations on the ethanol therapy of acute methanol poisoning in monkeys, Am. J. Ophthalmol. **48**:153, 1959.

Hepler, R. S.: Management of optic neuritis, Surv. Ophthalmol. **20**:350, 1976.

Lessell, S.: Toxic and deficiency optic neuropathies. In Smith, J. L., and Glaser, J. S., editors: Neuro-ophthalmology; Symposium of the University of Miami and the Bascom Palmer Eye Institute, vol. 7, St. Louis, 1973, The C. V. Mosby Co.

Lubow, M., and Adams, L.: The changing management of acute optic neuritis. In Smith, J. L., editor: Neuro-ophthalmology; Symposium of the University of Miami and the Bascom Palmer Eye Institute, vol. 6, St. Louis, 1972, The C. V. Mosby Co.

Phillips, C. I., Wang, M. K., and Van Peborgh, P. F.: Some observations on mechanism of tobacco amblyopia and its treatment with sodium thiosulfate, Trans. Ophthalmol. Soc. U.K. **90**:809, 1971.

Smith, J. L., and others: Sub-tenon steroid injection for optic neuritis, Trans. Am. Acad. Ophthalmol. Otolaryngol. **74**:1249, 1970.

Walsh, F. B., and Hoyt, W. F.: Clinical neuro-ophthalmology, vol. 1, ed. 3, Baltimore, 1969, The Williams & Wilkins Co.

CHAPTER 18

Therapy of diseases of the orbit

CELLULITIS

Cellulitis of the orbit is usually secondary to infection elsewhere in the body, most often of the paranasal sinuses, or is the result of trauma. It is always a serious disease and should be treated vigorously to avoid such complications as cavernous sinus thrombosis.

If the cellulitis is secondary to infection elsewhere in the body, therapy should be directed toward clearing the primary infection as well as treating the orbital process. Therapy consists of vigorous use of antibiotics administered systemically. If the causative organism is known, specific antibiotics against this organism should be used (Chapter 3). *Haemophilus influenzae* and *Diplococcus pneumoniae* have been found to be common pathogens in orbital cellulitis. If the causative organism has not been identified, treatment with broad-spectrum antibiotics or with a combination of penicillin and a broad-spectrum antibiotic is indicated. Therapy should continue until all signs of active inflammation have subsided, including the physical signs of inflammation, reduced white blood cell count, and normal temperature. In addition to the antibiotic therapy, hot compresses should be used almost continuously. Bed rest and general supportive measures should be prescribed.

In orbital cellulitis accompanied by cavernous sinus thrombosis, the treatment should be the massive use of antibiotics. If the causative organism is known, specific antibiotics are indicated. If the causative organism is unknown, it is well to institute treatment with broad-spectrum antibiotics. Some authors advise the intravenous administration of the newer synthetic penicillins in combination with the broad-spectrum antibiotics, plus the use of anticoagulants. Opinion seems to vary as to the actual value of anticoagulant treatment in this disorder. For the very ill patient, intravenous fluids and nasal oxygen should be used as supportive measures.

MYCOTIC INFECTIONS

Therapy against mycotic infections of the orbit should include the use of specific antifungus agents, the use of iodides, and possibly the use of radiation therapy. If the specific fungus organism is isolated, its sensitivity to the various chemotherapeutic agents should be determined. If the causative fungus cannot be isolated, fungistatic antibiotic therapy should be started with amphotericin

181

B, which is now the drug of choice in most of the orbital mycotic infections. The drug is given in an initial dose of 0.05 to 0.1 mg per kg of body weight, dissolved in 5% dextrose in water, by intravenous drip over a period of 3 to 6 hours. On the following day, or 48 hours later (depending on the severity of the infection), the dose of the drug is increased by 0.1 mg per kg of body weight, and this increase is repeated each day or every other day thereafter until a dosage of 1 mg per kg of body weight is reached. Generally, the total dose should not exceed 2 grams. The medication should be continued at that level until there is clinical response. In some patients this can be noted after a few days of treatment, but in others it may be necessary to continue the treatment for several weeks. The BUN level should be measured before treatment is started and at intervals while the patient is receiving the drug. If there is a sudden increase in the BUN level, the drug should be discontinued until the values are again within normal limits. Alternate-day therapy is much less toxic than daily therapy and should be used unless the infection is very severe, in which case daily therapy is advisable.

In addition to amphotericin B, flucytosine (Ancobon) and iodides are sometimes of value in the treatment of certain fungus infections. Flucytosine is effective against certain strains of *Candida, Cryptococcus, Torulopsis,* and *Aspergillus.* The medication is given orally in a daily dose of 50 to 200 mg per kg of body weight in three to four divided doses. Iodides are usually administered orally in the form of a saturated solution of potassium iodide, 5 to 10 drops in water three times a day, after meals. The concentration of the drug is gradually built up until the patient receives 20 drops three times a day. Once this drug level has been reached, the dose may be continued indefinitely, provided it is well tolerated. Sodium iodide, in doses of 15 grains three times a day, may be used instead of potassium iodide solution. With either iodide preparations, signs of iodism may occur at any time, and then the drug must be discontinued. If the patient shows no response to specific fungistatic antibiotics or to iodide therapy, x-ray treatment to the orbit may be of some value.

Orbital infections resulting from *Actinomyces* or *Nocardia* organisms should be treated with penicillin and sulfonamides. Strictly speaking, these are not true fungus infections, since these organisms fall somewhere between the fungi and the bacteria. These organisms usually respond to antibiotic therapy and are best treated with the penicillins or sulfonamide drugs, although often they are also responsive to broad-spectrum antibiotics.

MISCELLANEOUS GRANULOMATOUS DISEASES

Tuberculosis, syphilis, and sarcoidosis of the orbit are rare. Improvement of the disease of the orbit will follow successful treatment of the systemic disease. (See discussions of tuberculosis, syphilis, and sarcoidosis in Chapters 8 to 10, 12, and 16.)

PARASITIC INFECTIONS

The orbit may be involved in trichinosis, cysticercosis, echinococcosis, and onchocerciasis. The treatment of trichinosis in the chronic stage is purely symptomatic, with the use of salicylates or corticosteroids. Thiabendazole, an anthelmintic, has been reported to be effective in the treatment of trichinosis. A daily dose of 50 to 60 mg per kg of body weight is recommended. Cysticercosis and echinococcosis of the orbit are not amenable to medical therapy. Surgical removal of the lesions may become necessary. Onchocerciasis is treated by surgical removal of the involved areas, followed by the administration of diethylcarbamazine (Hetrazan) in an initial dose of 0.1 to 0.2 mg per kg of body weight. The dosage is gradually increased to 1 to 2 mg per kg of body weight over a period of 2 to 3 weeks. Allergic reactions that may develop as the microfilariae are killed can be controlled with antihistamines. Diethylcarbamazine applied topically has recently been demonstrated to penetrate the aqueous humor of rabbit eyes.

NONSPECIFIC INFLAMMATIONS
Pseudotumor

Pseudotumor of the orbit usually runs a limited course and will subside in time without any treatment. The problem in therapy is essentially that of making the correct diagnosis and differentiating the disease from other inflammatory or neoplastic conditions. The use of corticosteroids or corticotropic hormones seems to reduce the signs of inflammation for as long as the medication is continued. The response of the orbital inflammation to corticosteroid therapy is sometimes used to confirm the diagnosis. However, one must bear in mind that certain neoplasms, such as the lymphomas, might also regress under this form of therapy. X-ray therapy has been used for pseudotumor of the orbit but is now seldom prescribed. Response to x-ray therapy may be misleading in the management of this condition.

ENDOCRINE EXOPHTHALMOS
(GRAVES' DISEASE, MALIGNANT EXOPHTHALMOS)

Most cases of endocrine exophthalmos advance to a certain stage and then remain stationary or begin to resolve spontaneously. Mild forms of the disease can be treated with lubricant drops, and corticosteroid therapy is not indicated. Sleeping with the head elevated can reduce swelling and diplopia, which are usually exaggerated when the patient awakes. Wearing padded eye shields or taping the lids shut may alleviate lagophthalmos occurring during sleep.

The severe acute phases of this disease (severe proptosis with exposure keratitis, optic neuropathy, and glaucoma) can usually be managed with systemic corticosteroid therapy. Some patients show a response with doses of 40 to 60 mg of prednisone or its equivalent, but it is frequently necessary to employ doses of prednisone as high as 120 to 140 mg per day. It may be necessary to maintain a high steroid dosage for several weeks. Reduction of steroid dosage should be gradual. If flare-ups occur, it may be necessary to increase steroid dosage temporarily. With high doses of steroids, side effects are common (Chapter 2). Subconjunctival and retrobulbar injections of repository corticosteroids also have been successfully employed in some cases of progressive exophthalmos. Severe systemic reactions are reduced by this modality of drug administration. With steroid therapy the need for orbital decompression surgery has decreased, but this operation would still seem to have a place for patients unable to take or unresponsive to steroid therapy and for cosmetic purposes.

Systemic administration of such diuretics as hydrochlorothiazide (Hydrodiuril) may relieve some of the lid edema, conjunctival chemosis, and orbital swelling. They may be employed along with corticosteroids. Immunosuppressive therapy has been used successfully in a few cases of severe endocrine exophthalmos. As indicated elsewhere in this book, immunosuppressive therapy may produce serious complications, and the use of such drugs is not advisable for physicians unfamiliar with them.

Lid retraction associated with thyroid dysfunction may be temporarily relieved with the topical application of 5% to 10% guanethidine. The medication is instilled one to four times a day. Horner's syndrome is produced. While some patients respond to this therapy, many patients obtain little benefit from this treatment, and others discontinue the use of medication because of irritation. Unfortunately, no commercial preparation of guanethidine solution for topical ophthalmic use is available.

In the quiescent stage residuals of endocrine exophthalmia such as hypotropia, severe lid retraction, and orbital fat herniation may be treated surgically. Recession of the eyelid elevators often results in considerable improvement of lid retraction.

NEOPLASMS

Most neoplasms of the orbit are surgical or radiological conditions and are not successfully treated by any medical agents. In the treatment of primary or secondary orbital neoplasms, some of the chemotherapeutic agents are of value. These include the nitrogen mustards, chlorambucil (Leukeran), cyclophosphamide (Cytoxan), uracil nitrogen, actinomycin D, methotrexate, fluorouracil, vincristine, and androgenic and estrogenic hormones. Corticosteroids may be of value in the suppression of lymphomas of the orbit. In any event, consultation with an internist or a radiotherapist or both should be obtained if such agents are considered for the treatment of orbital lesions.

REFERENCES

Garber, M. I.: Methylprednisolone in the treatment of exophthalmos, Lancet **1**:958, 1966.
Gay, A. J., and Wolkstein, M. A.: Topical quanethidine therapy for endocrine lid retraction, Arch. Ophthalmol. **76**:364, 1966.
Henderson, J. W.: Orbital tumors, Philadelphia, 1973, W. B. Saunders Co.

Kramar, P.: Management of eye changes of Grave's disease, Surv. Ophthalmol. **18**:369, 1974.

Lazar, M., and others: Ocular penetration of Hetrazan in rabbits, Am. J. Ophthalmol. **66**:215, 1968.

Schimek, R. A.: Surgical management of ocular complications in Grave's disease, Arch. Ophthalmol. **87**:655, 1972.

Sneddon, J. M., and Turner, P.: Adrenergic blockade and the eye signs of thyrotoxicosis, Lancet **2**:525, 1966.

Trokel, S. L.: The orbit; annual review, Arch. Ophthalmol. **91**:223, 1974.

Watters, E. C., Wallar, H., Hiles, D. A., and Michaels, R. H.: Acute orbital cellulitis, Arch. Ophthalmol. **94**:785, 1976.

Werner, S. C.: Prednisone in emergency treatment of malignant exophthalmos, Lancet **1**:1004, 1966.

Werner, S. C., and Ingabar, S. H.: The thyroid; a fundamental and clinical text, ed. 3, New York, 1971, Harper & Row.

CHAPTER 19

Therapy of miscellaneous ophthalmic diseases

DISEASES OF THE EXTRAOCULAR MUSCLES

The treatment of extraocular muscle disorders is primarily outside the realm of medical agents. Mention is made here only of the drugs used in the treatment of strabismus and for the pharmacological tests for myasthenia gravis and of the possible value of topical anticholinesterase therapy for certain forms of ptosis.

Miotics and strabismus

Accommodative esotropia can sometimes be helped with miotic therapy. It is not generally advisable to substitute miotics for glasses or to continue miotic therapy indefinitely in the treatment of accommodative esotropia. However, there may be specific reasons for employment of miotics, which act by improving the accommodative convergence/accommodation ratio.

The stronger cholinesterase inhibitors are the most effective miotics in the treatment of strabismus. Isoflurophate (DFP) in a 0.025% solution may be used daily or every other day. Demecarium bromide (Humorsol) in 0.12% solution or echothiophate (Phospholine) iodide in 0.03% to 0.125% solution may be used daily or every other day instead of the DFP. There may be severe irritation of the eye after instillation. Many side reactions to this treatment have been noted, particularly headaches, ciliary spasm, and cysts of the iris in the form of pigment hypertrophy at the pupillary margin. The incidence of iris cysts after echothiophate iodide therapy may be greatly reduced by using 2.5% phenylephrine (Neo-Synephrine) as the diluent. Intermittent topical application of epinephrine reduces the incidence of cyst formation with DFP therapy. Sometimes there is enough absorption of the cholinesterase inhibitor to produce systemic signs of cholinesterase inhibition or an acetylcholinelike poisoning. These signs include sweating, tachycardia, nausea following stomach cramps, and diarrhea. It is important to realize that topical application of echothiophate iodide lowers systemic levels of pseudocholinesterase. This enzyme inactivates succinylcholine, which is a muscle relaxant used as an aid in intubation during general anesthesia. The use of succinylcholine in patients with lowered pseudocholinesterase levels may result in prolonged apnea. If strabismus surgery is planned for children treated with echothiophate iodide, succinylcholine should not be used; alternatively, the miotic should be discontinued 6 weeks before surgery.

Pharmacological test for myasthenia gravis

Edrophonium chloride (Tensilon) is the drug most commonly used to substantiate the diagnosis of myasthenia gravis. A test dose of 10 mg is given intravenously over a period of 1 minute. A positive test consists of improvement of the extraocular muscle strength, usually lasting for several minutes. Neostigmine, 0.5 mg, may be administered intravenously instead of edrophonium chloride.

Cholinesterase inhibitor to reduce ptosis of eyelid in myasthenia gravis

The use of strong cholinesterase inhibitors as eye drops has been reported to improve the ptosis of myasthenia gravis. Either DFP or demecarium bromide may be used. Of the two, demecarium bromide is preferable, since it is a specific antiacetylcholinesterase. The application of these agents has been suggested as a means of treating very mild cases of myasthenia gravis, in which the only significant muscular involvement is a minimal ptosis of the eyelids.

Lid retraction in Graves' disease

The application of topical 5% to 10% guanethidine one to four times a day will often temporarily relieve lid retraction in Graves' disease. Guanethidine is a sympatholytic agent, which, applied topically to the eye, relieves the increased sympathotonia of Müller's smooth muscle. A miosis also occurs. This treatment is less effective in patients who are still thyrotoxic or are receiving sympathomimetic drugs for their systemic disease.

PHARMACOLOGICAL TESTS FOR PUPILLARY ABNORMALITIES

Tonic pupil, known as Adie's syndrome when associated with hypoactive tendon reflexes, is characterized by decreased pupillary light reflexes. When 2.5% methacholine (Mecholyl) is instilled into the eye, pupillary constriction occurs. This drug does not produce miosis of the normal pupil. Similarly, the instillation of 0.0625% pilocarpine produces significant miosis of an Adie's pupil, whereas it produces little or no miosis of a normal pupil.

Horner's syndrome is characterized by ptosis, miosis, enophthalmos, and anhidrosis of the face on the involved inside. It is caused by a lesion of the sympathetic pathways. If the lesion occurs in the superior cervical ganglion or the fibers running to the pupil, mydriasis occurs after instillation of 1:1,000 epinephrine or 1% phenylephrine but not after instillation of 4% cocaine or 1% hydroxyamphetamine (Paredrine). The latter drug produces mydriasis only when the postganglionic neuron is intact. Cocaine mydriasis is absent with both pre- and postganglionic lesions but may be present with lesions of the brainstem and spinal cord.

TEMPORAL ARTERITIS (GIANT CELL ARTERITIS)

Treatment of temporal arteritis consists of the early use of high intensive doses of systemically administered corticosteroids or corticotropic hormones. These agents are seldom helpful in improving the condition in the involved optic nerve, but there is good evidence that they are of value in preventing the processes from involving the other eye. Therapy with corticosteroids should be continued as long as there is evidence of active arteritis, as indicated by elevated erythrocyte sedimentation rate. It should be appreciated that some patients may maintain high erythrocyte sedimentation rates without active arteritis.

JUVENILE XANTHOGRANULOMA (NEVOXANTHOENDOTHELIOMA)

Juvenile xanthogranuloma is a benign disorder occurring in infants and young children and is characterized by yellow, elevated, papular lesions of the skin mainly in the head and neck regions but also occurring less commonly on the trunk and extremities. The ocular involvement usually is in the form of an iris lesion, varying in color from salmon to tan or brown. Hyphema, uveitis, and glaucoma may occur.

The treatment employed for this disorder has varied considerably. Surgical excision of the lesion has been advocated, but this is probably unnecessary. Regression of the iris lesion occurs with low-dose irradiation. Good results recently have been reported with the topical and systemic use of corticosteroids.

MELANOMAS

Surgical excision is usually the treatment of choice for ocular melanomas. Some benefits have been reported from the use of photocoagulation in small melanomas. Bischloroethyl nitrosourea (BCNU) has been used in the treatment of uveal melanomas. Among other chemotherapeutic agents employed with some limited success in malignant melanoma are imidazole carboxamide and vincristine. Cobalt irradiation has been successfully used in the treatment of small choroidal melanomas.

VITREOUS DISORDERS
Degenerative conditions

Degenerative conditions of the vitreous may be secondary to chronic low-grade uveitis or systemic disease. If so, the basic problem should be treated. Efforts should be directed toward an overall improvement in the patient's general health and an attempts to reduce any inflammation present in the choroid or retina. Senile and myopic vitreous degenerations are not responsive to any therapy.

Hemorrhage

Vitreous hemorrhage may result from systemic diseases that affect the integrity of the retinal vessels, such as diabetes, hypertension, and blood dyscrasias.

It may also result from inflammation of the retinal vessels, arteritis, or phlebitis; it may also be seen in peripheral degenerations of the retina; and it may precede retinal detachment. There is no specific therapy for vitreous hemorrhage. Treatment must be directed toward the systemic disease, and proper surgical procedure should be done if retinal detachment has occurred. Photocoagulation is indicated for localized retinovascular anomalies (telangiectases, neovascularization, aneurysms) from which vitreous hemorrhages are occurring. Vitrectomy may be of benefit in selected cases where there has been no clearing of blood after prolonged time periods.

CATARACTS

Cataracts may develop secondary to many systemic diseases such as diabetes, myotonia atopia, idiopathic hypercalcemia, or galactosemia. If one of these conditions is present, the appropriate medical therapy should be undertaken. Specific metabolic disease is not known to be responsible for the development of senile or presenile cataracts. However, it is quite likely that lens changes result from altered metabolism. Many agents to improve lens metabolism have been suggested, including the topical use of irritants such as ethylmorphine hydrochloride (Dionin) and agents containing a high concentration of a sulfhydryl radical. There is little evidence that these agents are of any benefit.

MIGRAINE

Migraine is a common disorder characterized by paroxysms of headache, visual disturbance, nausea, and vomiting. There is often a family history of this disease. Migraine attacks may be prevented by the oral administration of methysergide (Sansert), 2 mg with each meal. This drug can be quite toxic and is not required by most patients. Continuous administration should not exceed 6 months. Mild attacks of migraine can be managed by sedatives and tranquilizers. Acute attacks may be relieved by the sublingual or oral administration of ergotamine tartrate (Gynergen) or ergotamine tartrate with caffeine (Cafergot), particularly if used early in the attack. Doses larger than 6 mg per day or 12 mg per week should be avoided because of toxicity. For the severe attack, intramuscular injections of ergotamine tartrate or dihydroergotamine tartrate or dihydroergotamine may be necessary. Recently two antihypertensive drugs, propranolol and clonidine, have been found to be effective for preventing attacks of migraine in some patients. Propranolol is used in a daily dose of 40 to 60 mg; clonidine dosage is $50\mu g$ to $100\mu g$ daily.

HEPATOLENTICULAR DEGENERATION (WILSON'S DISEASE)

Hepatolenticular degeneration is a disease of copper toxicity resulting from an inherited defect of copper metabolism. Various tissues of the body, particularly the brain and the liver, become saturated with copper, and the patient develops neurological manifestations. The chief ocular finding is a Kayser-

Fleischer ring, a yellow-brown ring in the periphery of the cornea that results from fine copper deposits in the deep stroma and Descemet's membrane.

Modern treatment consists of reducing copper intake and administering penicillamine, a chelating agent, in daily divided doses of 1 to 4 grams. With this therapy many of the manifestations of hepatolenticular degeneration, including the Kayser-Fleischer rings, may disappear.

TRIGEMINAL NEURALGIA

Phenytoin, in large doses of 300 to 400 mg daily, relieves trigeminal neuralgia in a few patients. The dose should be kept just below toxic levels.

Carbamazepine (Tegretol) is a recently introduced drug that is effective in the treatment of trigeminal neuralgia. The drug is more useful for the treatment of primary trigeminal neuralgia than for the treatment of secondary trigeminal neuralgias such as those following herpes zoster. A dosage of 600 to 1,200 mg daily is effective during acute attacks. Maintenance doses of 400 to 800 mg daily usually prevent further attacks. Occasionally serious hematological effects may occur with carbamazepine therapy (see section on therapeutic agents).

PROSTHETIC EYES

Many patients with prosthetic eyes are troubled with mucoid discharge and irritation. Primary consideration in the management of such symptoms should be the proper fitting of the prosthesis and the elimination of any infectious process.

The patient should be instructed in the care of the prosthesis. Lee Allen advises that the artificial eye be removed only for cleaning; this may be necessary once a week or once a month. If the lids close well at night, he recommends Enuclene eye drops three or four times a day for lubrication; if the eyes do not close well at night, silicone solutions, 100 centistokes, should be used. When the artificial eye becomes crusted, it should be removed and washed with soap and water. If the crust cannot be removed in this manner, soaking a plastic eye in a dentifrice for artificial teeth (Polident) for 30 minutes will remove the deposits effectively.

TRAUMATIC HYPHEMA

Treatment of traumatic hyphema is directed toward preventing recurrent or secondary hemorrhage, controlling intraocular pressure, preventing corneal blood staining, and treating iritis and associated ocular injuries. Classically, the treatment has consisted of hospitalization with bed rest and binocular patches for 5 days. If no secondary hemorrhage occurs and there has been some absorption of blood and if the intraocular pressure has remained normal, the patient is discharged and followed as an outpatient. Gonioscopy is performed at a later date to rule out angle recession, and a complete eye examination is performed, including indirect ophthalmoscopy, to rule out other possible co-existing injuries.

Disagreement exists regarding the value of bed rest and binocular patching. Some physicians contend that this treatment offers little or no advantage over no patching or unilateral patching and minor restriction of activity, while other physicians indicate many fewer complications with binocular patching and bed rest. Part of the differences in opinion probably result from the types of cases studied. The prognosis for hyphemas of less than one-half anterior chamber depth are excellent, while larger hyphemas have a poorer prognosis. Recent hyphemas (within 24 hours) have a better prognosis than older hyphemas. In small hyphemas, binocular patching and absolute bed rest may not be essential.

Some physicians have suggested the use of either miotics or mydriatics. Most recent studies have indicated that they are of no value in the treatment of small hyphemas and may be harmful in the treatment of larger hyphemas.

If glaucoma develops, it should be treated medically, preferably with osmotherapeutic agents, although carbonic anhydrase inhibitors may also be used (Chapter 13). If the intraocular pressure cannot be controlled with medical agents, surgical treatment may be undertaken, either by wide incision and irrigation or cryosurgical removal of the clot or by fibrinolysin irrigation of the anterior chamber. Surgical removal of the hyphema may also be indicated despite normal pressure if total hyphema persists for several days without some evidence of hemolysis. Blood staining of the cornea occurs rarely without elevated intraocular pressure.

Iritis can usually be managed with topical application of corticosteroids. Mydriatics should be avoided for the first 5 to 7 days of treatment.

Preliminary studies have suggested that secondary hemorrhages in traumatic hyphema can be reduced with the administration of aminocaproic acid, an antifibrinolytic agent. The rationale for the use of this drug is that it deters lysis of the initial clot until the primary ruptured vessels regain their integrity. The medication is given orally in a dose of 100 mg per kg every 4 hours for 5 days.

IRON DEPOSITS

Recently deferoxamine (Desferal) has been employed for the treatment of iron deposits in the eye. For the treatment of superficial iron deposits in the cornea, a 10% solution of deferoxamine in 1% methylcellulose is used four times a day for several weeks. Alternatively, the drug may be applied in a 5% concentration in any ointment base. For iron deposits in the deeper layers of the cornea and in the iris and lens, 0.5 ml of a 10% solution is injected subconjunctivally twice a week for 8 to 10 weeks.

REFERENCES

Allen, L.: Personal communication, 1966.

Amols, W.: A new drug for trigeminal neuralgia; clinical experience with carbamazepine in a large series of patients over 2 years, Trans. Am. Neurol. Assoc. 91:163, 1966.

Chin, W. B., Gold, A. A., and Breinen, G. B.: Iris cysts and miotics, Arch. Ophthalmol. 71: 611, 1964.

Cohen, D. N., and Zakov, Z. W.: The diagnosis of Adie's pupil using 0.0625% pilocarpine solution, Am. J. Ophthalmol. 79:883, 1975.

Crouch, E. R., and Frenkel, M.: Aminocaproic acid in the treatment of traumatic hyphema, Am. J. Ophthalmol. 81:355, 1976.

Galin, M. A., Harris, L. S., and Papariello, G. J.: Nonsurgical removal of rust stains, Arch. Ophthalmol. 74:674, 1965.

Gay, A. J., and Wolkstein, M. A.: Topical guanethidine therapy for endocrine lid retraction, Arch. Ophthalmol. 76:364, 1966.

Giles, C. L., and Westerberg, M. R.: Clinical evaluation of local ocular anticholinesterase agents in myasthenia gravis, Am. J. Ophthalmol. 52:331, 1961.

Lommatzsch, P.: Treatment of choroidal melanomas with [106]Ru, [106]Rh Beta-ray applicators, Surv. Ophthalmol. 19:85, 1974.

The Medical Letter on Drugs and Therapeutics, vol. 10, No. 13, June 28, 1968.

Pilger, I. S.: Medical treatment of traumatic hyphema, Surv. Ophthalmol. 20:28, 1975.

Schwartz, L. W., Rodrigues, M. M., and Hallett, J. W.: Juvenile xanthogranuloma diagnosed by paracentesis, Am. J. Ophthalmol. 77:243, 1974.

Stark, W. J., and others: Simultaneous bilateral uveal melanomas responding to BCNU therapy, Trans. Am. Acad. Ophthalmol. Otolaryngol. 75:70, 1971.

Sternlieb, I., and Scheinberg, H.: Penicillamine therapy for hepatolenticular degeneration, J.A.M.A. 189:146, 1964.

Thompson, H. S., and Mensher, J. H.: Adrenergic mydriasis in Horner's syndrome; hydroxy-amphetamine test for diagnosis of postganglionic defects, Am. J. Ophthalmol. 72:472, 1971.

Wise, J. B. Treatment of experimental siderosis bulbi, vitreous hemorrhage, and corneal bloodstaining with deferoxamine, Arch. Ophthalmol. 75:698, 1966.

THERAPEUTIC AGENTS

Attention is directed to the dosage
schedules for the drugs described in this
section. Unless otherwise stated, the
dosage given is for adults. Methods of
calculating pediatric dosage and
pediatric dosage tables of the commonly
used drugs are given at the end
of the section.

ANALGESICS

Analgesics are freqently classified as strong or mild depending on the severity of pain they relieve. Pain is a very subjective symptom, and individual response to drugs is highly variable. Analgesics produce their effect primarily by their action on the central nervous system; some drugs such as aspirin have additional peripheral effects that may reduce pain. In addition to raising the threshold of pain perception, strong analgesics may alter the patient's psychological response to pain.

STRONG ANALGESICS

Strong analgesics may be divided into two major groups: narcotic and non-narcotic. Drug dependence is produced by the narcotic group, and these agents are regulated under the Drug Abuse and Control Act.

Strong narcotics should not be used to treat mild pain that can be relieved with weaker drugs. All strong narcotics are compared with morphine, which is the prototype. Although strong narcotics are extremely valuable agents in relieving severe pain from a variety of causes, they produce many adverse reactions that limit their usefulness. These include respiratory depression, hypotension, bradycardia, nausea, vomiting, drug dependence, rise in intracranial pressure, spasm of the biliary and urinary tracts, and occasional hypersensitivity reactions (see individual agents).

Anileridine (Leritine)

Actions. Anileridine is a nonopiate-addicting analgesic with minimal sedative and hypnotic effects. The analgesic action is of relatively short duration. In equal amounts the drug is twice as potent as meperidine and one fourth as potent as morphine. The constipative effects common to the opiates are not observed with anileridine. The drug is useful in the relief of moderate pain, but it does not relieve severe pain as effectively as morphine does. Anileridine is used as an adjunct in general anesthesia to reduce the quantity of anesthetic required. It is also useful for the relief of postoperative pain. Addiction liability of anileridine is equivalent to that of morphine, and the drug is controlled by the federal narcotics law.

Adverse effects. Less nausea and vomiting occur with anileridine than with morphine in equianalgesic doses. Respiratory depression and circulatory depression occur to a much lesser degree than with morphine, although these do occur, especially in elderly patients or after too rapid injection. Undesirable side effects, especially undue respiratory depression, may be relieved by the administration of nalorphine.

Preparations. Preparations include the following: anileridine phosphate solution for injection, 25 mg in 1 ml, 50 mg in 2 ml, and 750 mg in 30 ml; anileridine hydrochloride for oral administration, tablets, 25 mg.

Dosage. The dosage for injection is as follows: if given intramuscularly or subcutaneously, initial dose is 25 to 50 mg, repeated in 4 to 6 hours as needed; if given intravenously, 50 to 100 mg, dissolved in 500 ml of 5% dextrose in water. Initially, this solution is given by slow infusion to provide 5 to 10 mg of the drug; this is followed by an intravenous drip to provide 0.6 mg of the drug per minute. Direct intravenous administration of concentrated solution should be accomplished with great caution, and no more than 10 mg should be injected at any one time.

Meperidine hydrochloride (Demerol)

Meperidine hydrochloride is a synthetic analgesic drug of the nonopiate narcotic type.

Actions. Meperidine is approximately one tenth as potent an analgesic as morphine. Analgesia is acompanied by euphoria, and the additive liability is high. Less sedation and less respiratory depression occur than with equianalgesic doses of morphine. Meperidine may exhibit summative effects with the ultrashort-acting barbiturates and gaseous anesthetics.

Adverse effects. Addiction to meperidine occurs after prolonged high dosage. Vertigo, nausea and vomiting, and occasional syncope with hypotension may be observed after administration of the drug. Overdosage may result in tremors, incoordination, and convulsions. Meperidine is contraindicated in patients suffering from shock, severe liver dysfunction, and increased intracranial pressure and after cholecystectomy.

Preparations. Preparations include the following: tablets, 50 and 100 mg; sterile solution, 50, 75, and 100 mg per ml; elixir, 10 mg per ml.

Dosage. The dosage is 50 to 150 mg for analgesia; doses larger than 100 mg are seldom necessary.

Morphine

Actions. The analgesic action of morphine is threefold: an increase in threshold of pain stimulation, a change in the appreciation of pain (euphoria), and sedation. Morphine is unsurpassed as an analgesic for moderate to severe pain.

Adverse effects. Side effects include respiratory depression, nausea and vomiting (especially in ambulatory patients), ureteral and common duct spasm, and constipation. These effects are not prominent in short-term use of analgesic dosage in the presence of pain. Nausea and vomiting occur frequently with oral administration, and parenteral use is almost always indicated. If morphine is to be used as a preoperative agent for patients undergoing intraocular surgery, a test dose should be given 1 or 2 days before surgery to ensure that the patient will not develop nausea and vomiting as a sensitivity reaction.

Very large doses of morphine for extremely severe pain must be administered cautiously if there is a possibility of sudden decrease in the severity of the pain, as in coronary occlusion or biliary colic. Depressant effects of morphine may be reversed in cases of overdosage by the administration of equivalent amounts of nalorphine, the demethylated allyl derivative of morphine.

Preparations. Preparations include the following: hypodermic tablets, 8, 10, 15, and 30 mg; for injection, 8, 10, 15, and 20 mg per ml.

Dosage. The dosage is 10 to 15 mg by injection as required to relieve pain.

MILD ANALGESICS

Mild analgesics include agents such as codeine and propoxyphene (Darvon), which are related to the stronger analgesics and the analgesic-antipruritic drugs such as aspirin. The mode of action of these two groups of drugs is quite diverse. In this section only the first group of drugs is presented. Aspirin and related drugs such as indomethacin and phenylbutazone, which possess anti-inflammatory effects, are considered under the section on anti-inflammatory drugs. Agents such as phenacetin and acetaminophin, which possess analgesic and antipruritic properties similar to aspirin but do not possess anti-inflammatory properties, are not listed since they are seldom used in ophthalmology.

Codeine

Codeine is a narcotic analgesic, a methylated derivative of morphine.

Actions. The analgesic action of codeine is approximately one sixth as potent as that of morphine. Codeine is effective against mild pain and is less addictive, less emetic, and less constipating than morphine. Codeine has an effective antitussive action. Its major uses are as an analgesic and as a depressant of the cough reflex.

Adverse effects. Codeine is more excitatory than morphine and may cause convulsive episodes in children. Addictive liability is much lower than with morphine, but addiction may occur after prolonged use. Rarely, exfoliative dermatitis may be observed.

Preparations. Preparations include the following: codeine sulfate or codeine phosphate, tablets and capsules, 8, 15, 30, and 60 mg; codeine phosphate solutions for injection, 15, 30, and 60 mg per ml; syrup, 2 mg per ml.

Dosage. The dosage for analgesia for adults is 10 to 60 mg given orally or hypodermically; for depression of cough reflex, 8 mg three to four times daily.

Pentazocine (Talwin)

Actions. Pentazocine is a synthetic analgesic with no significant anti-inflammatory or antipyretic effects. It appears to have approximately the same analgesic potency of codeine. The drug is useful for the relief of moderate pain of all types. It is not recommended for children under 12 years of age. The addiction potential of the drug is less than that of morphine and meperidine.

Adverse effects. Side reactions include dizziness, vertigo, nausea, and headache. Less frequent reactions include neuromuscular disturbances, sweating, weakness, and gastrointestinal disturbances. Like other analgesics, this drug must be used with caution in patients with intracranial disease.

Preparations. Pentazocine is prepared in the form of 50-mg tablets and in 1- and 10-ml ampuls containing 30 mg per ml.

Dosage. The usual oral dosage is 50 mg every 3 or 4 hours as needed. Doses of 100 mg may be necessary in some patients. The usual parenteral dose is 30 mg.

Propoxyphene hydrochloride (Darvon)

Actions. Propoxyphene hydrochloride is a synthetic nonantipyretic analgesic of approximately one half to two thirds of the analgesic potency of codeine. Because of its low analgesic potency, the drug is not suitable for use in moderate to severe pain. It does not depress respiration or circulation. It produces fewer gastrointestinal disturbances than codeine. It may be used in combination with anti-inflammatory agents for the treatment of rheumatoid arthritis. It is useful in patients in whom blood coagulation problems preclude the use of salicylates. Because propoxyphene hydrochloride will suppress abstinence symptoms in morphine addiction, it is regulated by the federal narcotics law, although its addictive liability is apparently less than that of codeine. The drug is administered only by the oral route because of local tissue irritation after parenteral use.

Adverse effects. The side effects are few. Occasional nausea, dizziness, and drowsiness may occur; infrequently, hypersensitivity and idiosyncrasy may be noted.

Preparations. It is prepared in the form of capsules, 32 and 65 mg, alone or combined with aspirin, phenacetin, and caffeine.

Dosage. The dosage is 32 to 65 mg as needed for relief of pain, either alone or with other medication.

ANESTHETICS

Local anesthetics produce a transient and reversible loss of sensation in the area where they are administered. (For further information see Chapter 6.) Local anesthetics may interfere with nerve conduction in one or more ways. Basically they block nerve conduction by interfering with depolarization so that threshold potential is not reached and nerve action potential does not occur. The apparent primary mechanism for this is a reduction of the permeability of the cell membrane to sodium ions.

Local anesthetics have effects on the cardiovascular and central nervous systems. They are sometimes used to treat cardiac arrythmias. At toxic levels vasodilatation and decreased myocardial contractility occur. Hypotension, depressed cardiac conduction, and cardiac arrest may occur.

Toxicity to the central nervous system may initially take the form of stimulation, which is manifested by tremors, shivering, and convulsions. With higher doses, depression of the central nervous system with subsequent respiratory depression may occur.

Epinephrine is frequently added to local anesthetics to prolong their duration of action. The vasoconstrictive action of epinephrine decreases absorption of anesthetic solutions and thus prolongs their effect. Hyaluronidase may be added to anesthetic solutions to enhance the infiltration of the anesthetic.

The pharmacological activitiy of topical anesthetics is similar to that of other local anesthetics. Some injectable agents such as tetracaine and lidocaine have surface anesthetic activity, whereas other drugs such as procaine have no significant topical anesthetic effects. The most common topical agents in ophthalmology are proparacaine 0.5% (Ophthaine, Ophthetic, and Alcaine), benoxinate 0.4% (Dorsacaine), tetracaine 0.5% (Pontocaine), and cocaine 0.5%. The amount of the drug absorbed after topical application is so small that systemic side reactions do not occur. However, local side effects may occur and include allergic reactions of the conjunctiva and eyelid, corneal epithelial edema, and initial discomfort after instillation.

LOCAL ANESTHETICS
Bupivacaine (Marcaine)

Bupivacaine is a long-acting amide-type anesthetic.

Actions. Like all local anesthetics, bupivacaine stabilizes the neural membrane and decreases and prevents transmission of nerve impulses. The onset of action is slightly slower than that of procaine or lidocaine, but it persists much longer, for periods of 3 to 6 hours or more. The addition of epinephrine 1:200,000 prolongs the anesthetic time. The drug does not diffuse into tissues as readily as does procaine or lidocaine, and placement of the injection of the drug must be more precise when used as an ophthalmic local anesthetic. Bupivacaine produces some pain when injected. Some ophthalmologists have combined the use of bupivacaine with other local anesthetics such as mepivacaine (Carbocaine) in an endeavor to achieve the desirable properties of each.

Adverse effects. Reactions to bupivacaine are usually due to overdosage. Central nervous system toxicity may take the form of depression but more commonly presents as excitement and convulsions. Short-acting barbiturates or muscle relaxants should be administered intravenously for the treatment of convulsions. Cardiovascular manifestations of hypotension, bradycardia, and even cardiac arrest require prompt supportive measures—intravenously administered fluids, vasopressor drugs, oxygen, and cardiac massage. Local allergic reactions may occur.

Preparations. Solutions are available in single- and multiple-dose containers in concentrations of 0.25%, 0.50%, and 0.75%, with and without epinephrine 1:200,000.

Dosage. The lowest dosage that provides satisfactory anesthesia should be employed. The 0.75% solution has been used most frequently in ophthalmology. The maximum safe dose in an adult is 250 mg with epinephrine and 200 mg without epinephrine.

Lidocaine hydrochloride (Xylocaine)

Lidocaine is a rapid-acting, general-purpose local anesthetic approximately twice as potent as procaine and of equal toxicity in low concentrations.

Actions. Lidocaine imparts a prompt and extensive local anesthetic action upon infiltration or nerve block or upon topical application to mucous membranes. Although the toxicity of the drug is equivalent to that of procaine at 0.5% concentration, it is 50% more toxic than procaine at 2% concentration. No vasoconstriction accompanies the anesthetic action of lidocaine. Thus epinephrine may be added to reduce the role of absorption and toxicity and to prolong the anesthetic action. Lidocaine is effective when employed without a vasoconstrictor. It is especially useful in individuals sensitive to epinephrine and other pressor amines or to procaine and related anesthetics.

Adverse effects. The incidence of side effects is very low, and very few systemic reactions have been observed. Patients often show signs of drowsiness after they have been given lidocaine without epinephrine for regional or nerve block anesthesia. Toxicity, which usually develops only with overdosage, is manifested by hypotension, nausea, hyperhidrosis, muscular twitching, and convulsions. Hypotension may occur during spinal anesthesia induced with lidocaine.

Cardiovascular collapse may occur as an idiosyncratic reaction and demands immediate supportive therapy—oxygen, vasopressor drugs, intravenous fluids, and cardiac massage if indicated. Central nervous system toxicity should be treated with short-acting, intravenously administered barbiturates.

Preparations. Preparations include: solution used parenterally, 0.5%, 1%, 1.5%, 2%, and 4%; and 0.5%, 1%, 1.5%, and 2% with epinephrine 1:100,000 or 1:200,000; solution used intravenously, 2%; solution used topically, 4%; jelly, 2%; ointment, 2.5% and 5%; suppositories, 100 mg.

Dosage. The dosage for infiltration anesthesia is 0.5% with or without epinephrine 2 to 50 ml; for nerve block anesthesia, 1% or 2% solution, 1 to 30 ml, with or without epinephrine; for topical anesthesia to mucous membranes, 1% or 2% solution, 4% only when lower concentrations are ineffective. Maximum safe dosage is 7.5 mg per kg of body weight when used with epinephrine; without epinephrine maximum safe dosage is 5 mg per kg of body weight.

Mepivacaine (Carbocaine) hydrochloride

Actions. Mepivacaine hydrochloride is a local anesthetic structurally related to lidocaine. It is about equal in potency and toxicity to lidocaine but has a longer effect than lidocaine. Epinephrine is not needed to provide longer duration of effect, and this agent may be useful when epinephrine is not advisable.

Adverse effects. The incidence of side rections is low, and reactions probably occur with the same frequency as with lidocaine. They include nausea, vomiting, muscular contractions, convulsions, hypotension, and respiratory failure. Convulsions should be treated with an ultrashort-acting barbiturate such as thiopental or a muscle relaxant such as succinylcholine. The hypotensive reaction is treated with vasopressor drugs. Oxygen should be administered for respiratory distress.

Preparations. Preparations include the following: solution for injection, 1%, 1.5%, 2% and 3%; solution for spinal anesthesia, 4%; 2% with vasoconstrictor levonordefrin 1:20,000.

Dosage. For infiltration anesthesia the dosage is 1% solution, 15 to 30 ml; 1.5% solution, 10 to 15 ml; 2% solution, 10 to 20 ml. Not more than 8 mg per kg of body weight should be injected in a single dose.

Prilocaine (Citanest) hydrochloride

Actions. Prilocaine hydrochloride is a local anesthetic chemically related to lidocaine. Prilocaine has a somewhat longer latent period than lidocaine, but it has a considerably longer duration of effect. The drug does not diffuse into tissues as well as lidocaine; therefore, some anesthesiologists believe it is not as useful for infiltration anesthesia as lidocaine. Epinephrine is not needed to provide longer duration of effect, and the agent may be useful when epinephrine therapy is not advisable.

Adverse effects. Prilocaine is relatively less toxic than lidocaine. The side reactions include nausea, drowsiness, tremors, nervousness, convulsions, hypotension, and respiratory failure. Management of convulsions consists of the intravenous injection of an ultrashort-acting barbiturate such as thiopental or a muscle relaxant such as succinylcholine. Vasopressor drugs are indicated if severe hypotension occurs. Oxygen therapy should be given for respiratory distress.

Methemoglobinemia may occur with prilocaine from a metabolite of the drug o-toluidine. At the usual dosage this is generally of no significance. However, in patients with idiopathic methemoglobinemia, anemia, or cardiac failure, the possibility of potential danger should be considered. The symptoms of methemoglobinemia can be reversed with intravenous injection of 1% methylene blue in a dose of 1 to 2 mg per kg of body weight.

Preparations. Preparations include solution for injection, 1%, 2%, and 3%.

Dosage. For infiltration anesthesia the dosage is 1% or 2%, 20 to 30 ml. For nerve block anesthesia the dosage is 1% or 2%, 3 to 5 ml. The maximum recommended single dose is 8 mg per kg of body weight.

Procaine hydrochloride (Novocain)

Procaine hydrochloride is one of the most effective and least toxic local anesthetics. It is not surface active.

Actions. Procaine hydrochloride induces a local anesthetic action of short to moderate duration upon infiltration or introduction into the spinal canal, epidural space, or paravertebral area. Because of its low penetrating power, the drug is not active on topical application. Epinephrine is usually employed with procaine to produce a local vasoconstriction in order to slow the absorption of procaine from the tissues. As a result, the duration of the analgesic action is extended, and the potential toxicity of the anesthetic is reduced. Vasoconstrictors are sometimes administered to reduce the vasodepression that may result from the use of procaine as a spinal anesthetic. Procaine and sulfonamide derivatives are mutually antagonistic. Procaine has also been employed intravenously for systemic analgesia, but the merits of this type of therapy are currently in doubt.

Adverse effects. Toxicity of procaine is expressed as central nervous system stimulation followed by depression. This effect may be prevented or ameliorated by short-acting barbiturates. Cardiovascular collapse can occur as an idiosyncratic reaction in unduly sensitive patients. Such a reaction requires immediate supportive therapy: oxygen, vasopressor drugs, intravenous fluids, and cardiac massage if indicated.

Procaine probably should not be used for analgesia in situations requiring effective utilization of sulfonamides.

Preparations. Preparations include the following: ampuls containing sterile crystals, 50, 150, 200, 300, and 500 mg, and 1 gram; solutions used parenterally, 0.5%, 1%, 1.5%, 2%, 1% with ephedrine 2.5%, 1% with ephedrine 5%, 1.5% with epinephrine 1:200,000 or 1:750,000, 2% with epinephrine 1:20,000 or 1:50,000 or 1:75,000; solution for spinal anesthesia, 10%.

Dosage. The dosage is as follows: for infiltration anesthesia, solutions of 0.25% to 0.5% with epinephrine; for nerve block, 1% or 2% solution with epinephrine; for spinal anesthesia, 50 to 200 mg; maximum safe dose equals 15 mg per kg of body weight.

TOPICAL ANESTHETICS
Benoxinate (Dorsacaine)

Benoxinate, a benzoic acid derivative, is a surface-active local anesthetic.

Actions. Benoxinate is an effective local anesthetic. The onset of surface anesthesia in the eye is rapid, and the duration is approximately 20 minutes. The toxicity of benoxinate is similar to that of tetracaine (Pontocaine) hydrochloride. The drug is employed exclusively as a topical agent in the eye.

Ophthalmic uses. The rapid onset and relatively short duration of the effective anesthesia produced by this drug contribute to its usefulness in ophthalmology. Short operative procedures, tonometry, removal of foreign bodies, and gonioscopy may be accomplished using benoxinate as the analgesic agent.

Adverse effects. The incidence of side reactions after topical application to the eye is very low. Only slight irritation follows topical instillation. Mild superficial corneal edema occurs rarely. Accommodation, pupil diameter, and pupillary reaction to light are not affected. In patients with cardiac disease, thyroid disease, or allergies, the drug should be employed with caution, and the lowest possible dose should be used.

Preparation. Benoxinate is prepared in ophthalmic solution, 0.4%.

Dosage. The dosage for tonometry is 1 drop of 0.4% solution. For removal of a foreign body from the eye, 2 drops are instilled at 90-second intervals for several doses.

Cocaine

Cocaine is a potent, highly toxic local anesthetic with important side effects.

Actions. Cocaine is a potent inhibitor of nerve conduction and induces a strong, prolonged local anesthetic action after infiltration, nerve block, or topical application to mucous membranes and the eye. Cocaine blocks the reabsorption of the effector substance norepinephrine from the receptor site back into the terminal sympathetic nerve fiber; prolonged sympathetic stimulation is produced (for example, pupillary mydriasis). Use of the drug is limited to topical application; cocaine should never be injected. A strong vasoconstriction is induced by topical application of cocaine.

Ophthalmic uses. Cocaine is not recommended for general ophthalmic use. For cataract surgery, cocaine is occasionally used topically in a 2% to 4% solution as an adjunct to infiltration anesthesia with other agents. Cocaine, 0.2 ml of 4% solution, is sometimes injected subconjunctivally, in equal parts with 1:10,000 epinephrine and 5% homatropine, to break posterior synechiae and to produce mydriasis. Side reactions may occur from this procedure. Topical instillation of cocaine has been reported to deepen the anterior chamber in patients who have had recent cataract surgery and contact of the anterior face of the vitreous to the corneal endothelium.

Adverse effects. In the eye, cocaine induces mydriasis and partial cycloplegia. There may be slight retraction of the upper lid. The corneal epithelium may become dry and pitted and may slough, partly because of the loss of protective eyelid reflexes. A variable effect on intraocular pressure occurs. Acute attacks of narrow-angle glaucoma have been precipitated by the drug.

Cocaine is a very potent stimulator of the cortex of the central nervous system. The addictive properties of the drug are well known. Systemic absorption of the drug from mucous membranes may result in toxic manifestations, including hyperreflexia, restlessness, delirium, tachycardia, irregular respiration, chills, and fever, all of which are referable to central nervous system stimulation and may terminate in convulsions. Acute cocaine intoxication may pursue a rapid course and result in immediate death due to a concurrent toxic action of the drug on the myocardium. If central nervous system toxic reactions occur, the short-acting barbiturates, thiopental or pentobarbital, should be given intravenously. Cardiovascular collapse requires immediate supportive therapy—oxygen, vasopressor drugs, fluids and blood given intravenously, and cardiac massage if necessary.

Preparations. Cocaine alkaloid, NF, cocaine hydrochloride, USP; compounding is necessary for prescription.

Dosage. The dosage is as follows: topical application in the eye, 1% to 4% solution; mucous membrane anesthesia, 5% to 10% solution; these may be mixed with 1:1,000 epinephrine solution.

Proparacaine hydrochloride (Ophthaine, Alcaine, Ophthetic)

Proparacaine hydrochloride is an effective surface local anesthetic.

Actions. Proparacaine is a strong local anesthetic approximately equal to tetracaine (Pontocaine) hydrochloride in potency. The onset of analgesia is rapid, and the duration of action is about 20 minutes. The drug produces minimal irritation in the eye, and there is very little hyperemia, lacrimation, or drying.

Ophthalmic uses. Proparacaine is useful for short-term local anesthesia in the eye. Tonometry, removal of foreign bodies, conjunctival scraping, and other procedures of short duration may be performed with adequate analgesia produced by this drug. Retrobulbar injection of local anesthetics is facilitated by the prior application of proparacaine.

Adverse effects. Proparacaine is a highly toxic drug if significant amounts enter the systemic circulation. Local instillation in the eye rarely produces side effects. Mild transient corneal edema may occur but is unusual. Isolated corneal immune reactions have been reported with proparacaine. Allergic contact dermatitis is extremely rare.

Preparation. Preparation includes the following: a 0.5% solution that is applied topically.

Dosage. For removal of foreign bodies the dosage is 1 or 2 drops of 0.5% solution 2 minutes before the procedure; for tonometry the dosage is 1 or 2 drops of 0.5% solution instilled immediately before measurement; for deep anesthesia the dosage is 1 drop every 5 minutes for a total of 5 to 7 drops.

Tetracaine (Pontocaine) hydrochloride

Tetracaine hydrochloride is a member of the local anesthetic group that is ten times as potent as cocaine and ten times as toxic as procaine.

Actions. Tetracaine is a long-acting, surface-active local anesthetic when applied to mucous membranes and the eye. The drug induces a prolonged spinal anesthesia and may be used as a continuous caudal analgesic agent. It is sometimes used in combination with procaine in spinal anesthesia. No vasoconstriction occurs after its application to the eye or to mucous membranes.

Ophthalmic uses. Tetracaine is employed topically for the induction of analgesia in the cornea. An excellent long-lasting local anesthetic action is induced. Intraocular pressure is not elevated, accommodation is not paralyzed, and no mydriasis occurs. An 0.5 solution is generally employed for instillation into the eye.

Adverse effects. Topical application into the eye causes mild irritation. Transient corneal edema may occur. Local drug sensitivity reactions are uncommon. The drug is quite toxic if accidentally introduced into the bloodstream. The primary manifestation of toxicity is central nervous stimulation that may proceed to convulsive activity followed by depression. Short-acting barbiturates may be employed as a preventive measure before the use of tetracaine. A vasodepressor action may follow introduction of the drug into the spinal canal. Ephedrine or phenylephrine may be employed to combat the vasodepressor effect. Rapid absorption from mucous membranes must be avoided. Tetracaine should not be used on surfaces that are to be extensively traumatized.

Preparations. Preparations include the following: ampuls containing 10, 15, 20, and 250 mg of the salt as a powder; solutions given parenterally, 0.2% and 0.3% with 6% dextrose; solutions, 0.15%, 1%, and 2%; ophthalmic ointment, 0.5% in white petrolatum; ophthalmic solution, 0.5%.

Dosage. The dosage is as follows: for ophthalmic use, 0.5% solution or 0.5% ointment applied topically; for spinal anesthesia, 10 to 20 mg total; for caudal anesthesia, initial dose, 30 ml of 0.15% with epinephrine solution; for mucous membrane analgesia, 2% solution given topically.

NOTE: One milliliter of tetracaine hydrochloride is equal to 10 ml of procaine hydrochloride. Maximum safe dose, by injection, is 1 mg per kg of body weight.

ANTIANXIETY DRUGS

See also section on antihistamines.

Antianxiety drugs are widely used to control mild and moderate states of anxiety and tension in normal patients and in patients with neuroses. These drugs are sometimes classified as minor tranquilizers to distinguish them from drugs such as most phenothiazines, which are considered major tranquilizers. The antianxiety agents have to a large degree replaced the use of barbiturates as sedatives. It is held that antianxiety agents have a more selective action of the subcortical centers of the brain than do the sedative-hypnotics and are less apt to produce drowsiness and lethargy than the barbiturates.

These drugs have been used to treat withdrawal symptoms in alcoholism and to reduce symptoms of toxic psychoses. Skeletal muscle spasticity related to anxiety and tension may be relieved with these drugs.

There are not sufficient data to judge the comparative effectiveness of these agents. Accordingly, some representative individual agents are described below.

MINOR TRANQUILIZERS
Chlordiazepoxide (Librium)

Chlordiazepoxide is an effective tranquilizing agent that is chemically unrelated to the phenothiazines.

Actions. Chlordiazepoxide has tranquilizing effects similar to those of chlorpromazine, although it does not produce the autonomic blocking effect that chlorpromazine does. It produces sedative, anticonvulsant, and muscle relaxant effects. It does not act interneuronally, as does meprobamate. Chlordiazepoxide is used in a wide variety of psychiatric disorders, including anxiety and tension states. It is also administered to relax skeletal muscle spasticity.

Adverse effects. Drowsiness and ataxia may occur in some patients receiving chlordiazepoxide. Other side reactions include syncope, headache, skin rashes, menstrual irregularities, altered libido, and constipation. Occasional paradoxical excitement reactions occur in psychiatric patients. The side reactions usually disappear after the dose is reduced. The drug should be used with caution in alcoholics and in patients with impaired hepatic or renal function.

Preparations. Preparations include the following: capsules and tablets, 5, 10, and 25 mg; ampuls, 100 mg dry powder in a 5-ml ampul with a 2-ml ampul of diluent.

Dosage. The dosage for relief of mild or moderate anxiety is 10 mg three or four times a day; for relief of severe anxiety the dosage is 20 to 25 mg three or four times a day.

Diazepam (Valium)

Diazepam is a benzodiazepine derivative.

Actions. Diazepam apparently acts at the limbic and subcortical levels of the central nervous system, producing sedative, skeletal muscle relaxant, and anticonvulsant effects. It does not appear to block peripheral autonomic action. The drug has been used for relief of anxiety and tension, in the treatment of psychoneurotic states, as adjunctive therapy in relief of skeletal muscle spasm, and as preoperative medication for patients undergoing surgery.

Adverse effects. Side effects include drowsiness, dizziness, fatigue, dysarthria, and ataxia. Hypotension, headaches, diplopia, confusion, depression, nausea, and jaundice have been reported. The possibility of hepatic and renal dysfunction and blood cell depression should be considered with long-term therapy. Dependence may occur with long-term high dosage therapy.

Preparations. Preparations include the following: tablets, 2, 5, and 10 mg; injection, 5 mg per ml.

Dosage. Doses of 2 to 10 mg two to four times a day are given for the treatment of psychoneurotic reactions, treatment of muscle spasm, and as an adjunct to anticonvulsants. As a preoperative medication, diazepam is administered intramuscularly 1 to 2 hours before surgery in a dose of 10 mg.

Droperidol (Inapsine)

Droperidol is a butyrophenone derivative that is structurally related to haloperidol.

Actions. Droperidol produces effects similar to haloperidol and the phenothiazines. It acts primarily at the subcortical level in the central nervous system. It also produces a partial block of alpha-adrenergic receptor sites; consequently, the cardiovascular response to sympathomimetic amines is increased. The drug is used for preoperative medication for its antianxiety, sedative, and antiemetic effects.

Adverse effects. Extrapyramidal symptoms including dystonia, oculogyric crises, extended neck, and flexed limbs can occur. Hypotensive effects may be transitory or persist for several hours.

Preparations. Preparations include the following: injection, 2.5 mg per ml.

Dosage. The usual adult dosage for premedication ranges from 2.5 to 10 mg by intravenous or intramuscular route, 30 to 60 minutes before anesthesia.

MAJOR TRANQUILIZERS: PHENOTHIAZINES

Although phenothiazines frequently are classified as major tranquilizers, they have varying multiple pharmacological effects, including antihistamine action, antiemetic action, analgesia, antipruritic action, adrenergic potentiation, alpha-adrenergic blockade, and sedation. The degree of tranquilizing effects produced is somewhat variable with different phenothiazines.

Phenothiazines are primarily prescribed for the treatment of psychoses. They are most valuable in controlling severe tension, agitation, and psychomotor excitement. They have been used with some success in controlling behavioral problems in mentally retarded patients. Phenothiazines are also prescribed as antiemetic agents, particularly in postoperative patients, as preoperative agents to potentiate other hypnotics, and as adjuncts in the treatment of severe, chronic pain.

The pharmacological effects and adverse reactions of the phenothiazines vary widely, as do the indications for their clinical use. Descriptions of some individual representative agents follow.

Chlorpromazine (Thorazine)

Chlorpromazine is the prototype of phenothiazine compounds.

Actions. The exact mechanism of action of chlorpromazine is unknown. Psychotropic actions are produced by chlorpromazine, and it has been used for many years in the acute and chronic management of schizophrenia, in senile, organic, and toxic psychoses, and in the manic phase of manic-depressive psychoses. Although chlorpromazine is still widely prescribed for these purposes, today other drugs are commonly substituted because of fewer side reactions. In addition to its calming effect, chlorpromazine is effective in the management of postoperative nausea and vomiting. It has been widely used in the past for preoperative sedation.

Adverse effects. With long-term administration or high doses, extrapyramidal reactions may develop. Additionally, orthostatic hypotension, cholestatic jaundice, and various blood dyscrasias may occur. Pigmentation of the posterior surface of the cornea and anterior polar cataracts have been found in patients receiving long-term chlorpromazine.

Preparations. Preparations include the following: rectal suppositories, 25 and 100 mg; injection; solution, 25 mg per ml in 1-, 2-, and 10-ml containers; oral; time-released capsules, 30, 75, 150, 200 and 300 mg; tablets, 10, 25, 50, 100, and 200 mg; syrup, 10 mg per 5 ml.

Dosage. For control of nausea and vomiting, usual adult doses are 10 to 25 mg every 4 to 6 hours orally or intramuscularly until symptoms are relieved. The medication may also be given by rectal suppositories in a dosage of 100 mg every

6 to 8 hours. For treatment of psychoses the dosage is highly variable and must be individualized.

Prochlorperazine (Compazine)

Prochlorperazine is a phenothiazine derivative approximately five times as potent as chlorpromazine.

Actions. Prochlorperazine is employed as a tranquilizing agent in a wide variety of conditions ranging from mild emotional disorders and neuroses to severe psychiatric disturbances. It produces less adrenergic blockade and hypotension than chlorpromazine. Minimal additive effects occur with other central nervous system depressants. The drug also exerts a strong antiemetic effect.

Adverse effects. Sedation, dizziness, tachycardia, and xerostomia are the more common side reactions. Orthostatic hypotension and jaundice occur rarely. Neurological disturbances, particularly extrapyramidal involvement resembling parkinsonism, are frequently observed. Prochlorperazine should not be employed in children weighing less than 20 pounds.

Preparations. Preparations include the following: prochlorperazine suppositories, 2.5, 5, and 25 mg; prochlorperazine edisylate solution given parenterally 5 mg per ml; syrup, 1 and 10 mg per ml; sustained-release prochlorperazine maleate capsules, 10, 15, 30, and 75 mg; tablets, 5, 10, and 25 mg.

Dosage. The use and dosage for prochlorperazine is as follows: rectally, one 25-mg suppository twice daily; orally, 15 to 40 mg daily divided into three or four doses, which may be increased to 75 to 125 mg daily in psychotic patients; for nausea and vomiting, parenterally, 5 to 10 mg intramuscularly every 3 to 4 hours to a maximum of 40 mg total for any 24-hour period.

Triflupromazine (Vesprin)

Triflupromazine is a phenothiazine derivative with a chemical structure closely related to that of chlorpromazine. It is approximately twice as potent as chlorpromazine.

Actions. This drug is a tranquilizer employed for a wide variety of psychotic disorders. It is also an antiemetic, useful in controlling nausea and vomiting. It produces additive effects when used in combination with central nervous system depressants. This agent is employed as a preanesthetic medication in combination with analgesics and sedatives.

Adverse effects. The most common side effect of triflupromazine is a temporary parkinsonian syndrome, which disappears when the drug is discontinued. Hypotension and tachycardia occur after parenteral administration. Other side effects include the following: excessive drowsiness, blurred vision, weakness, and gastrointestinal disturbances. Jaundice is a rare complication.

Preparations. Preparations include the following: tablets, 10, 25, and 50 mg; solution for injection, 10 to 20 mg per ml; emulsion (oral), 10 mg per ml.

THERAPEUTIC AGENTS **209**

Dosage

FOR TRANQUILIZING EFFECTS: Given orally, the dosage is 10 to 25 mg two or three times a day; by injection the dosage is 20 to 50 mg two or three times a day.

FOR RELIEF OF NAUSEA AND VOMITING: Given orally, the prophylactic dose is 20 to 30 mg; the dose for intramuscular injection is 5 to 10 mg every 4 to 6 hours as needed.

FOR PREOPERATIVE MEDICATION: Ten milligrams are given orally or intramuscularly in combination with analgesics and sedatives.

ANTICOAGULANTS

The value of anticoagulant therapy in cardiac and vascular surgery is well established. The value of anticoagulant therapy in many pathological disorders for which it has been employed is controversial. Among these are coronary artery disease, cerebrovascular disease, polycythemia, peripheral vascular disease, pulmonary hypertension, and peripheral arterial thrombosis. The value of anticoagulants in ophthalmological vascular disorders is also somewhat controversial (Chapter 15).

Whenever anticoagulants are used, it is important to monitor the effects with laboratory procedures. Response of individual patients to the anticoagulants is quite variable. Furthermore, there may be increased or decreased effects resulting from concurrent use of other medications (Chapter 15). Whole-blood clotting times are determined to measure the effects of heparin; however, rarely the correlation between blood clotting times and plasma heparin activity is not good.

The one-stage prothrombin time is used to regulate the dosage of orally administered anticoagulants. This test actually measures factors other than prothrombin (Factor II), which are depressed with anticoagulant therapy. These include Factors V (proaccelerin), VII (proconvertin), and X (Stuart-Prower factor).

Heparin sodium

Heparin is a high molecular weight polymer consisting of disaccharide units that include glucosamine and glucuronic acid in combination with sulfuric acid.

Actions. Heparin is obtained from animal tissues of the liver and lungs. In the body the material is also found in the mast cells. As a therapeutic agent, heparin is employed as an anticoagulant. The primary action is antithrombotic and requires a cofactor. Thrombin is inactivated by heparin before the action of thrombin on fibrinogen. The drug is inactive by mouth and must be administered by the intravenous or deep subcutaneous route. Heparin also exerts a lipid-clearing action in the blood, converting lipoproteins of low density to lipoproteins of high density. Heparin possesses some anti-inflammatory and anti-fibrin activity. The drug is used in various types of thrombotic disease to prevent thrombosis. The anticoagulant effect is proportional to the quantity of heparin in the blood. It is also employed in the preparation of blood for certain types of transfusions.

Ophthalmic uses. Heparin sodium is employed either alone or in combination with the coumarin drugs in the treatment of partial or impending central retinal venous occlusions. Because of its lipid-clearing properties, it has been tried in the treatment of macular degeneration. Its effectiveness in this disease is doubtful.

Adverse effects. The principal side effect of heparin sodium is a hemorrhagic tendency caused by inhibition of the normal clotting mechanisms. Excessive bleeding at operative sites, purpura, ecchymosis, or hematuria necessitates discontinuance of the drug. In cases of overdosage, hexadimethrine bromide (Polybrene) or protamine sulfate may be useful as equivalent antagonists of heparin.

Preparations. Preparations are as follows: injection, 1,000, 5,000, 10,000, 20,000, and 40,000 units per ml; gel, 20,000 units per ml (1 USP unit equals 0.01 mg heparin sodium).

Dosage. Dosage is as follows: Intermittent intravenous injection, 5,000 to 10,000 units initially, followed by 2,500 to 10,000 units every 4 to 6 hours; continuous intravenous infusion, 10,000 units in 1,000 ml of physiological saline solution or 5% dextrose at a rate of 25 drops per minute; deep subcutaneous injection, 10,000 to 12,500 units every 12 hours. Doses are governed by frequent determinations of clotting time, which should be maintained between 20 and 30 minutes. For treatment of atherosclerosis and hyperlipemia there is no well-defined dose; usually 20,000 units are given twice a week. Subcutaneous doses of 5,000 units of heparin every 12 hours have been used to prevent venous thrombosis and pulmonary embolism in postoperative patients.

Bishydroxycoumarin (Dicumarol)

Bishydroxycoumarin is a synthetic compound, dimethylenebishydroxycoumarin.

Actions. Bishydroxycoumarin is an anticoagulant that acts by the inhibition of prothrombin formation and involves an antagonism to vitamin K. It is used in the management of various embolic and thrombotic conditions. A latent period of 24 to 72 hours precedes the full therapeutic effect. The drug is cumulative, and a maintenance dose must be determined for each patient. Control of dosage is achieved by prothrombin time determinations. A latent period also precedes the diminution of the anticoagulant effect after discontinuance of the drug. Vitamin K and its analogues are effective antidotes for bishydroxycoumarin overdosage and may be useful for rapid reduction of the anticoagulant effects of the coumarin drugs.

Ophthalmic uses. Bishydroxycoumarin is used in combination with heparin for the treatment of partial or impending central retinal venous occlusions. It is also used for prophylaxis against central retinal venous occlusion in the unaffected eye when a retinal venous occlusion has occurred in the fellow eye.

Adverse effects. The primary side effect of therapeutic dosage is a hemorrhagic tendency. Hemorrhagic diathesis is a constant possibility when accurate dosage is not attained. Transaminase determinations are distorted when coumarin drugs are present in the bloodstream. With careful dosage and adequate control by serial prothrombin determinations, the drug has a low order of toxicity. The drug is contraindicated in patients with hemorrhagic disease, blood dyscrasias, ulcerative disease of the gastrointestinal tract, or liver disease.

Preparations. Preparations include the following: capsules, 25, 50, and 100 mg; tablets, 25, 50, and 100 mg.

Dosage. Bishydroxycoumarin is administered by the oral route only, 300 mg in the first 24 hours (in older patients an initial daily dose of 200 mg is advisable), 200 mg in the next 24 hours, and from 0 to 100 mg the following day as indicated by the prothrombin level. Maintenance dose is between 25 and 100 mg daily. The usual therapeutic range of prothrombin levels is 20% to 40%. (See Chapter 15 for new theories of drug dosage.)

NOTE: Salicylates, quinine, quinidine; phenylbutazone, and corticosteroids may exert an additive effect on the depression of coagulation by coumarin drugs. Broad-spectrum antibiotics that suppress bacteria-producing vitamin K may also increase the anticoagulant effects.

Warfarin sodium (Coumadin)

Warfarin sodium is a hydroxycoumarin derivative.

Actions. Warfarin sodium effects an anticoagulant action by depression of prothrombin formation in the liver. An antivitamin K action is the basis for the inhibition of prothrombin. The drug may be administered intravenously as well as orally. Vitamin K and its analogues are effective as antidotes for overdosage. Warfarin is used to inhibit intravascular clotting. It action is rapid in onset and prolonged in duration. It is thirty to forty times as potent as bishydroxycoumarin.

Ophthalmic uses. Warfarin sodium has been used in combination with heparin for the treatment of partial or impending central retinal venous occlusions. When retinal venous occlusion has occurred in one eye, warfarin sodium is sometimes used for prophylaxis against central retinal venous occlusion in the contralateral eye.

Adverse effects. The primary side effect of warfarin sodium is a tendency toward excessive bleeding, which is almost always caused by overdosage. The drug should be used with extreme caution in patients with liver or kidney disease and in pregnant patients. Adequate control is achieved by means of frequent prothrombin activity determinations.

Preparations. Preparations are as follows: for injection, 50 mg of powder with 2-ml ampul of sterile water; 75 mg of powder with 3-ml ampul of sterile water; tablets, 2, 2.5, 5, 7.5, 10, and 25 mg.

Dosage. The oral or intravenous dose is 25 to 50 mg initially; the average daily maintenance dose is 5 to 10 mg, depending on the prothrombin level; usual therapeutic ranges of prothrombin levels are 20% to 40%. See Chapter 15 for new theories of drug dosage.

ANTIHISTAMINES

Antihistamines act by blocking the action of histamine at the cellular level; they do not affect the formation or release of histamine. The effects of histamine in producing contraction of smooth muscle, increasing capillary permeability, and stimulating nerve endings are effectively antagonized by antihistamines. The vasodilatation and hypotension produced by histamine are only partially blocked by antihistamines; the stimulation of gastric acid is not affected. Some antihistamines diminish motion sickness and relieve nausea and vomiting, probably as a result of affecting neuropathways from the labyrinthine. Most antihistamines produce some sedation and drowsiness, although some have a central nervous system excitatory effect. In varying degrees, most antihistamines have some local anesthetic and anticholinergic properties.

The principal use of antihistamines is in the treatment of allergic disorders. They are particularly effective in the management of hay fever and acute allergic urticaria. They are less useful for the treatment of chronic urticaria or allergic rhinitis. They are of little value in the treatment of bronchial asthma. The value of antihistamines in relieving symptoms of common colds is questionable. Antihistamines have been used with some success in the treatment of parkinsonism. Because of their sedative and antiemetic effects, some antihistamines have been used in combination with other drugs as preoperative agents, particularly when surgery is performed with the patient under local anesthesia.

Ophthalmic uses. See also the individual agents that follow. Antihistamines are employed for treatment of acute allergic reactions of the eyelids and conjunctiva. They are most effective when given systemically. The topical application of antihistamines in the treatment of allergic conjunctivitis is of questionable value. Antihistamines may be used to relieve or prevent postoperative nausea and vomiting. Because of their sedative and antiemetic effects, they are sometimes used as preoperative agents.

Adverse effects. The incidence and severity of reactions to antihistamines vary considerably between different drugs and among individuals. The most common side effect is central nervous system depression, including drowsiness, dizziness, and ataxia. Dryness of the mouth is also common. With large doses, blurred vision, urinary retention, and tachycardia may occur. Occasionally central nervous system stimulation with symptoms of tremors, insomnia, and irritability occurs. Rarely blood dyscrasias have been reported in patients receiving antihistamines. Skin sensitization may occur with antihistamines, particularly if they are used topically.

Antazoline

Antazoline is an antihistamine that has been used as a topical agent in the treatment of ocular disorders.

Actions. As a histamine antagonist, this drug will reduce, to a variable degree, the effects of histamine released in allergic reactions. Consequently, antazoline has been found useful in nasal allergies, hay fever, and allergic reactions to drugs. The action is palliative, and the drug is useful primarily as an adjunct to specific methods of treatment in allergies. Antazoline also has sedative and local analgesic activity.

Ophthalmic uses. Antazoline phosphate is occasionally useful in the management of ocular allergies when used topically. The drug is much less irritating to ocular tissues than are other members of the histamine antagonizing group. All topical antihistamine solutions may be sensitizing, consequently they are rarely employed.

Adverse effects. After topical application in the eye, few, if any, side effects occur.

Preparations. Preparations include ophthalmic solution, phosphate, 0.5%.

Dosage. The dosage is 1 or 2 drops as an 0.5% isotonic solution in each eye every 3 or 4 hours as required to relieve symptoms.

Chlorpheniramine (Chlor-Trimeton)

Chlorpheniramine is an effective histamine antagonist.

Actions. As a histamine antagonist, chlorpheniramine will partially alleviate the effects of histamine released in allergic reactions. Consequently, it has been found useful in nasal allergies, hay fever, and allergic reactions to drugs. The action is palliative, and the drug is useful primarily as an adjunct to specific methods of treatment in allergies. It also has sedative and local analgesic effects. It is therapeutically efficient and induces a low incidence of side effects. It may be administered in very low dosage with effects comparable to those achieved with much higher doses of other antihistamines.

Adverse effects. Side effects are similar to those induced by other antihistamines. Incidence of side effects produced by chlorpheniramine, however, is low.

Preparations. Preparations include the following: tablets, 4 mg; repeat action tablets, 8 and 12 mg; solution given parenterally, 10 and 100 mg per ml; syrup, 0.4 mg per ml.

Dosage. The dosage is as follows: given orally, 2 to 4 mg; given parenterally, intravenously, or intramuscularly, 5 to 20 mg.

NOTE: Chlorpheniramine is not compatible in solution with allergenic substances or oil-containing materials.

Cyclizine (Marezine)

Cyclizine is an antihistamine prepared as the hydrochloride or the lactate salt.

Actions. Cyclizine is employed primarily for its effect against motion sickness. It is effective in the control of vertigo, nausea, and vomiting resulting from motion and from vestibular dysfunction. Sedation occurs to a variable degree, more frequently with high doses. The value of this compound in allergic states has not been established.

Adverse effects. In therapeutic doses for motion sickness, cyclizine induces relatively few of the side effects usually associated with antihistaminic compounds. Drowsiness and dryness of the mouth may occur with higher doses.

Preparations. Preparations include tablets, 50 mg, and suppositories, 50 and 100 mg.

NOTE: Cyclizine lactate is prepared as a solution for intramuscular injection only, 50 mg per ml.

Dosage. The hydrochloride is administered orally or rectally. For motion sickness the dosage is 50 mg orally 30 minutes before exposure to motion and then 50 mg three times daily before meals. For vestibular dysfunction the dosage is 50 to 100 mg three times daily. For severe vomiting, 50 mg is given intramuscularly three to four times a day. Dosage for children 6 to 10 years is one half of the adult dose, and for children under 6 years, one fourth of the adult dose.

Cyproheptadine hydrochloride (Periactin)

Actions. Cyproheptadine is an antagonist of histamine and serotonin. The functions of serotonin are unknown; it is a vasoconstrictor, has a stimulating effect on the gastrointestinal tract, and is thought to be important as a neurohumoral agent in the transmission of impulses to the brain. Cyproheptadine is used chiefly as an antipruritic agent; it has been used only in the treatment of acute and chronic allergies.

Adverse effects. Drowsiness is the chief side effect of cyproheptadine. Drug rash, nausea, and dizziness have also been reported after its use.

Preparations. It is prepared in the form of tablets, 4 mg, and a syrup, 0.4 mg per ml.

Dosage. The dosage for adults is 4 mg three to four times a day, and for children 2 to 4 mg one to four times a day, depending on the size and condition of the patient.

Dimenhydrinate (Dramamine)

Dimenhydrinate is the chlorotheophylline salt of diphenhydramine (Benadryl), with actions similar to those of other antihistamines.

Actions. Dimenhydrinate has a potent effect against motion sickness and is used for the prevention or treatment of motion sickness and for the management of other conditions involving vertigo, nausea, and vomiting. It has been employed in the treatment of Meniere's syndrome, labyrinthitis, radiation sickness, and vestibular dysfunction resulting from streptomycin therapy. Dimenhydrinate also exerts a moderately strong antihistamine action and mild sedative effects.

Adverse effects. Prolonged and chronic use of dimenhydrinate may result in toxic effects common to all antihistaminic preparations, including hematopoietic depression.

Preparations. Preparations include the following: tablets, 50 mg; elixir, 3.1 mg per ml; solution given parenterally, 50 mg per ml; suppositories, 100 mg.

Dosage. The dosage for prevention of nausea and vomiting resulting from motion sickness or other causes is 50 to 100 mg administered orally every 4 hours or 50 mg administered intramuscularly.

Diphenhydramine hydrochloride (Benadryl)

Diphenhydramine hydrochloride is an antihistaminic drug, widely used in the management of certain allergic conditions.

Actions. As a histamine antagonist, this drug will partially alleviate the effects of histamine released in allergic reactions. Consequently, it has been found useful in nasal allergies, hay fever, and allergic reactions to drugs. The action is palliative, and the drug is useful primarily as an adjunct to specific methods of treatment of allergies. It also has sedative and local analgesic activity.

Adverse effects. All antihistamines produce toxic side effects that include sedation, tremors, nervousness, anorexia, and dryness of mucous membranes. Blood dyscrasias occur rarely after prolonged use. Local sensitivity to the drug may develop after topical administration.

Preparations. Preparations include: capsules, 50 mg; liquid, 12.5 mg per 4 ml; solution given parenterally, 50 mg per ml.

Dosage. The dosage is as follows: given orally, 50 mg three to four times daily; given parenterally for severe symptoms, 10 to 50 mg every 4 hours.

Hydroxyzine (Atarax, Vistaril)

Hydroxyzine is a diphenylmethane derivative and is similar in chemical structure and pharmacological actions to some drugs of the antihistamine group.

Actions. Hydroxyzine has a wide range of actions, including antihistaminic, local anesthetic, sedative, antispasmodic, and ataractic effects. The primary use for the drug is as a tranquilizer. It acts centrally but exerts no hypnogenic effect. It has been shown to be effective as a tranquilizer in psychoneuroses, tension states, and nonorganic hypertension and when used as a preoperative medication. The drug is also employed in dermatological therapy.

Adverse effects. Pruritus, urticaria, drowsiness, and dryness of the oropharynx have been observed. When coumarin-type drugs are used concurrently, the requirement for the anticoagulant may be greatly reduced, and patients on combined therapy must be checked carefully to prevent bleeding. Hydroxyzine may potentiate the action of barbiturates and narcotics. The toxicity of hydroxyzine is low, and many of the side effects are transient.

Preparations. Hydroxyzine hydrochloride is prepared as a parenterally administered solution, 25 and 50 mg per ml; tablets, 10, 25, and 100 mg; syrup, 2 mg per ml. Hydroxyzine pamoate is prepared as capsules, 25, 50, and 100 mg; suspension given orally, 5 mg per ml.

Dosage. Dosage is usually highly individualized. When it is given orally for tranquilization, 25 to 100 mg is given three to four times a day. When it is given parenterally for emergency use when a more rapid onset of action is desired, the intramuscular dose is 50 to 100 mg every 4 to 6 hours. As a preanesthetic agent, 25 to 50 mg is given intramuscularly 30 to 45 minutes before surgery.

Promethazine (Phenergan)

Promethazine is one of the most potent antihistamine drugs available. It is a phenothiazine derivative and is prepared as the hydrochloride.

Actions. The primary use of promethazine has been in the therapy of allergic states amenable to antihistamines. Its additional pharmacological effects form the basis for other clinical applications. It has been useful in the control of motion sickness, nausea, and vomiting and possesses a strongly sedative effect that reduces apprehension and produces light sleep. It is frequently employed in combination with barbiturates and analgesics preoperatively when surgery is to be performed with the patient under local anesthesia. When it is given with central nervous system depressants, promethazine produces summative effects that reduce the required dosage of the central nervous system depressants.

Adverse effects. Drowsiness and vertigo related to sedation may be produced. Hypotension, muscular weakness, lassitude, and gastrointestinal disturbances are also occasionally observed. Patients show wide variations of sensitivity and side effects. Sometimes side reactions are transient, but at times they are so persistent that another drug must be substituted.

Preparations. Preparations include the following: tablets, 12.5, 25, and 50 mg; solution given parenterally, 25 and 50 mg per ml; syrup, 1.25 and 5 mg per ml; suppositories, 25 and 50 mg.

Dosage. The dose should be the smallest amount of the drug consistent with relief of symptoms. The usual oral dose is 25 mg before retiring, or 12.5 mg three or four times daily before meals and upon retiring. Usual injection is 12.5 to 25 mg.

For motion sickness the dosage is 25 mg twice daily; for nausea and vomiting, 25 mg is given orally, rectally, or by injection, repeated every 4 to 6 hours; for sedation, 25 to 50 mg is given orally or by injection.

Because of its additive effect with morphine, meperidine, and other depressant analgesics, the dose of these other medications should be reduced by one fourth to one half.

ANTI-INFECTIVE CHEMOTHERAPEUTIC AGENTS

Anti-infective agents are chemotherapeutic drugs that are employed clinically for their antibacterial activity. Unlike antibiotics, they are not synthesized by living microorganisms. They are distinguished from antiseptics and disinfectants, which may eradicate infections when applied topically but cannot be administered systemically because of toxicity. Anti-infective agents may act by several mechanisms: by inhibition of either bacterial wall synthesis, protein synthesis, or nucleic acid synthesis or by antagonism of the metabolites of micro-organisms.

Aminosalicylic acid (PAS, para-aminosalicylic acid)

Aminosalicylic acid is an anti-infective agent. It is a derivative of salicylic acid and contains an amino group in the *para* position.

Actions. PAS has an action against the tubercle bacillus that is quantitatively weaker than that of the streptomycins. It is used as an adjuvant to other drugs in the treatment of tuberculous infections primarily because of its additive effect and also to achieve a reduction in the rate of development of drug-resistant bacilli. It is also useful in patients in whom streptomycin is contraindicated. The drug has had some use in the treatment of tuberculous infections of the eye.

Adverse effects. Anorexia, nausea, and vomiting are common side effects. Dermatoses and drug fever are occasional toxic manifestations.

Preparations. Preparations include the following: tablets, and capsules, 500 mg, 1 and 2 grams; powder, 1 gram; various sized packets, 4 and 8 grams.

Dosage. PAS is administered orally, 8 to 16 grams daily in four divided doses.

Boric acid

Boric acid is a weak organic acid.

Actions. Boric acid is an antiseptic with weak germicidal potency. The compound is widely used because of the general opinion that it does not injure the tissues. However, at concentrations of 2% or greater, boric acid may exert a phagocytolytic effect that may depress a primary defense mechanism against bacterial invasion. This deleterious effect may be circumvented by keeping boric acid solutions under refrigeration, which reduces the solubility of the compound to less than 2%.

Ophthalmic uses. Boric acid solution is widely used as an eyewash. Boric acid is also employed in a 2% concentration as the buffering agent for many ophthalmic solutions. Boric acid compresses are used in the treatment of many eruptive, oozing, dermatological lesions of the eyelids.

Adverse effects. Although boric acid is relatively nontoxic, its absorptions from burned skin or open lesions of the skin may result in poisoning that can be fatal. Manifestations of local toxicity are stomatitis, eczematous rash, and edema.

Preparation. Boric acid is prepared in powder form.

Dosage. Solutions for topical applications should not exceed 2% concentration.

Isoniazid (INH, Niconyl, Nydrazid, Tyvid)

Isoniazid is an anti-infective agent derived from nicotinic acid.

Actions. Isoniazid is a potent inhibitor of the tubercle bacillus. It is effective in relatively small doses and may be employed alone or in combination with other antituberculosis agents. Combination therapy is desirable to retard the development of resistance to each drug in the combination. Isoniazid is useful in patients in whom resistance or hypersensitivity to other antituberculous drugs has developed.

Adverse effects. Peripheral neuropathy may develop, particularly in malnourished patients. The effect results from the action of isoniazid against pyridoxine and may be prevented by administering 50 to 100 mg of pyridoxine daily. Other toxic effects include drowsiness, febrile reactions, vertigo, muscular twitching, ataxia, optic neuritis, and psychotic episodes. Recently hepatitis has been attributed to isoniazid therapy.

Preparations. Preparations include the following: tablets, 100 and 300 mg; solution for injection, 100 mg per ml; syrup, 10 mg per ml.

Dosage. The dosage given orally is 5 to 20 mg per kg of body weight in one to three doses; given intramuscularly, 5 to 20 mg per kg of body weight daily in one to three doses; given topically, 10 ml of 100 mg per ml of solution applied three times a week.

Pyrimethamine (Daraprim)

Actions. Pyrimethamine is a synthetic antimalarial drug that is a folic acid antagonist. It has its greatest antimalarial effect on the erythrocytic stages of malarial infections. However, it is also active against the exoerythrocytic phases. It arrests sporogony in the mosquito and consequently is helpful in preventing transmission of malaria. It is also effective against intracellular, dividing *Toxoplasma* parasites. It is probably ineffective against the encysted forms of the parasite.

Ophthalmic uses. Pyrimethamine is used in combination with sulfonamide drugs in the treatment of uveitis and retinitis caused by *Toxoplasma*.

Adverse effects. The side effects include bone marrow depression, thrombocytopenia, megaloblastic anemia, and leukopenia. In addition, vomiting and diarrhea may occur.

Pyrimethamine is contraindicated in pregnant patients because it may interfere with normal embryonic development.

Preparation. It is prepared in 25-mg tablets.

Dosage. For uveitis and retinitis caused by *Toxoplasma*, the dosage is 50 mg along with 4 grams of sulfadiazine or triple sulfonamides daily, in divided doses, for 1 to 3 weeks, depending on response and drug toxicity. Thereafter the dosage is 25 mg daily, with 2 grams of sulfadiazine for 4 to 8 weeks. Priming doses of 50 mg two to four times a day for 1 to 2 days have been recommended by some physicians.

NOTE: Blood counts should be obtained at intervals of 3 to 4 days during early treatment with pyrimethamine. Thereafter weekly blood counts should be obtained. If blood cell depression occurs, calcium leucovorin (folinic acid), 5 to 15 mg daily, should be administered until the blood count has reached safe levels.

Sulfonamides

The sulfonamides are effective against many gram-positive organisms as well as some gram-negative bacilli and diplococci. This group of drugs acts against bacteria by virtue of competitive inhibition of the utilization by bacteria of *p*-aminobenzoic acid. It is further postulated that certain bacteria require *p*-amino-benzoic acid for the synthesis of folic acid, a necessary growth factor, and that the sulfonamides prevent the synthesis of folic acid by substrate competition.

The tubercle bacillus, fungi, and spirochetes are resistant to the sulfonamide drugs.

Adverse effects. Undesirable side effects common to this group of drugs include dermatitis, leukopenia, hemolytic anemia, and drug fever, all of which may be related to acquired sensitivity, that is, "drug allergy."

Renal lesions may result from precipitation of crystals of the drug in the renal

Table 22. Dosage for commonly used sulfonamides*

Drug	Trade name	Use	Dose Initial	Dose Maintenance
Phthalylsulfathia-zole	Sulfathalidine	Intestinal anti-septic	50 to 100 mg/kg body weight	3 to 7 grams daily in four divided doses
Sulfachloro-pyridazine	Sonilyn	Urinary anti-infective	2 to 4 grams	0.5 to 1 gram q6h
Sulfadiazine	Sulfadiazine	Systemic anti-infective	2 to 4 grams	0.5 to 1 gram q4-6h
Sulfadimethoxine	Madribon	Systemic anti-infective	1 gram	500 mg q24h
Sulfameter	Sulla	Urinary anti-infective	1.5 grams	500 mg q24h
Sulfamethoxazole	Gantanol	Systemic anti-infective	2 grams	1 gram q8-12h
Sulfamethoxypy-ridazine	Midicel acetyl	Systemic anti-infective	1 gram	500 mg daily
Sulfa-trimetho-prim and sulfa-methoxazole combination	Bactrim, Septra	Urinary anti-infective	160 mg trimetho-prim and 800 mg sulfa-methoxazole	160 mg trimetho-prim and 800 mg sulfamethox-azole q12h
Sulfisoxazole	Gantrisin	Systemic anti-infective	4 to 6 grams	1 to 2 grams q4h
Trisulfapyrimi-dines (contains equal amounts of sulfadiazine, sulfamethazine, and sulfamera-zine)	Multiple preparations	Systemic anti-infective	2 to 4 grams	1 gram q4-6h

*The commonly used topical ocular preparations are sulfisoxazole (Gantrisin) as a 4% solution or ointment and sulfacetamide as a 10%, 15%, or 30% solution and as a 10% ointment.

tubules or, rarely, from a direct toxic reaction on the tubule cells. Newer members of the sulfonamide group are more soluble, but crystal formation remains a potential side effect. Hepatic damage and peripheral neuritis have been observed as toxic reactions to sulfonamides. Some sulfonamide derivatives such as succinylsulfathiazole (Sulfasuxidine) and phthalylsulfathiazole (Sulfathalidine) are poorly absorbed from the intestine and are activated by hydrolysis in the intestinal tract. This type of drug may be employed as an intestinal antiseptic.

Newer drugs of this class are characterized by a low renal clearance, resulting in more sustained blood levels achieved by administration of lower doses. Sulfamethoxypyridazine (Midicel acetyl) and sulfadimethoxine (Madribon) are examples of the newer sulfonamides. The long-acting sulfonamides may produce a higher incidence of erythema multiforme reactions than other sulfonamides.

Dosage. See Table 22 for the dosage of commonly used sulfonamides.

ANTIFUNGAL AGENTS

Antifungal agents may be divided into two groups: antibiotic antifungal agents and nonantibiotic antifungal agents. Many nonantibiotic antibacterial agents, including antiseptics and disinfectants, have some fungistatic or fungicidal properties.

Amphotericin B (Fungizone)

Amphotericin B is an antibiotic agent obtained from *Streptomyces nodosus* that is used for the treatment of mycotic infections.

Actions. Amphotericin B exerts a variable fungistatic action against a broad spectrum of fungi and yeast, including *Histoplasma, Blastomyces, Cryptococcus, Coccidioides,* and some species of *Candida.* The drug is not fungicidal. Amphotericin B is almost always administered by the parenteral route and is used in the treatment of deep-seated mycoses. Although the drug is not completely effective in all cases of mycotic infections caused by the fungi just mentioned, it represents a promising advance in the therapy of mycotic infection.

Ophthalmic uses. This drug is used for the treatment of mycotic infections of the eyes and ocular adnexa. Cultures should be obtained and the effectiveness of amphotericin determined. For involvement of the cornea the drug is administered topically; in addition, subconjunctival injections may be given. Anterior intraocular infections are treated by subconjunctival injection and intravenous administration. Anterior chamber irrigations may be necessary and valuable. Intravenous therapy is used for posterior intraocular and orbital infections. The intraocular penetration of amphotericin B by topical administration is poor.

Subconjunctival therapy provides only modest therapeutic levels.

Adverse effects. The toxicity of amphotericin B is appreciable at therapeutic dose levels. Initial side effects include headache, chills, fever, and anorexia. Renal toxicity is indicated by increased levels of BUN and creatinine during prolonged courses of treatment, and it limits the amount of the drug that may be administered. This effect is usually reversible on discontinuance of the drug. Renal function must be checked at intervals during prolonged use of the drug. Thrombophlebitis may result at infection sites because of irritation of the venous endothelium. Other side effects include gastrointestinal distress, diarrhea, and anemia.

The drug is contraindicated in patients in whom a mycotic infection by a susceptible organism has not been accurately and properly diagnosed. Because of the appreciable toxicity, the use of the drug should be limited to hospitalized patients.

Preparations. Preparations include buffered powder for injection, 50 mg.

Dosage. The dosage, by intravenous infusion, is 0.1 mg per ml in 5% dextrose in water; the initial dose, 0.1 to 0.25 mg per kg of body weight, may be increased gradually up to 1 mg per kg of body weight or until toxicity intervenes; maximum total dose is 1 mg per kg of body weight when the drug is given daily and 1.5 mg per kg of body weight when the drug is given on alternate days; the dosage should be adjusted to the response of the patient. Therapy may be given daily or on an alternate-day basis. The total dose of amphotericin B for the average-sized adult should not exceed 2 grams. For topical application in the eye, 1.5 to 8 mg per ml is used; for subconjunctival injection, 2 to 5 mg in a volume of 0.5 ml; for anterior chamber irrigation, 20 to 30 μg in a volume of 0.1 to 0.2 ml.

NOTE: Do not dissolve or dilute with saline solution, since saline solution will precipitate amphotericin B.

Flucytosine (Ancobon)

Flucytosine is a fluorinated pyrimidine related to fluorouracil and floxuridine.

Actions. Flucytosine is converted by fungal cells (but not by mammalian cells) to fluorouracil, which is a metabolic antagonist. Flucytosine has inhibitory activity against *Candida* and *Cryptococcus*. It has been reported to also have some effect against certain strains of *Aspergillus* and *Torula* but is ineffective against *Histoplasma, Blastomyces,* and *Coccidioides*. It is well absorbed after oral administration.

Ophthalmic uses. Flucytosine has been employed in the treatment of *Candida* endophthalmitis.

Adverse effects. Bone marrow suppression may occur, which can lead to anemia, leukopenia, and thrombocytopenia. Elevated BUN and creatinine levels may occur. Other side effects include nausea, vomiting, diarrhea, vertigo, headaches, and hallucinations.

Preparations. The drug is available in capsules containing either 250 mg or 500 mg.

Dosage. The dosage is 50 to 150 mg per kg of body weight per day divided into six interval doses.

Griseofulvin (Fulvicin-U/F, Grifulvin V, Grisactin)

Griseofulvin is a fungistatic agent derived from the mold *Penicillium griseofulvin*.

Actions. Griseofulvin has a highly selective fungistatic action against certain superficial fungus infections. It is administered systemically and is effective in the eradication of infections caused by the dermatophytes, *Trichophyton, Microsporum,* and *Epidermophyton*. Tinea capitis, tinea corporis, tinea unguium, and chronic tinea pedis resulting from the organisms just mentioned may be treated effectively with systemically administered griseofulvin. It is the first drug to become available that allows adequate treatment of fungus infections of the skin by systemic administration. Griseofulvin is effective against only the fungi mentioned, and it is essential that the correct diagnosis be made as to the causative organism. The effectiveness of the drug may be increased by the concomitant application of standard dermatological topical and surface agents.

Adverse effects. Serious side effects are infrequently observed but may include headache, leukopenia, skin eruptions, allergic reactions, nausea, diarrhea, and fatigue. The drug is contraindicated in patients with fungus infections caused by organisms other than the sensitive dermatophytes and with infections that are amenable to ordinary topical measures.

Preparations. Griseofulvin is available in tablets, 125, 250, and 500 mg.

Dosage. The dosage is as follows: adults, initially, 500 mg to 1 gram daily in a single dose or divided doses after meals; reduced to 500 mg daily or less as infection clears; children, 10 mg per kg of body weight in a single dose or divided doses after meals; dosage should be continued until replacement of infected skin structures occurs.

Nystatin (Mycostatin, Nilstat)

Nystatin is an antifungal agent derived from *Streptomyces noursei*.

Actions. Nystatin is active primarily against *Candida albicans*. The drug is not absorbed from the gastrointestinal tract or through the skin via mucous membranes. It has a variable degree of effectiveness in many forms of moniliasis. Topical administration has proved effective in thrush and cutaneous moniliasis. Oral therapy is useful in intestinal moniliasis, but systemic effects are unlikely because the drug is poorly absorbed. Nystatin is not satisfactory for parenteral administration.

Ophthalmic uses. Nystatin is used in the treatment of certain mycotic infections of the cornea. The selection of this drug should be determined by fungus cultures and sensitivity tests. Nystatin is usually applied topically. Subconjunctival injection is somewhat irritating but may be employed along with topical administration. The intraocular penetration of nystatin by systemic or topical administration is poor. Subconjunctival injection is effective.

Adverse effects. Nystatin is essentially nontoxic, and few side effects result from its use. Transitory and mild diarrhea, vomiting, and nausea may occur.

Preparations. Preparations are as follows: applied topically, cream, 100,000 units per gram; ointment, 100,000 units per gram; powder, 100,000 units per gram; tablets, 500,000 units; suspension, 100,000 units per ml.

Dosage. Dosages are as follows: for intestinal moniliasis, 500,000 to 1,000,000 units orally three times daily; for thrush, 100,000 units applied topically once or twice daily; for cutaneous moniliasis, 100,000 units applied topically once to several times daily; oral dosage for children, 100,000 units three or four times daily; for topical ophthalmic administration, solution, 25,000 to 100,000 units per ml or ointment, 100,000 units per gram.

ANTIVIRAL AGENTS

In the past few years considerable progress has been made in the development of effective antiviral drugs. Inhibitors of nucleic acid synthesis such as idoxuridine have been available for topical use in the eye. Other inhibitors of nucleic acid synthesis such as Vidarabine (Vira-A, adenine arabinoside, ARA-A) and trifluorothymidine (TFT) have proved effective for the treatment of ophthalmic disease. Vidarabine has recently become available as a 3% ointment (Chapter 11).

Idoxuridine (IDU, IUDR, Herplex, Stoxil)

Idoxuridine is an antimetabolic analogue of thymidine. The utilization of thymidine in the synthesis of deoxyribonucleic acid (DNA) is inhibited by IDU. Viral synthesis of DNA is suppressed; the effects may also extend to host cells.

Ophthalmic uses. IDU is used topically in the treatment of herpes simplex and vaccinia keratitis. The drug is most effective in the epithelial forms of herpes simplex infections. Its effectiveness in stromal herpes keratitis is not fully established. It is sometimes used in combination with corticosteroids in the treatment of the combined forms of superficial and deep herpes simplex keratitis and in the treatment of herpetic iritis; in this instance the IDU helps to offset the harmful effects of corticosteroids on the superficial infection. Strains of herpes simplex virus may develop resistance to IDU.

Adverse effects. No serious side effects or contraindications are known when IDU is used as an ophthalmic solution. Mild irritation of the eyelids and conjunctiva, mild corneal edema, small punctate defects in the corneal epithelium, and corneal anesthesia can occur. Healing of the corneal stroma may be impaired.

Stomatitis, leukopenia, alopecia, nausea, vomiting, and diarrhea have occurred when the drug was administered intravenously for the treatment of cancer.

Preparations. IDU is prepared in ophthalmic solution, 0.1%, and in ophthalmic ointment, 0.5%. In solution it is unstable when exposed to heat and light. Refrigeration of the solution is advisable. Old solutions should be discarded.

Dosage. One drop is instilled into the eye every hour during the day and every 2 hours at night. Alternatively, the drops may be given every minute for ten doses four times a day. Ointment is instilled into the eye four to five times a day. The drops may be used during the day, and the ointment may be used at bedtime.

ANTI-INFLAMMATORY AGENTS

Anti-inflammatory agents are commonly divided into two groups: the corticosteroids and ACTH, and the noncorticosteroids. For the ophthalmologist the corticosteroid agents are by far the most valuable, although some serious side effects may accompany their use (Chapter 2). The nonsteroidal anti-inflammatory agents are occasionally employed in the treatment of mild inflammations such as uveitis and episcleritis. Some of these agents have analgesic, antipyretic, and antirheumatic properties and are used therapeutically for these purposes.

Corticotropin (ACTH, Actest, Acthar, Actrope, Cortigel, Cortrophin, Depo-ACTH, Solacthyl)

ACTH is a compound of principles obtained from the anterior lobe of pituitary glands from farm animals.

Actions. ACTH preparations stimulate the adrenal cortex to produce and secrete all of the cortical steroid hormones endogenous to that gland with the exception of aldosterone. The stimulatory effect of ACTH is effective only in the presence of functional adrenocortical tissue. The effects of the drug are rapid and, in general, resemble those from hydrocortisone administration. Because of its protein content, ACTH is active only after parenteral dosage.

Ophthalmic uses. ACTH is used for the therapy of a wide variety of nonspecific inflammations of the globe and orbit. Included among these are anterior and posterior uveitis, sympathetic ophthalmia, traumatic retinal edema, optic neuritis, temporal arteritis, and pseudotumor of the orbit (Chapter 2).

Adverse effects. The side effects of ACTH are similar to those resulting from the therapeutic use of adrenocortical steroids. Hypertension, hirsutism, metabolic aberrations, and electrolyte imbalance may occur. Hypersensitivity reactions have been observed. Long-term use of the drug is contraindicated in patients with diabetes mellitus, congestive cardiac disease, chronic renal disease, and hypertension.

Preparations. Preparations include the following: powder for preparation of injection solutions, 25 and 40 USP units; solutions for injection, 20, 40, and 80 units per ml. Corticotropin is also available as a gel, 20, 40, 80, and 100 ml.

Dosage. The dosage is as follows: given intramuscularly, 40 to 80 units of the solution per day in four divided doses or in a single dose of gel; given intravenously, 40 to 80 units in 1,000 ml of 5% dextrose by slow infusion over a period of 12 to 24 hours.

Acetylsalicylic acid (aspirin)

Actions. Aspirin is the most important representative drug of the antipyretic, nonnarcotic analgesics. The analgesic action is believed to occur by virtue of a selective depressant action on the central nervous system. Low-intensity pain, particularly headache, myalgia, and neuralgia, is most likely to be amenable to relief by the ingestion of aspirin. The mechanism of analgesia induced by aspirin appears to be different from that induced by the narcotics. In large doses, aspirin also exerts a prothrombinopenic effect and a uricosuric action. The antipyretic action of aspirin occurs only in the presence of fever. Large doses of acetylsalicylic acid exert an anti-inflammatory, antirheumatoid effect and a complex, poorly understood influence on carbohydrate metabolism. Aspirin decreases prostaglandin levels and also reduces platelet aggregation.

Ophthalmic uses. Aspirin is used for the relief of mild ocular pain of any origin. Before the development of the corticosteroids, aspirin was frequently employed for its anti-inflammatory effects in the treatment of uveitis. It is still used occasionally for this disease, either alone or in combination with the corticosteroids. Aspirin has also been used for the treatment of retinovascular occlusive disorders affecting small vessels, as in diabetes mellitus.

Adverse effects. No serious side effects arise from analgesic, antipyretic doses of aspirin. Massive dosage requires consideration of its antiprothrombin effects and the effects it has on the gastrointestinal tract and acid-base balance. Aspirin may be administered orally or rectally but is too irritating for parenteral use.

Preparations. Preparations include the following: tablets, 5 grains (pediatric, 1, 1.5, and 2.5 grains); capsules, 5 grains; suppositories, 1, 1.5, 2, 2.5, and 5 grains.

Dosage. The dosage is 5 to 10 grains as required. For severe uveitis 90 to 100 grains per day, or until tinnitus develops, are divided into doses at 4-hour intervals. For less severe uveitis 60 to 75 grains are given per day.

Indomethacin (Indocin)

Indomethacin is 1-(p-chlorobenzoyl)-5-methoxy-2-methylindole-3-acetic acid.

Actions. Indomethacin is an antirheumatic drug that has anti-inflammatory, analgesic, and antipyretic actions. It has no effect on pituitary or adrenal function. Indomethacin appears to inhibit prostaglandin synthesis. It is effective in reducing fever, swelling, and tenderness and in relieving pain in patients with rheumatic diseases. It is used in the treatment of rheumatoid arthritis, rheumatoid spondylitis, osteoarthritis, and gout.

Ophthalmic uses. Indomethacin has been used in the treatment of nongranulomatous uveitis, particularly in that type associated with rheumatoid disorders. It has also been used for the treatment of postoperative inflammation, including cystoid maculopathy.

Adverse effects. Indomethacin may cause gastrointestinal irritation and peptic ulcers. It should not be used in patients with peptic ulcers or ulcerative colitis. Indomethacin may aggravate psychiatric disturbances, epilepsy, and parkinsonism; in some patients it produces dizziness and lightheadedness. Also reported are hepatic toxicities, hypersensitivities, hearing disturbances, hematological reactions, alopecia, edema, and hypertension. Corneal deposits and pigmentary macular changes have been described.

Preparations. It is prepared in 25-mg capsules.

Dosage. For rheumatoid arthritis, rheumatoid spondylitis, and osteoarthritis, the dose initially is 25 mg two or three times a day; if no response occurs, the daily dose is increased 25 mg a day at weekly intervals. A daily dose of 150 to 200 mg must not be exceeded. For acute attacks of gout, 50 mg is given three times a day until symptoms are relieved.

Phenylbutazone (Butazolidin)

Phenylbutazone is a synthetic derivative of pyrazolone, related chemically to aminopyrine.

Actions. In addition to analgesic and antipyretic effects, phenylbutazone produces a strong anti-inflammatory effect. It also reduces the serum uric acid. Because of its analgesic and anti-inflammatory actions, it is useful in the management of gout and psoriasis with arthritis and rheumatoid arthritis. It has also been recommended for use in acute superficial thrombophlebitis in carefully selected patients.

Ophthalmic uses. Phenylbutazone has been reported to be useful in the treatment of certain cases of uveitis, particularly those associated with the arthritides.

Adverse effects. Side effects occur in 40% of patients receiving phenylbutazone, and it may be necesary to discontinue its use in some patients. The most commonly observed side effects are edema, rash, epigastric pain, vertigo, and stomatitis. Central nervous system stimulation, lethargy, gastrointestinal bleeding, various blood dyscrasias, and cardiac arrhythmias are less commonly observed. Increased activity of the coumarin type of anticoagulants occurs. Because of the numerous and serious toxic side effects, patients receiving this drug require constant medical supervision.

Use of the drug is contraindicated in patients with edema, cardiac decompensation, or a history of peptic ulcer. The medication should be discontinued if a significant reduction in the formed elements of the blood occurs.

Preparation. Preparation is in the form of 100-mg tablets.

Dosage. The dosage initially is 300 to 600 mg daily in three or four divided doses until the desired effect is obtained. Maintenance dose is 100 to 200 mg. Doses of larger than 600 mg should not be employed. High doses should not be used for more than 10 days.

Typhoid vaccine for nonspecific protein therapy

Actions. Typhoid vaccines, as nonspecific protein agents, produce a febrile response after intravenous injection. As a result of this hyperpyrexia, a certain "shock" reaction occurs in which the defensive mechanisms of the body are stimulated. Initially, there may be a chill; this is followed by fever, usually occurring 3 to 4 hours after injection and lasting for several hours. Muscular aches and malaise sometimes follow.

Leukopenia may occur soon after typhoid vaccine administration, followed in a few hours by leukocytosis. The adrenal cortices are probably stimulated, and there is a general response of the immune processes.

Ophthalmic uses. Typhoid vaccines are employed in the treatment of uveitis. Before the introduction of ACTH and the corticosteroids, typhoid vaccines were commonly used. They are now seldom employed for this purpose.

Adverse effects. Excessive fever, with a temperature over 106° F, may occur in patients who are particularly sensitive to the typhoid antigen. The patient's temperature should be checked frequently, and cold sponging and other heat dispersion techniques should be applied if excessive fever develops. The drug should not be used in patients with advanced arteriosclerosis, cardiac disorders, active tuberculosis, anemia, or renal and hepatic insufficiency, or in elderly persons.

Preparations. Solutions for intravenous delivery must be prepared from USP vaccines.

Dosage. The techniques of administration vary considerably. Single intravenous injections may be given, 10 to 25 million organisms. Repeated injections on alternate days are given two or three more times. The dose is increased up to 20 to 50 million organisms, depending on the patient's response. Some physicians prefer to give 5 million organisms initially and a second intravenous injection of 5 to 10 million organisms after several hours, depending on the febrile reaction. A temperature response of 103° to 105° F for 3 to 5 hours is desirable.

NOTE: Typhoid vaccines should not be employed after the systemic administration of corticosteroids. These vaccines shock the adrenal cortex, and if adrenal atrophy has occurred from corticosteroid therapy, adrenal collapse may occur.

IMMUNOSUPPRESSIVE (ANTINEOPLASTIC) AGENTS

Developed primarily for the treatment of neoplastic disease, these cytotoxic drugs have also been employed in the treatment of autoimmune disease. They have been used successfully in the treatment of many autoimmune disorders, including arthritis, systemic lupus erythematosus, nephrosis, glomerulonephritis, psoriasis, ulcerative colitis, autoimmune hemolytic anemias, and homograft reactions. In ophthalmology they have been used with some success in the treatment of severe forms of uveitis resistant to other therapy. They have been used in occasional patients with the ophthalmopathy of Graves' disease and in patients with pseudotumors of the orbit. Certain drugs such as triethylenemelamine (TEM) have been used as adjunctive treatment of retinoblastoma. Nitrogen mustards and other alkylating agents have also been used for treatment of ocular neoplastic disease. Triethylenethiophosphoramide (Thio-TEPA) has been used to retard pterygium recurrence after surgical excision.

The antineoplastic agents have been classified into alkylating agents, antimetabolites, antibiotics, Vinca alkaloids, and radioactive isotopes. Readers are referred to other sources for detailed description of the pharmacological action of these drugs. Brief descriptions of only some of the agents more commonly used in ophthalmology are given below.

Basically these drugs act by blocking protein synthesis at different levels—precursor stages leading to RNA-DNA synthesis or subsequent activity of RNA and DNA. However, their exact mechanism of action in autoimmune disease remains obscure.

The most commonly used agents for treatment of immune disease are azathioprine (Imuran), cyclophosphamide (Cytoxan), chlorambucil (Leukeran), and methotrexate. Although therapy with these drugs may be successful in controlling the inflammatory-immune process, recurrences and flare-ups are common when the drugs are discontinued or the dosage is reduced. Furthermore, very serious side effects occur with these drugs, including infections, suppression of bone marrow activity and hematopoiesis, gastrointestinal disturbances, and cutaneous reactions. Teratogenic effects may also occur. Malignancies have been associated with the use of these drugs in whole organ transplantation. Because of these various serious side effects, these agents should not be employed by physicians unfamiliar with them.

Azathioprine (Imuran)

Azathioprine is a derivative of 6-mercaptopurine in which substitution of the sulfhydryl group has been achieved to impede degradation of the compound in vivo.

Actions. Like 6-mercaptopurine, azathioprine is an antimetabolite that acts by interfering with nucleic acid synthesis. It has been used in the treatment of thrombocytopenic purpura, autoimmune hemolytic anemias, glomerulonephritis, lupus erythematosus, and rheumatoid arthritis. Antibody formation is inhibited by azathioprine; for this reason the drug has been used in suppressing immune reactions after whole organ transplantation.

Ophthalmic uses. Azathioprine has been used experimentally and in a limited number of clinical cases to suppress immune reactions in the cornea and uvea.

Adverse effects. Azathioprine may produce nausea, vomiting, leukopenia, and bone marrow depression. Increased susceptibility to many common infections develops.

Preparation. Azathioprine is prepared in tablets, 50 mg.

Dosage. For treatment of inflammatory disorders, the initial dose is 50 mg per day, which is increased by 50 mg weekly to a maximum of 150 mg. For treatment of graft rejection, 1 to 4 mg per kg of body weight is given daily.

Chlorambucil (Leukeran)

Actions. Chlorambucil is a derivative of nitrogen mustard. It is cytotoxic and has been used in the treatment of chronic lymphatic leukemia, lymphomas, lymphosarcomas, and Hodgkin's disease. It is thought to be less toxic to the hemopoietic system than is nitrogen mustard.

Ophthalmic uses. Chlorambucil has been used in the treatment of severe immune inflammatory intraocular disorders such as uveitis and retinal vasculitis that have been unresponsive to cortical steroid therapy.

Adverse effects. Bone marrow depression, including leukopenia, thrombocytopenia, and anemia, often occur. This toxicity appears to be dose related and is usually reversible. Patients receiving chlorambucil should be monitored with regular blood counts. The drug is teratogenic and should not be used during the first trimester of pregnancy.

Preparations. Chlorambucil is prepared in 2-mg tablets to be given orally.

Dosage. Usual adult dosage is 0.1 to 0.2 mg per kg of body weight for 3 to 6 weeks. Further treatment is defined by the response of patient and toxic reactions.

Cyclophosphamide (Cytoxan)

Cyclophosphamide is an antineoplastic drug related to nitrogen mustards. It is classified as an alkylating agent.

Actions. The exact mechanism of action of cyclophosphamide is unknown; it is probable the drug acts by interfering with DNA replication and cell division. It is useful in the treatment of Hodgkin's disease, lymphosarcomas, reticulum cell sarcoma, multiple myeloma, and some forms of leukemia. It has a palliative effect on some solid carcinomas. The drug has also been used to suppress severe immune reactions, including those after whole organ transplant and severe disabling rheumatoid arthritis.

Ophthalmic uses. Cyclophosphamide has been used to suppress severe immune reactions of the uvea that are unresponsive to other drugs. It has also been used in the treatment of retinoblastoma.

Adverse effects. Alopecia is a common side reaction; this is reversible. Leukopenia and bone marrow depression generally occur. Other side reactions include nausea, vomiting, anorexia, weight loss, diarrhea, and mucosal ulceration. The drug is highly teratogenic.

Preparations. Preparations include the following: vials of 100 and 200 mg for injection; tablets, 50 mg.

Dosage. For anti-inflammatory therapy, 50 mg are given daily and increased by 50 mg every 4 weeks until there is clinical improvement. The maintenance dose is 50 to 100 mg daily. For treatment of graft rejection, the initial dose is 20 to 40 mg per kg of body weight given over a 1- to 4-day period. The oral maintenance dose is 1 to 3 mg per kg of body weight. The intravenous maintenance dose is 10 to 15 mg per kg of body weight every 7 to 10 days. A blood count should be obtained weekly and the leukocyte count maintained between 2,000 and 5,000 per mm^3.

Mechlorethamine hydrochloride (Mustargen, nitrogen mustard)

Actions. Mechlorethamine hydrochloride is a cytotoxin that has an affinity for cancer cells and other rapidly growing cells. The precise action of the drug is unknown. However, it interferes with growth and mitotic cell division.

It is also used as a palliative agent in patients with Hodgkin's disease, lymphosarcoma, reticular cell sarcoma, and bronchogenic carcinoma.

Ophthalmic uses. Mechlorethamine hydrochloride has been used in combination with x-ray therapy for the treatment of retinoblastoma. However, it has not been used as extensively in the treatment of this disorder as has triethylenemelamine (TEM).

Adverse effects. Nausea, vomiting, anorexia, and thrombophlebitis are the common side effects; others are lymphocytopenia, granulocytopenia, thrombocytopenia, and anemia. Extravasation outside the vein leads to severe local inflammation and sometimes to sloughing of the overlying tissues.

Preparation. The preparation for injection is powder, 10 mg.

Dosage. The dosage is 0.1 mg per kg of body weight by intravenous injection daily for 4 days.

Mercaptopurine (Purinethol)

Mercaptopurine is an analogue and metabolic antagonist of adenine, a nucleic acid constitutent, and hypoxanthine, a purine base.

Actions. Mercaptopurine interferes with nucleic acid synthesis. It is used in the treatment of acute leukemia and chronic myelocytic leukemia. Mercaptopurine suppresses antibody synthesis and has been used in the treatment of serious immune reactions.

Ophthalmic uses. Mercaptopurine has been used to treat severe cases of uveitis unresponsive to corticosteroid and ACTH therapy.

Adverse effects. Mercaptopurine is a cytotoxic agent and can produce many serious side reactions, including bone marrow depression, liver damage with jaundice, gastrointestinal irritation and ulceration, nausea, vomiting, and anorexia. This drug can produce abortion and teratogenetic effects; whenever possible, it should be avoided during the first trimester of pregnancy.

Preparation. It is prepared in the form of 50-mg tablets.

Dosage. The dosage is 2.5 to 5 mg per kg of body weight per day. Low doses should be used initially and increased if no clinical improvement occurs. Larger doses are used in the treatment of nonhematological malignancies.

Triethylenemelamine (TEM)

Actions. TEM is a cytotoxic antineoplastic agent that has an action similar to that of the nitrogen mustards. The exact mechanism of action is unknown, but it is probably by an antienzymatic action and therefore interference with cell mitosis. Rapidly growing cells and cancer cells are selectively affected.

Ophthalmic uses. TEM is used along with x-ray therapy for the treatment of retinoblastoma.

Adverse effects. TEM frequently produces anemia, leukopenia, thrombocytopenia, and bone marrow depression, and frequent hemograms should be obtained on patients receiving this medication. Diarrhea, vomiting, and anorexia may occur, particularly if the drug is administered orally.

Preparations. Preparations include the following: tablets, 5 mg; for injection, vials of sterile powder.

Dosage. The dosages for retinoblastoma are as follows:

ORALLY: Initial dose, under 12 months of age, 2.5 mg; between 12 and 18 months of age, 3.5 mg; administered before x-ray therapy and at conclusion of therapy; subsequent doses are given at intervals, depending on the patient's response and tolerance to drug and on blood cell counts. A total dose of 15 mg is recommended.

INTRAMUSCULARLY: 0.082 to 0.1 mg per kg of body weight, one dose before x-ray therapy and a second dose after x-ray therapy is concluded.

INTRA-ARTERIALLY: 0.06 to 0.08 mg per kg of body weight into the internal carotid artery as a single dose before x-ray treatment and repeated when the hemogram is normal. Alternately, a catheter may be inserted into the carotid artery via the superior thyroid artery, and TEM may be given in a daily dose of 0.03 mg per kg of body weight concurrently with x-ray therapy.

Triethylenethiophosphoramide (Thio-TEPA)

Triethylenethiophosphoramide is an alkylating agent related to nitrogen mustard.

Actions. The drug is used as a palliative agent in the treatment of neoplastic diseases. Its action is believed to result from the release of ethylenimine radicals and their effects on dividing cells. The drug may be injected into local sites or given intravenously for the treatment of neoplasms.

Ophthalmic uses. Triethylenethiophosphoramide has been applied topically to prevent recurrence of pterygium after surgical removal. It has also been used topically to prevent corneal vascularization after chemical burns.

Adverse effects. The drug is radiomimetic and is highly toxic to the hematopoietic system when given systemically. Other possible side effects include vomiting, anorexia, headache, and allergic reactions. There are no significant systemic side effects with topical therapy. Changes in skin pigmentation of eyelids have occurred in Blacks.

Preparation. The drug is prepared in 15-mg vials.

Dosage. As prophylaxis against recurrence of pterygium, a 1:2,000 solution is applied to the eye every 3 hours during the day for 6 to 8 weeks. Treatment is started within a few days after surgical removal of the pterygium.

CHELATING AND EPITHELIOLYTIC AGENTS
Ethylenediamine tetra-acetate sodium (EDTA, sodium edetate, Endrate, Versenate Sodium)

Ethylenediamine tetra-acetate sodium is the sodium salt of the chelating agent EDTA.

Actions. EDTA chelates various metallic ions into a soluble complex that is rapidly excreted by the kidneys. Calcium ions are preferentially removed by sodium EDTA. Intravenous administration of sodium EDTA removes calcium from the bloodstream, whereas local application of the drug reduces regional tissue calcium.

Ophthalmic uses. Solutions of sodium EDTA are applied topically for the removal of calcium deposits in the cornea that occur in such diseases as band keratopathy.

Adverse effects. The most common side effects of systemically administered EDTA are malaise, fever, headache, and arthralgia. Hypocalcemia and possible significant changes in calcium balance may occur with overdosage. Hypocalcemic tetany may also occur. The systemic use of this compound is extremely dangerous and requires expert attention. Renal tubular necrosis has been observed as a sequel to systemic administration of this agent.

After topical application to the eye, conjunctival redness and chemosis occur. Stromal corneal edema, usually transient but occasionally permanent, has also been observed.

Preparations. No commercial ophthalmic preparations are presently available. Disodium edetate (Endrate) is available in a 15%, 150-mg ampul of 20 ml. This may be used to prepare solutions for ophthalmic use. Five milliliters of disodium edetate may be injected in 120 ml of a standard ophthalmic isotonic irrigating solution without calcium, such as Dacriose. This yields a 0.02M solution.

Dosage. For removal of calcium from the cornea, the eye is anesthetized with cocaine, and the corneal epithelium is completely removed. Several milliliters of the EDTA solution are applied in an iontophoresis cup fitted to the cornea for 15 to 20 minutes. Occasional slight movement of the cup will improve the circulation of the fluid. After removal of the cup the eye is irrigated with physiological saline solution, an antibiotic is instilled, and a tight bandage is applied.

Alternatively, after the removal of epithelium, the EDTA solution may be applied by continuous drip or constant irrigation for 15 minutes. This application plus rubs of the cornea with a cotton applicator is usually successful in removing most calcium bands. The EDTA may also be delivered by the application of a Weck Cel sponge to the cornea after epithelial debridement.

For most calcium infiltration of the cornea 0.02M (0.70%) solutions of EDTA are satisfactory. Occasional higher concentrations, 0.05M (1.85%), may be required.

NOTE: This agent should not be confused with calcium-disodium edetate, which is administered systemically for the treatment of lead and other metallic poisoning.

Epitheliolytic agents: iodine and ether

Actions. After topical application, epitheliolytic agents cause destruction of the corneal epithelium. They are most effective against necrotic epithelium. Studies indicate that they do not remove viruses or enter live cells. However, viable corneal epithelium may be removed by vigorous scrubbing with an applicator.

Ophthalmic uses. Iodine and ether scrubs of the cornea are used in the treatment of herpes simplex keratitis. They are most effective in the superficial dendritic forms of the disease. When these agents are employed, it is well to remove all of the corneal epithelium.

Adverse effects. There are no significant side reactions to the local application of epitheliolytic agents. Pain, conjunctival injection, and chemosis often follow their use. These agents should not be applied to deep corneal lesions, since chemical keratitis and permanent scarring may result.

Preparations. Preparations include the following: tincture of iodine, 2% to 5%; ether, USP.

Dosage. Iodine solutions and ether are applied with an applicator after topical application of corneal anesthesia.

NOTE: Cocaine inactivates iodine. It should not be used for corneal anesthesia before iodine scrubs.

ENZYMES
Alpha-chymotrypsin (Alpha Chymar, Quimotrase, Zolyse)

Alpha-chymotrypsin is a proteolytic enzyme prepared from mammalian pancreas. It is the most stable and diffusible of the four varieties of chymotrypsin.

Ophthalmic uses. Alpha-chymotrypsin is used to facilitate cataract extraction. The lens zonules are lysed after a short contact time with alpha-chymotrypsin. The drug has also been employed topically in the treatment of dendritic keratitis.

Adverse effects. Transient glaucoma may occur in the immediate postoperative period after alpha-chymotrypsin has been used. No attempt should be made to perform intracapsular cataract surgery in individuals under 20 years of age. Vitreal lens adhesions present in young individuals are not dissolved with alpha-chymotrypsin.

Preparations. Preparations include the following: powder, 750 units with 10 ml diluent; dilution with 5 ml yields a 1:5,000 solution; dilution with 10 ml yields a 1:10,000 dilution.

Dosage. The posterior chamber is irrigated with 1 to 3 ml of a 1:5,000 to 1:10,000 solution. After 2 to 4 minutes the posterior chamber is irrigated with diluent alone or with saline solution. Techniques vary considerably with individual surgeons.

Fibrinolysin, human (Thrombolysin)

Actions. Fibrinolysin is a proteolytic enzyme prepared by activating a fraction of the blood plasma with streptokinase. It lyses fibrin and is of some help in the dissolution of freshly formed clots. Once organization of the blood clot has occurred, however, fibrinolysin is not of value. The drug is not an anticoagulant, and concomitant therapy with anticoagulating agents is necessary to prevent additional thrombus formation.

Ophthalmic uses. Fibrinolysin may be tried in patients with recent occlusions of the central retinal vein. It is usually given in combination with anticoagulants. Fibrinolysin has been advocated for the removal of large, partially organized hyphemas producing secondary glaucoma. The anterior chamber is opened and irrigated with a solution of fibrinolysin containing 1,250 units per ml. This solution is injected and aspirated until the clot is dissolved and the anterior chamber is free of blood, which usually requires 30 minutes.

Adverse effects. The side effects of systemic therapy with fibrinolysin include fever, chills, abdominal and chest pain, nausea, vomiting, and dizziness. Either hypotension or hypertension may occur. The undesirable effects on the ocular tissues from local irrigation into the eye are not yet well evaluated. There is no systemic reaction from local use.

Fibrinolysin is contraindicated in patients with any hemorrhagic diathesis, hypofibrinogenemia, and severe liver dysfunction.

Preparations. Preparation is as follows: Thrombolysin, vials, 50,000 units.

Dosage. The dosage varies with the preparation. Before using, the physician should study the brochure enclosed with the preparation.

Hyaluronidase (Alidase, Hyazyme, Wydase)

Actions. Hyaluronidase is an enzyme that hydrolyzes hyaluronic acid, an essential component of the connective tissue cement substance. As a result, tissue permeability is increased, and injected solutions and local accumulations of fluid spread more rapidly and are absorbed faster.

Ophthalmic uses. Hyaluronidase is added to the local anesthetic solutions used for ocular surgery.

Adverse effects. There are no significant side effects. Since the drug might cause the spread of an infection, it should not be injected into sites of infection.

Preparations. Preparations are as follows: (lyophilized powder, 150 USP units and 1,500 USP units per vial); solution for injection, 150 USP units per ml.

Dosage. The dosage in local anesthesia for ocular surgery is 150 USP units per 30 ml of anesthetic solution (5 to 6 units per ml).

MIOTICS

Miotics (Chapter 4) may be divided into two major pharmacological groups: the direct-acting cholinergic (muscarinic) agents, which stimulate the sphincter muscle of the iris, and the indirect-acting cholinesterase inhibitors, which potentiate the action of acetylcholine by inhibiting acetylcholinesterase, the enzyme catalyzing the hydrolysis of acetylcholine.

DIRECT-ACTING AGENTS

All drugs in the direct-acting category have muscarinic effects, that is, stimulation of structures innervated by the postganglionic parasympathetic fibers. These drugs stimulate secretion by many glands, including the lacrimal, salivary, bronchial, gastric, and intestinal glands. They also stimulate contraction of the smooth muscle of the gastrointestinal tract and urinary bladder, thus resulting in increased peristalsis and evacuation of the bladder. Smooth muscles of the bronchial tract are also stimulated. Muscarinic drugs produce variable cardiovascular effects, including generalized vasodilatation, fall in blood pressure, bradycardia, and increased skin temperature.

In the eye these drugs produce contraction of the sphincter muscle of the iris, thus causing miosis. They also stimulate contraction of the circular muscle of the iris and thereby produce accommodation. Increased facility of aqueous humor outflow and consequent fall in the intraocular pressure, particularly in patients with glaucoma, follow the application of these agents into the eye. In addition, there may be some alteration in aqueous humor secretion. Vasodilatation of the iris and episcleral vessels may occur.

Ophthalmic uses. Direct-acting cholinergic agents are used in the treatment of glaucoma. Pilocarpine is used principally in the treatment of primary glaucoma, either the narrow-angle or open-angle type. It is also used to produce miosis after pupillary dilatation. Carbachol is useful in the treatment of open-angle glaucoma. It is often helpful in patients in whom pilocarpine therapy is ineffective. It should not be used in acute narrow-angle glaucoma, since it produces significant vasodilatation of the iris and episcleral vessels.

Adverse effects. Prolonged use of these miotic drops may result in the formation of follicles in the conjunctiva. Rarely is contact dermatitis seen. Headaches and accommodative spasm may follow the use of these drugs; these symptoms are more pronounced in the early treatment with the drug. For pilocarpine, these symptoms are minimized by the use of the Ocusert delivery system. Refractiveness to the ocular hypotensive actions of these agents, particularly pilocarpine, may develop after prolonged use.

Systemic reactions to the topical use of these drugs are rare and usually occur from overdosage. Such reactions resemble muscarine poisoning and include symptoms of gastrointestinal cramping, vomiting, diarrhea, sweating, and occasionally cardiac arrhythmias. These effects may be partially antagonized with the administration of atropine.

Carbachol (Carbacel, Carcholin, Doryl, Mistura C)

Preparations. Preparations include the following: ophthalmic solutions and sprays, 0.75%, 1.5%, and 3% with benzalkonium chloride (simple aqueous solutions do not penetrate the cornea); ophthalmic ointment, 1.5%; 0.1% solution in 1.5-ml vials for instillation into the anterior chamber after cataract surgery.

Dosage. The dosage is 1 drop of solution or one mist application one to four times a day or application of ointment twice a day for the treatment of open-angle glaucoma.

Pilocarpine

Preparations. Preparations include the following: nitrate and hydrochloride ophthalmic solutions and sprays, 0.25% to 10%; ophthalmic ointment, 1% and 2%; spray 0.5% to 4%; Ocuserts P-20 (release pilocarpine at a rate of 20μg per hour for 1 week) and P-40 (release pilocarpine at rate of 40μg per hour for 1 week).

Dosage. The dosage is 1 to 2 drops or spray application instilled into the eye two to six times a day or Ocusert inserted into conjunctival cul-de-sac once a week for the treatment of open-angle glaucoma. In acute angle-closure glaucoma, 2% to 4% pilocarpine drops should be instilled into the eye every 10 minutes for an hour and then every 1 to 2 hours until the pressure is controlled.

CHOLINESTERASE INHIBITORS

Cholinesterase inhibitors (Chapter 4) achieve their pharmacological effects by inhibition of the enzyme acetylcholinesterase, thus permitting the accumulation of excessive amounts of acetylcholine. Effects occur wherever acetylcholine is found, namely, at the parasympathetic postganglionic endings, the neuromuscular junctions, the autonomic ganglia, and the central nervous system. Depression of the enzyme pseudocholinesterase (butrylcholinesterase), also may occur with administration of certain of these agents.

Individual cholinesterase inhibitors react with acetylcholinesterase in somewhat different manners. Reversible enzyme-inhibitor complexes are formed by certain inhibitors that may be quite rapidly reversible over a period of minutes, as exemplified by edrophonium chloride (Tensilon). The enzyme-inhibitor complex formed with inhibitors such as physostigmine and neostigmine are slowly reversible over a period of hours. The organophosphate anticholinesterases such as echothiophate form an irreversible complex with acetylcholinesterase, which is highly resistant to hydrolysis. The duration of action may be several weeks and is governed by the rate of enzymatic synthesis. Administration of a reversible inhibitor may block the effect of subsequent administration of an irreversible inhibitor by binding the enzyme receptor site.

In small doses anticholinesterases have little effect on neuromuscular transmission. With increasing doses neuromuscular block of the depolarizing type can occur. Some cholinesterase inhibitors such as edrophonium and neostigmine produce direct stimulation of the neuromuscular junction and are used in the treatment of myasthenia gravis. Initial central nervous system stimulation followed by depression may occur with administration of cholinesterase inhibitors.

Topical application of cholinesterase inhibitors into the eye results in miosis and stimulation of accommodation. Improved aqueous humor outflow with a fall in intraocular pressure occurs in eyes with open angles. There is some vasodilation of the conjunctival and iris vessels.

Ophthalmic uses. The anticholinesterases are used in the management of open-angle glaucoma. Their use should generally be restricted to those patients who have failed to respond to other weaker miotics. Some patients with aphakia and other secondary types of glaucoma may respond to anticholinesterases. These drugs may also be helpful in the treatment of accommodative esotropia since they decrease the accommodative convergence/accommodation ratio.

Adverse effects. Spasm in the ciliary body is a frequent side effect of anticholinesterases, resulting in pain intensified by accommodation to light and accompanied by congestion of the eye. These effects are most severe during the initial phases of treatment and may subside as treatment continues. Because of the congestion produced, these drugs should not be used in the treatment of narrow-angle glaucoma. In some patients, persistence of ciliary spasm may necessitate discontinuance of the drugs. Both anterior cortical and posterior subcapsular lens opacities apparently may result from long-term topical application of anticholinesterases. Retinal detachments have also rarely been reported as a complication of therapy with the strong anticholinesterase agents. Stenosis of the lacrimal puncta also has occurred.

Hyperplasia of the pigment epithelium of the iris ("iris cysts") may develop after prolonged use of anticholinesterases. These usually disappear upon withdrawal of the drug. Iris cysts may be prevented by the use of 2.5% phenylephrine (Neo-Synephrine) as the diluent for agents such as echothiophate. Alternatively weak solutions of epinephrine given concurrently in the eye may prevent iris cyst formation.

Systemic cholinergic stimulation including salivation, nausea, vomiting, and diarrhea may follow local instillation of anticholinesterase agents. All are quickly controlled upon withdrawal of the drug. The antidote for accidentally produced acute toxicity is the systemic administration of atropine and pralidoxime (Protopam) chloride.

Demercarium bromide (Humorsol)

Preparation. This agent is prepared in 0.125% and 0.25% solution in 5-ml vials.

Dosage. The dosage is 1 to 2 drops of either 0.125% or 0.25% solution once or twice a day.

Echothiophate (Phospholine) iodide

Preparation. The agent is prepared in the form of a powder, 1.5, 3, 6.25, and 12.5 mg supplied with sterile diluent to make a 5-ml solution.

Dosage. The dosage is 1 drop of 0.03% to 0.25% solution, once or twice a day.

Isoflurophate (DFP; Floropryl)

Preparations. Preparations include the following: ophthalmic solution, 0.1% in anhydrous peanut oil (isoflurophate is hydrolyzed by contact with water); ophthalmic ointment, 0.025%, in polyethylene mineral oil gel.

Dosage. The dosage for glaucoma is 1 drop of 0.1% solution every 12 to 72 hours and for strabismus, 1 drop (¼-inch strip of ointment) at bedtime.

Neostigmine (Prostigmin)

Preparations. Preparations include the following: neostigmine bromide ophthalmic solutions, 5%; ampuls, methylsulfate, 0.25, 0.5, and 1 mg per ml; tablets, bromide, 15 mg.

Dosage. The dosage is 1 or 2 drops of 2.5% or 5% solution two to six times a day for postoperative distention and urinary retention; 0.25 mg is administered by injection.

Physostigmine, Eserine

Preparations. Preparations include the following: ophthalmic solutions, 0.25% and 0.5%; ophthalmic ointment, 0.25%.

Dosage. The dosage is instillation of solution or ointment one to four times a day.

Edrophonium chloride (Tensilon)

Edrophonium chloride is a curare antagonist related chemically to neostigmine.

Actions. In myasthenic patients, edrophonium administered intravenously will induce a rapid but transient increase in muscular strength. It may be used as a diagnostic agent in myasthenia gravis and to determine the relative effectiveness of other treatment. As an antidote to curare, the drug acts rapidly, but effects are weaker than with neostigmine. Edrophonium has a mild anticholinesterase action, but the neuromuscular effects are probably direct.

Adverse effects. In very large doses edrophonium has a curariform action that can lead to apnea. Bronchiolar spasm and increased salivation have been observed in patients with asthma or cardiac disease treated with this drug, and it should be used in these patients with extreme care.

Preparation. It is prepared in a solution for injection, 10 mg per ml.

Dosage. The dosage as an antidote to curare is 10 mg intravenously, given slowly, maximum, 40 mg; as a diagnostic aid in myasthenia gravis, 10 mg given intravenously—2 mg is given slowly and the remainder is administered after 45 seconds if no untoward reaction has occurred.

MYDRIATICS AND CYCLOPLEGICS

Mydriasis may be produced by stimulation of the dilator muscle of the iris or by paralysis of the pupillary sphincter muscle of the iris (Chapter 4). Sympathomimetic or adrenergic agents produce mydriasis by direct stimulation of the iris dilator muscle. They do not affect the sphincter muscle of the iris or the circular muscle of the ciliary body. They do not produce any significant weakness of accommodation (cycloplegia).

Other agents such as hydroxyamphetamine (Paredrine) produce mydriasis by releasing norepinephrine from the sympathetic nerve terminals. Potentiation of the effect of norepinephrine with consequent mydriasis is achieved with cocaine, which blocks the resorption of norepinephrine back into the terminal sympathetic fibers.

Parasympatholytic (anticholinergic) agents act by blocking the action of acetylcholine on the iris sphincter and ciliary muscles. Thus they produce mydriasis as well as cycloplegia. All cycloplegics produce mydriasis. On the other hand, mydriatic agents produce little or no cycloplegia.

The mydriatic and cycloplegic agents are employed for many purposes in ophthalmology (see individual agents below). They are used frequently to permit measurement of refractive errors, as aids in ophthalmoscopy and retinal photography, in the treatment of anterior uveitis, and in the management of preoperative and postoperative patients undergoing intraocular surgery. Certain agents, such as epinephrine, may be valuable in the treatment of open-angle glaucoma. Strong cycloplegics such as atropine are used in the treatment of malignant glaucoma.

Both local and systemic side effects can occur with the use of these drugs (see individual agents below).

Epinephrine (Adrenalin); levoepinephrine (Adrenatrate, Epifrin, Epinal, Epitrate, Eppy, Glaucon, Lyophrin, Mistura E, Mytrate)

Actions. Epinephrine is a sympathomimetic agent with primarily adrenergic action. The drug duplicates most of the actions of stimulation of the sympathetic nervous system. The pharmacological actions include an increase in heart rate, vasoconstriction in the visceral areas, vasodilatation in the muscles, and an elevated blood pressure. Epinephrine is useful in the management of serious asthmatic attacks and severe hypersensitivity reactions. In the eye, topical administration of epinephrine produces vasoconstriction and slight pupillary mydriasis. Intraocular pressure is reduced as a result of decreased aqueous production and improvement in aqueous outflow.

Ophthalmic uses. The levoepinephrine preparations are used as adjuncts in the control of open-angle glaucoma. They are used in combination with other antiglaucoma medications, miotics, and carbonic anhydrase inhibitors. Hypersecretion glaucoma may be improved with the use of the levoepinephrine products.

Epinephrine, USP, is used with local anesthetics to delay absorption of the anesthetic. It is also used in weak solutions as a conjunctival decongestant.

Adverse effects. The side effects include pain and stinging sensation after instillation into the eye. Rebound hyperemia and melanin deposits in the cornea and conjunctiva may also occur. Macular edema has occurred in aphakic eyes. Palpitation and increased pulse rate may occur after topical use. The drug should be used with caution in patients with hypertensive cardiovascular disease.

Preparations. Preparations are as follows: Adrenatrate (epinephrine bitartrate, 1% and 2%); Epifrin (epinephrine hydrochloride, 0.25%, 0.5%, 1%, and 2%); Epinal (epinephrine borate complex, 0.25%, 0.5%, and 1%); Eppy (epinephryl borate, 0.5% and 1%); Epitrate (epinephrine bitartrate, 2%); Glaucon (epinephrine hydrochloride, 0.5%, 1%, and 2%); Lyophrin (epinephrine bitartrate, 2%) and Mytrate (epinephrine bitartrate, 1% and 2%) in bottles that are 5, 7.5, 10, or 15 ml; epinephrine, USP 1:1,000 solution; Mistura E (epinephrine hydrochloride, 0.25%, 0.5%, 1%, and 2%) as a spray.

Dosage. The dosage for glaucoma is 1 drop or one mist application of a levo-epinephrine product once or twice a day. For conjunctival decongestion the dosage is 25 minims of 1:1,000 epinephrine added to 30 ml of ophthalmic collyria. For use with local anesthetics the dosage is 1:50,000 to 1:200,000 dilution of epinephrine in the anesthetic solution.

Hydroxyamphetamine hydrobromide (Paredrine)

Actions. Hydroxyamphetamine hydrobromide is a synthetic sympathomimetic amine. It is an adrenergic drug that is more stable than epinephrine and has only a fraction of the vasopressor effect of epinephrine. Unlike epinephrine, it produces little central nervous system stimulation. In the eye it produces mydriasis with little, if any, cycloplegia. The drug acts by releasing norepinephrine from sympathetic nerve terminals.

Ophthalmic uses. Hydroxyamphetamine hydrobromide is used as a mydriatic chiefly as an aid in ophthalmoscopy. It is sometimes used in combination with homatropine as an aid in refraction.

Adverse effects. No significant side effects result from topical application. The drug should be used with caution in patients with narrow angles.

Preparation. It is prepared in ophthalmic solution, 1%.

Dosage. The dosage is 1 or 2 drops instilled topically, which may be repeated in 10 minutes. For refraction the dosage is 1 or 2 drops instilled into the eye in combination with 4% or 5% homatropine, repeated in 10 minutes.

Phenylephrine (Neo-Synephrine) hydrochloride

Actions. Phenylephrine hydrochloride is a synthetic sympathomimetic compound with actions predominantly on the cardiovascular system. A sustained pressor action occurs that is of longer duration than that obtained by epinephrine administration. The pressor action is accompanied by a consistent and significant bradycardia related to a rise in the diastolic blood pressure. Although the stroke volume is increased, the bradycardia results in a small reduction of the minute volume of the cardiac output. There is minimal cardiac stimulation. It appears, therefore, that the significant bradycardia must be related to reflex vagal action.

Instilled into the eye, phenylephrine produces mydriasis without cycloplegia. This effect lasts up to 2 to 3 hours. A fall in intraocular pressure may occur in normal- and open-angle glaucomatous eyes.

Ophthalmic uses. Phenylephrine is used principally for its mydriatic effects. When employed in a 10% concentration, rapid complete mydriasis occurs. The drug is valuable in breaking posterior synechiae and as an aid in ophthalmoscopy and retinal photography. Solutions containing 0.125% phenylephrine are used as a conjunctival decongestant. The 2.5% solution is used as a diluent for echothiophate iodide.

Adverse effects. Side effects from topical instillation are uncommon but include systemic cardiovascular effects with elevated blood pressure and tachycardia. Phenylephrine should not be used in patients with narrow-angle glaucoma.

Preparations. Preparations include the following: solutions for topical application, 0.125%, 0.25%, 0.5%, and 2.5%, and 10%; emulsion, 10%; solution for injection, 1%.

NOTE: Contact with metal should be avoided. Cloudy solutions should be discarded. The container must be tightly stoppered. The drug is incompatible chemically with butacaine.

Dosage. The dosage for mydriasis is 1 or 2 drops of 2.5% or 10% solution, which may be repeated in 10 to 15 minutes. For conjunctival decongestion the dosage is 1 to 2 drops of 0.125% solution.

CYCLOPLEGICS
Atropine

Actions. Atropine blocks the action of certain parasympathetic nerves and cholinergic drugs. There is no reduction in the liberation of acetylcholine, but the tissues are rendered insensitive to the action of acetylcholine. Most of the body secretions (salivary, sweat, mucous, and alimentary tract) are decreased. The action of the vagus nerve on the bronchial muscles, alimentary tract, and heart is blocked with atropine.

In the eye there is pupillary dilatation and paralysis of accommodation that may last for as long as 2 or 3 weeks. In the normal eye no significant rise in intraocular pressure is produced. In the glaucomatous eye, particularly with the narrow-angle variety of glaucoma but also in some eyes with open-angle glaucoma, a rise in intraocular pressure may occur after the use of atropine, either topically or systemically.

Ophthalmic uses. Atropine is employed for its mydriatic and cycloplegic effects. It is used as an aid in refraction, particularly in young children in whom accommodation is very active. It is also used in the treatment of all forms of iritis to prevent the formation of posterior synechiae, to relieve iris and ciliary pain, and to put the inflamed tissue at rest. It is used topically both preoperatively and postoperatively in many types of intraocular surgery. It is used systemically as a preoperative agent when surgery is to be performed with the patient under general anesthesia.

Adverse effects. Contact dermatitis involving the lids and conjunctiva is frequently seen after the topical use of atropine. In addition, dryness and flushing of the skin, thirst, and acceleration of the heart may occur after topical application, particularly in infants with fair complexions. Toxic reactions may be seen after the systemic administration of as little as 0.6 mg. Each drop of a 1% solution of atropine contains 0.5 mg of atropine. To decrease the amount of systemic absorption from topically instilled atropine, pressure should be applied over the lacrimal sac after instillation, or the head should be tipped so that the excess medication runs out the lateral side of the eye. Atropine should not be used in patients with narrow-angle glaucoma or with anatomical predilection toward this disease.

Preparations. Preparations include the following: ophthalmic solution, 0.5% to 4%; usual strength is 1%; ophthalmic ointment, 0.5%, 1%, and 2%; atropine sulfate for injection, 0.3, 0.4, 0.5, 0.6, and 1.2 mg per ml in 1-, 20-, and 30-ml ampuls; tablets, hypodermic, 0.3, 0.4, and 0.6 mg; tablets, oral, 0.4 mg.

Dosage. The dosage is as follows: 1 or 2 drops of solution or ointment instilled into the eye one to three times a day; for refraction in children under the age of 30 months, 1 drop of 0.5% solution three times a day for 3 days before refraction and on the morning of refraction; from 30 months to 5 years of age, 1 drop of 1% solution three times a day for 3 days before refraction and on the morning of refraction; for preanesthesia, 0.25 to 1 mg.

Cyclopentolate (Cyclogyl)

Actions. Cyclopentolate is a synthetic spasmolytic agent that produces mydriasis and cycloplegia upon instillation into the eye. The onset of action is rapid (20 to 30 minutes), and the duration of action is short (2 to 24 hours).

Ophthalmic uses. Cyclopentolate is employed chiefly as an aid in refraction. It is also used when a short-acting cycloplegic is desired, as in relief of ciliary spasm and as a preoperative and postoperative mydriatic agent.

Adverse effects. Occasional transient neurotoxic effects are observed after local instillation. These reactions are characterized by incoherence, visual hallucinations, slurred speech, and ataxia, seizures also have been noted. These reactions are more common with the 2% solution. The drug should be employed with caution in patients suffering from glaucoma, particularly the narrow-angle variety.

Preparations. Cyclopentolate is prepared in solutions, 0.5% to 2%.

Dosage. The dosage is 1 to 3 drops of 0.5% or 1% solution at 5-minute intervals 20 to 30 minutes before refraction. In heavily pigmented individuals, 2% solution may be required.

Eucatropine (Euphthalmine) hydrochloride

Actions. Eucatropine hydrochloride is a weak cholinergic blocking agent. It is an effective mydriatic but produces very little cycloplegia. Its duration of action is usually only 2 to 4 hours.

Ophthalmic uses. Eucatropine hydrochloride is useful as an aid in ophthalmoscopy. Because it is not a vasoconstrictor and its duration of action is brief, it is often used as a provocative mydriatic test agent in patients suspected of having narrow-angle glaucoma.

Adverse effects. There are no significant side effects from the topically instilled medication. This drug should not be used in patients who are known to have narrow-angle glaucoma.

Preparations. No commercial preparations are available. Compounding is necessary for prescription.

Dosage. One or two drops of a 5% or 10% solution are instilled into the eye and repeated in 10 to 15 minutes if necessary.

Homatropine

Actions. Homatropine is a synthetic alkaloid resembling atropine in its action. It is a weaker drug than atropine, and its cerebral effects are less distinct.

In the eye, homatropine produces mydriasis and cycloplegia, which last up to 72 hours.

Ophthalmic uses. Homatropine is used as an aid in refraction. It is also used in the treatment of iritis and iridocyclitis and for relief of ciliary spasm. It is frequently employed as a cycloplegic and mydriatic in preoperative and postoperative conditions.

Adverse effects. There are very few side effects from the topical use of homatropine. The dryness of the skin and mouth encountered with atropine is much less frequent with homatropine. Homatropine should not be used in patients with narrow-angle glaucoma.

Preparations. Preparations are in the form of homatropine hydrobromide ophthalmic solutions, 1%, 2%, 4%, and 5%.

Dosage. The dosage is 1 or 2 drops of 2% to 5% solution two or three times a day. For refraction the dosage is 1 or 2 drops of 2% homatropine every 10 to 15 minutes for 5 doses, or 1 or 2 drops of 4% or 5% homatropine (sometimes combined with hydroxyamphetamine hydrobromide) repeated in 15 minutes.

Scopolamine, hyoscine

Actions. Scopolamine closely resembles atropine in action. It blocks the action of certain parasympathetic nerves and cholinergic drugs by rendering tissues insensitive to the action of acetylcholine. The action of scopolamine is of shorter duration than that of atropine. Scopolamine also differs from atropine in that it usually produces a hypnotic effect.

In the eye, scopolamine produces mydriasis and cycloplegia, which may last up to 7 days. In the normal eye there is no significant rise in intraocular pressure. In glaucomatous eyes, particularly the narrow-angle variety, a rise in intraocular pressure may occur after the use of scopolamine, either topically or systemically.

Ophthalmic uses. Scopolamine is employed for its mydriatic and cycloplegic effect. It is occasionally used as an aid in refraction. It is frequently used in the treatment of iritis and iridocyclitis, particularly in patients sensitive to atropine. The drug is also used systemically as a preoperative agent when surgery is to be performed with the patient under general anesthesia.

Adverse effects. Contact dermatitis of the eyelids is less common with scopolamine than with atropine. Dryness of the mouth and flushed skin are the most common side effects of scopolamine. Idiosyncratic reactions are more likely to occur with scopolamine than with atropine, and ordinary doses occasionally induce severe reactions. Central nervous system excitement may follow the topical or systemic administration of scopolamine. Systemic absorption of topically applied eye drops is reduced if pressure is applied over the lacrimal sac after instillation or if the head is tipped so that the excess medication runs out the lateral side of the eye.

Scopolamine should not be used in patients with narrow-angle glaucoma. If the drug is necessary as a preoperative medication in such patients, topical instillation of pilocarpine should be employed.

Preparations. Preparations include the following: scopolamine hydrobromide ophthalmic solutions, 0.2% and 0.25%; hyoscine for injection; 300, 400, 500, and 600 μg per ml; tablets, 300, 400, and 600 μg and 1.2 mg.

Dosage. The dosage is as follows: 1 to 2 drops of solution instilled into the eye one to three times a day; preanesthetic medication, 300 to 600 μg.

Tropicamide (Mydriacyl)

Actions. Tropicamide is an effective mydriatric and short-acting cycloplegic agent. Its onset of action is rapid (15 to 30 minutes), and its duration of action is short (30 minutes to 4 hours).

Ophthalmic uses. Tropicamide is an aid in refraction. It is also valuable when rapid mydriasis and cycloplegia are desired, as in retinal photography, breaking of posterior synechiae, and rapid pupillary dilatation in preoperative and postoperative conditions.

Adverse effects. No significant side reactions occur after topical use of tropicamide in the eye. This drug should not be instilled into the eye of patients with narrow-angle glaucoma.

Preparations. It is prepared in 0.5% and 1% solutions.

Dosage. One to 2 drops are instilled at 5-minute intervals for two to three doses. Refraction must be performed within 30 to 45 minutes after application because the cycloplegic effect wears off rapidly.

PRESERVATIVE-ANTISEPTICS

In general pharmacology, antiseptics are defined as drugs that may be applied to tissues to kill bacteria or inhibit their growth. Disinfectants are agents that are applied to nonliving tissue for bactericidal purposes. Preservatives are agents that are added to prevent decomposition. In ophthalmology the term "preservatives" has been used to designate agents that are added to a preparation or product for the purpose of inhibiting the growth of micro-organisms in the preparation, thereby helping to maintain sterility during use.

Benzalkonium (Zephiran) chloride

Benzalkonium chloride is a quaternary ammonium antiseptic with a nitrogenous cationic radical in an ionized molecule.

Actions. Benzalkonium chloride is an effective inhibitor of bacterial growth of both gram-positive and gram-negative organisms. Cationic surfactants such as benzalkonium are fairly strong detergents as well as antiseptics, and the detergent action contributes to the effectiveness of the antiseptic effect. Ordinary soaps should not be used on the skin surface before application of benzalkonium, since soaps inactivate cationic surfactants. Benzalkonium acts as a bacteriostatic and bactericidal agent by virtue of decreasing surface tension, with a resultant change in the permeability of the bacterial cell membrane. As a result, bacteria are unable to remain in equilibrium with the environment, lose vital intracellular materials, and fail to reproduce and survive.

Ophthalmic uses. Aqueous solutions of benzalkonium chloride, 1:10,000, are applied topically for the treatment of mild and nonspecific conjunctivitis. This agent is also added to solutions of carbachol to enhance the corneal penetration of carbachol by decreasing the surface tension of the cornea. It is also used as the preservative-antiseptic in many commercial eye preparations in weak concentrations (1:10,000 to 1:50,000).

Adverse effects. Concentrations of benzalkonium chloride stronger than 0.1% may produce skin irritation. Solutions of benzalkonium to be employed for prolonged instrument sterilization must contain sodium nitrate to prevent corrosion of the instruments. The storage of cotton balls for skin disinfection in benzalkonium should be discouraged because *Pseudomonas*-type organisms have been found to flourish in this environment, with consequent contamination of the skin and neutralization of the antiseptic action of the benzalkonium solution. Containers to be used for short-term storage and sterilization of instruments in benzalkonium should be sterilized carefully before being filled with the antiseptic.

Preparations. Preparations include the following: concentrate 17% aqueous solution; aqueous solution, 1:750; tincture, 1:750.

Dosage. For topical use on intact skin, minor wounds, and abrasions, 1:750 tincture or aqueous solution; for use on mucous membranes and broken skin, 1:5,000 to 1:20,000 aqueous solution; for topical use in the eye, aqueous solutions should be prepared in concentrations of 1:10,000 to 1:20,000. Concentrations of 1:5,000 are used for ophthalmic preparations that are not directly instilled into the eye, such as contact lens cleaning solutions.

Chlorobutanol (chlorbutol)

Chlorobutanol is a potent sedative and hypnotic.

Actions. Chlorobutanol acts similarly to chloral hydrate but is more toxic. Its chief use is as an antiseptic preservative for various types of solutions, including ophthalmic preparations. Solutions varying from 0.15% to 0.6% are utilized for this purpose.

SEDATIVES AND HYPNOTICS

The sedative-hypnotic agents are usually classified into two major pharmacological groups: barbiturates and nonbarbiturates. These drugs act by producing varying degrees of central nervous system depression. This ranges from sedation to hypnosis to respiratory depression with increasing dosage.

In small doses, anxiety and emotional tension may be relieved without causing drowsiness or lethargy. The most common use of sedative-hypnotics is to treat uncomplicated insomnia.

BARBITURATES

Barbiturates are classified by their duration of action, which varies with their distribution, metabolism, and excretion. Phenobarbital is described as a long-acting barbiturate. Examples of intermediate- and short-acting barbiturates are amobarbital (Amytal), pentobarbital (Nembutal), and secobarbital (Seconal). An example of an ultrashort-acting barbiturate is thiopental (Pentothal).

Adverse reactions. Adverse reactions to barbiturates are relatively uncommon unless excessive doses are taken or unless the patient is unusually sensitive to these medications. Drowsiness and lethargy occur in such instances. Residual hangover is common after hypnotic doses. Other side reactions include nausea and vomiting and skin rashes. In some patients, particularly the elderly, restlessness and excitement may occur. Barbiturates are contraindicated in patients with porphyria since this disease is aggravated by barbiturates.

Dependence and tolerance to barbiturates may occur. Abrupt withdrawal of barbiturates in chronic users may result in delirium and convulsions. Overdosage can cause hypotension, tachycardia, respiratory distress, coma, and death. Because of drug interactions, barbiturates must be reduced when they are given with other central nervous system depressants.

Pentobarbital sodium (Nembutal)

Pentobarbital is the ethyl, 1-methylbutyl derivative of barbituric acid.

Actions. Pentobarbital is a hypnotic and sedative with short to moderate duration of effect. It is used to induce sleep or sedation and as a preanesthetic sedative. It is also effective as an antidote for the central nervous system stimulation induced by local anesthetics. Adequate sedation is obtained within 20 to 30 minutes after ingestion.

Adverse effects. Pentobarbital should not be employed in patients who react with excitement. Restlessness and excitement may be caused when the drug is administered in the presence of severe pain. Respiratory and circulatory depression result from large doses. Skin eruptions, nausea and vertigo, headache, and lassitude are additional side effects. The drug is contraindicated in patients with severe liver disease.

Preparations. Preparations include: elixir, 4 mg per ml; capsules, 30, 50, and 100 mg; tablets, 100 mg; injection, 50 mg per ml; suppositories, 30, 60, 120, and 200 mg.

Dosage. It is given orally, 25 to 100 mg for sedation and hypnosis; 50 to 200 mg for preanesthetic sedation 30 to 60 minutes before surgery.

Phenobarbital sodium

Phenobarbital is the ethyl-phenyl derivative of barbituric acid.

Actions. Phenobarbital is a potent, long-acting hypnotic and sedative. It is employed in the management of insomnia and many other conditions requiring the use of a long-acting sedative. Because the phenyl ring in the compound imparts a specific depressant action on the motor cortex, phenobarbital is valuable as an anticonvulsant.

Adverse effects. The most common side effect of sedation with phenobarbital is hangover. Large doses may cause respiratory and circulatory depression. In some patients, excitement rather than sedation may be induced. Hypersensitivity, apparently allergic in nature, may occur, manifested by dermatitis, cutaneous lesions, and swelling of the eyelids, cheeks, and lips. Addiction to phenobarbital may occur, but little or no tolerance to the drug develops.

The drug is contraindicated in persons with known idiosyncrasy, in patients with parkinsonism, psychoneuroses, and significant renal disease, and in extremely elderly persons.

Preparations. Preparations include the following: elixir, 4 mg per ml; tablets, 16, 32, 50, 64, and 100 mg; capsules, 65 and 100 mg; solutions, 130 and 160 mg per ml.

NOTE: Aqueous solutions are unstable and heat labile.

Dosage. Phenobarbital is administered orally, 15 to 30 mg, repeated two to four times a day for sedation; for hypnosis, 60 to 200 mg.

Secobarbital (Seconal) sodium

Secobarbital is the allylmethylbutyl derivative of barbituric acid.

Actions. Secobarbital sodium is a short-acting sedative and hypnotic. It is easily absorbed from the gastrointestinal tract, and therefore its onset of action is rapid. In the presence of severe pain it may cause excitement rather than sedation.

Adverse effects. Skin eruptions, vertigo, nausea, diarrhea, and headache may occur as side effects. Addiction is possible with prolonged use. High dosage at toxic levels may result in severe respiratory depression, peripheral vascular collapse, and coma. Because secobarbital sodium is metabolized in the liver, caution should be exercised in its administration to patients with significant impairment of liver function.

Preparations. Secobarbital is prepared in the following forms: elixir, 4.4 mg per ml; capsules, 30, 50, and 100 mg; tablets, enteric coated, 50 and 100 mg; solution, injection, 50 mg per ml; suppositories, 30, 65, 130, and 200 mg.

Dosage. The dosage is as follows: for sedation, 50 to 100 mg; for hypnosis, 100 to 200 mg orally; for preanesthetic medications, 50 to 200 mg, 30 to 60 minutes before surgery.

NONBARBITURATES
Chloral hydrate

Chloral hydrate is a chlorinated derivative of ethyl alcohol.

Actions. Chloral hydrate is an effective sedative and soporific agent. It produces sedation and sleep smoothly and rapidly. The sleep that follows the administration of chloral hydrate is physiological. The patient can be aroused easily and awakens alert and usually without hangover. As with other hypnotics, no analgesia occurs.

Adverse effects. In therapeutic doses the most prominent side effect is irritation of the gastric mucosa, which can be minimized if the drug is administered with water or milk. Large doses result in deep stupor, vasodilatation, hypotension, cyanosis, and respiratory depression. Combination with alcohol results in rapid and severe depression.

The use of chloral hydrate is contraindicated in patients with serious liver or renal dysfunction. The drug should be employed with caution in patients with severe cardiac disease.

Preparations. Preparations include the following: capsules, 250 and 500 mg, and 1 gram; solution and syrup, 100 mg per ml; suppositories, 500 and 650 mg, and 1.3 grams.

Dosage. Chloral hydrate is administered orally, 0.5 to 2 grams; for sedation in infants and children, 25 to 40 mg per kg of body weight (total dose not to exceed 1 gram); for hypnotic effect, 50 mg per kg of body weight, orally or rectally, in three to four divided doses.

Glutethimide (Doriden)

Glutethimide is widely prescribed as a hypnotic, particularly in patients unable to tolerate other drugs. Many patients do not have a hangover with this medication as they experience with barbiturates.

Adverse effects. Skin reactions may occur. Nausea, paradoxical excitement, blood dycrasias, and blurred vision have been reported. Prolonged use may result in dependence, and withdrawal symptoms may be severe.

Preparations. Preparations include the following: capsules, 500 mg; tablets, 125, 250, and 500 mg.

Dosage. The dosage is as follows: adults and children over 12 years of age, as a sedative, 125 to 250 mg three times a day after meals; as a hypnotic, 250 to 500 mg at bedtime.

VACCINES
Staphylococcal vaccine (staphylococcal phage lysate, staphage lysate)

Actions. Staphylocococcal phage lysate is prepared by lysing parent cultures of coagulase-positive *Staphylococcus aureus* (serologic types I and II) with Gratia polyvalent bacteriophage. The lysate is filtered; no preservative is added. The product contains an antigenic fraction of *Staphylococcus aureus* and active staphylococcus bacteriophage. Administration of staphylococcal phage lysate appears to decrease cellular hypersensitivity to *Staphylococcus aureus* and increase the capability of macrophages to inactivate staphylococci. Additionally, the bacteriophage is able to lyse staphylococci. The drug has been used for the treatment of chronic and recurrent staphylococcal infections in all parts of the body.

Ophthalmic uses. Staphylococcal phage lysate is an adjunct in the treatment of recurrent staphylococcic infections of the eyelids, including folliculitis, blepharitis, and hordeola. Epithelial erosions of the cornea secondary to staphylococcic infections of the eyelid margins are also improved after staphylococcal phage lysate therapy.

Adverse effects. Patients should be given skin tests with small amounts (0.01 to 0.05 ml) of the vaccine and the reaction graded. Caution should be used in administration of this agent to any patient with a known history of allergy to this type of protein.

Preparations. Preparations are as follows: 1-ml ampuls for subcutaneous injections; 10-ml vials for aerosol, topical, and oral administration.

Dosage. The usual initial dosage for subcutaneous injection is 0.05 to 0.1 ml. This is increased in increments of 0.1 ml every 1 to 4 days until a maximum dose of 0.5 ml is reached. Maintenance dosage is dependent on patients response. The medication also has been instilled topically into the eye.

Vaccinia immune globulin (VIG)

Actions. VIG is human antivaccinia serum obtained by fractionating the gamma globulin from donated blood of military recruits who have been vaccinated 4 to 8 weeks before donation. VIG provides passive antibody against the vaccinia virus. This medication has been reported to be successful in prophylaxis of vaccinia in eczematous patients and in the treatment of various complications of vaccinia, including accidental autoinoculation, eczema vaccinatum, generalized vaccinia, and vaccinia gangrenosum.

Ophthalmic uses. VIG has been used successfully in the treatment of the various forms of ocular vaccinia lesions, including lesions of the lids and conjunctiva. It should not be used for treatment of corneal lesions.

Adverse effects. No significant side reactions to VIG have been reported.

As with ordinary gamma globulin, there is no danger of transmission of the virus of serum hepatitis. The administration of VIG does not interfere with the development of active immunity created by smallpox vaccination.

Preparation. It is prepared in 5-ml vials; each milliliter contains 1.69 mg of gamma globulin. This drug is distributed free by the American Red Cross. It can be obtained through the regional blood centers.

Dosage. Dosage is 0.12 to 0.24 ml per kg of body weight, administered intramuscularly in the gluteus or lateral thigh muscle. In children, no more than 5 ml should be injected into any one site. The dose may be repeated if no response occurs in 24 to 48 hours.

VASODILATORS
Nitroglycerin

Nitroglycerin is a smooth muscle relaxant.

Actions. The action of primary interest is the relaxant effect of this drug on the musculature of the coronary arteries. It is used in the management of angina pectoris and affords immediate relief from attacks of anginal pain as well as adequate prophylaxis against the occurrence of anginal pain. The mechanism of action is not known completely, but experimental evidence has been accrued indicating that improved blood flow through the coronary arteries with a reduction in cardiac ischemia results from the action of nitroglycerin. Meningeal vessels and vessels in the skin of the blush area are also dilated. Mention has been made of the smooth muscle relaxing quality of nitroglycerin in conditions other than angina pectoris, but other and more effective agents are available for these problems.

Ophthalmic uses. Nitroglycerin has been used for the treatment of retinal arterial spasm. Its effectiveness in producing dilatation of the retinal vessels is equivocal.

Adverse effects. Excessive dosage or unusual susceptibility of the patient can result in syncope, hypotension, headache, and elevated gastrointestinal disturbances. Methemoglobinemia may result from chronic overdosage. Headache and dizziness may occur during initial exposure to the drug, but tolerance to these side effects is quickly developed. Nitroglycerin is contraindicated in patients with early myocardial infarction.

Preparations. Preparations are in the form of tablets, 0.15, 0.3, 0.4, and 0.6 mg; capsules (time released), 2.5 and 6.5 mg.

Dosage. The dosage is 0.4 to 0.6 mg sublingually.

Tolazoline hydrochloride (Priscoline)

Tolazoline hydrochloride is an adrenolytic and sympatholytic agent.

Actions. Tolazoline blocks sympathetic nerves at the effector cell-nerve junction. It inhibits the vasoconstrictor action of epinephrine and levarterenol and exerts a vasodilating effect on small blood vessels, apparently by direct action. It is employed in the management of peripheral vascular disease for the purpose of increasing the flow of blood in the peripheral vessels. It is effective against peripheral vascular occlusion resulting from vasospasm and is used in the treatment of arteriosclerosis obliterans, Buerger's disease, Raynaud's phenomenon, and other disorders in which vasospasm is a prominent factor. The vasodilatation effected by the drug has a duration of several hours.

Ophthalmic uses. Tolazoline has been administered both orally and by retrobulbar injection for the treatment of central retinal artery occlusions, both partial and total. Although it is one of the few agents that can dilate retinal vessels, improvement after use of this agent is rare because of the disease process.

Adverse effects. Side effects frequently include sensations of warmth or chilliness, flushing, and gooseflesh. A variable hypotensive effect may occur, and tolazoline should be administered with caution to patients with coronary artery disease.

Preparations. Preparations include the following: tablets, 25 mg, sustained release, 80 mg; solution, injection, 25 mg per ml.

Dosage. Dosage is as follows: given orally, 25 mg four to six times daily; given parenterally, 10 to 50 mg four times daily. Dosage must be individualized and may be increased gradually until the desired response is obtained.

VITAMINS

A list of the estimated daily adult requirements and therapeutic dosage of the vitamins in the treatment of deficiency states is given in Table 23.

Vitamin K

Vitamin K is an essential fat-soluble element involved in the production of prothrombin in the liver. Replacement therapy may be required in the presence of various hepatic diseases in which formation of prothrombin is depressed.

Table 23. Vitamins

Vitamin	Name	Estimated daily adult requirement	Therapeutic dose for deficiency states
A	Oleovitamin A	5,000 units	15,000 to 25,000 units daily
B_1	Thiamine	1 to 2 mg	10 to 40 mg daily
B_2	Riboflavin	1 to 2 mg	5 to 10 mg daily
Nicotinic acid	Niacin	10 to 20 mg	Highly variable—50 to 500 mg daily
B_6	Pyridoxine	1 to 2 mg	10 to 100 mg daily
B_{12}	Cyanocobalamin, pantothenic acid	$5\mu g$ to $6\mu g$*	$15\mu g$ to $30\mu g$ twice weekly, weekly, or biweekly
C	Ascorbic acid	40 to 60 mg	100 to 200 mg daily
D_2	Calciferol	400 to 800 units	1500 to 4000 units daily
D_3	7-Dehydrocholesterol	400 to 800 units	1500 to 4000 units daily
E	Alpha-tocopherol	5 to 30 units*	50 to 100 units daily

*Exact requirements not known.

Table 24. Vitamin K and analogues

Drug	Trade names	Dosage	Preparations
Phytonadione (K₁)	Mephyton, Konakion	Orally, 5 to 25 mg Intramuscularly, 5 to 25 mg	Tablets, 5 mg Solution, injection, 2 mg/ml
	Aqua mephyton	Intramuscularly or intravenously, 10 to 50 mg	Solution, injection, 2 mg/ml
Menadione (K₃)	Menadione	2 to 10 mg daily	Tablets, 1, 2, 5, and 10 mg Solution, injection, 2 and 10 mg/ml
Menadiol sodium diphosphate	Kappadione, Synkayvite	5 to 10 mg daily Antidote for coumarin overdosage: 75 mg intramuscularly	Injection, 5 and 10 mg/ml Tablets, 5 mg
Menadione sodium bisulfite	Hykinone	Orally, intramuscularly, or intravenously, 2.5 to 10 mg Antidote for coumarin overdosage: 50 to 100 mg by slow intravenous infusion	Solution, injection, 10 mg/ml Tablets, 5 mg Solution, oral, 5 mg/ml
Methylamine naphthol HCl (K₅)	Synkamin	Orally, 4 mg daily Injection, 1 to 5 mg	Capsules, 4 mg Solution, injection, 1 mg/ml

Vitamin K compounds are also useful as antidotes against the action of anticoagulants of the coumarin type, which act by inhibiting prothrombin formation.

The two naturally occurring vitamins are vitamin K₁ and vitamin K₂. Several synthetic analogues of vitamin K are also available, with a wide range of activity. These compounds are essentially nontoxic, except in newborn infants, in whom large doses, particularly in premature infants, may lead to hyperbilirubinemia and kernicterus.

Vitamin K compounds may be administered by the oral, intramuscular, or intravenous route, depending on the circumstances in the individual case.

See Table 24 for the dosage and preparations of vitamin K and analogues.

MISCELLANEOUS
Carbamazepine (Tegretol)

Carbamazepine is an iminostilbene derivative used in the treatment of trigeminal neuralgia.

Actions. The drug provides symptomatic relief of pain associated with primary trigeminal neuralgia in a high percentage of patients. It is less effective in other facial neuralgias and in secondary trigeminal neuralgia as, for example, the type that follows herpes zoster.

Adverse effects. The drug may have adverse hematological effects; aplastic anemias, agranulocytosis, thrombocytopenia, and leukopenia have occurred. Patients receiving carbamazepine should have base-line blood counts taken, repeated at weekly or biweekly intervals during treatment. Other side effects include dizziness, drowsiness, gastrointestinal disturbances, abnormalities in liver function, urinary distress, and allergic reactions.

Preparation. Carbamazepine is prepared in 200-mg tablets.

Dosage. The drug is administered in an initial dose of 100 mg twice a day with meals, with increments of 100 mg every 12 hours until relief. Doses range from 200 to 1,200 mg daily. Maintenance dose is 400 to 800 mg daily.

Fluorescein sodium

Fluorescein sodium is a phthalein dye that has an intense fluorescence in dilute solutions.

Actions. Fluorescein stains tissues not protected by living epithelium. When applied topically, solutions of this drug will penetrate the intact cornea. When injected intravenously, the dye appears rapidly throughout the vessels of the body in sufficient concentration to be recognized by its yellow-green appearance.

Ophthalmic uses. Fluorescein solutions are applied topically to aid in the diagnosis of abrasions and foreign bodies of the cornea. They are also used to check the fit of corneal contact lenses. This stain is used in measuring ocular tensions with an applanation tonometer. It has also been injected intravenously in a 5% or 10% solution to study aqueous secretion of the ciliary body and to aid in the diagnosis of internal carotid artery insufficiency. Delayed appearance of the dye in the retinal vessels of one eye indicates decreased internal carotid blood flow. The pattern of blood vessels in the ocular fundus may also be studied by the intravenous administration of fluorescein.

This agent may be used to determine lacrimal system patency. Appearance of the dye in nasal secretions after topical application into the eye indicates an open passageway.

Adverse effects. The toxicity of this dye is low, and no side effects result from the topical use of this material. Transient nausea occurs in a significant number of patients receiving intravenous fluorescein. Brief febrile reactions have occurred that were possibly caused by contamination of the fluorescein with pyrogens. Urticaria and other allergic phenomena have occurred in a small number of patients; cardiovascular collapse has been reported in very rare instances.

Solutions of fluorescein may become contaminated with *Pseudomonas* organisms. Only fresh solutions or impregnated filter strips should be used.

Preparations. Preparations include the following: paper strips, impregnated; ophthalmic solution, USP, 2% in 3% sodium bicarbonate; sterile ampuls for injections, 5% and 10%.

Dosage. For detection of foreign bodies and corneal abrasions, 1 or 2 drops are instilled into the eye, followed by irrigation. Ten milliliters of the 5% solution or 5 ml of the 10% solution is injected intravenously.

Zinc sulfate

Actions. Zinc sulfate is a soluble salt possessing both astringent and antiseptic properties. It is thought that the zinc ion can precipitate protein. Zinc sulfate irritates the gastric mucosa and induces vomiting when given orally. For this reason the drug has been employed as an emetic.

Ophthalmic uses. Zinc sulfate is used in the treatment of nonspecific and mild forms of conjunctivitis and is quite effective against Morax-Axenfeld conjunctivitis. It is thought that zinc sulfate counteracts the enzyme effects of the bacteria. Vasoconstrictors are often added to zinc sulfate ophthalmic preparations.

Adverse effects. There are no significant side reactions to the local application of zinc sulfate.

Preparations. It is prepared in solution, 0.2% and 0.25%, and ointment, 0.5%.

Dosage. Application of the solution or ointment is required two to four times a day.

PEDIATRIC DOSAGE DETERMINATION

All drugs should be used with great caution in children, and the dosage should be individualized. The dosages for newborn children have not been as accurately determined as they have been for older children. Drug should be used in early infancy only for significant disorders. In newborn infants, metabolism and excretion of drugs may be deficient because of inadequate detoxifying enzymes or inefficient renal function. Drug permeability of blood-tissue membranes and drug-protein binding may be altered.

In general, small children have increased metabolic rate, and consequently the relative dosage may need to be increased. Dosage may have to be adjusted for body temperature (increased metabolism), edema (dependent on whether the drug is primarily in extracellular fluid), and the types of illness (kidney and liver disease may decrease drug metabolism). Older children should never be given a dose greater than an adult dose.

The determination of pediatric dosages has been based on proportions of adult doses. Many rules and formulas have been developed that are not entirely satisfactory but may serve as a rough guide. Dosage determined on the basis of surface area is a more accurate method of estimating the pediatric dose (Table 25).

$$\text{Child dose} = \frac{\text{Surface area of child in m}^2 \times \text{Adult dose}}{1.75}$$

or

$$\text{Surface area in m}^2 \times 60 = \text{Percentage of adult dose}$$

The formula for calculating approximate surface are in children is

$$\text{Surface area (m}^2) = \frac{4W + 7}{W + 90}$$

where W is weight in kg.

Table 25. Determination of drug dosage from surface area*

| Weight | | | | Percentage of |
kg	lb	Approximate age	Surface area (m²)	adult dose
3	6.6	Newborn	0.2	12
6	13.2	3 months	0.3	18
10	22	1 year	0.45	28
20	44	5.5 years	0.8	48
30	66	9 years	1	60
40	88	12 years	1.3	78
50	110	14 years	1.5	90
65	143	Adult	1.7	102
90	154	Adult	1.76	103

*From Kempe, C. H., Silver, H. K., and O'Brien, D., editors: Current pediatric diagnosis and treatment, ed. 4, Los Altos, Calif., 1976, Lange Medical Publications.

Other rules based on proportion of adult dose are:

CLARK'S RULE: Based on weight, for children over 2 years.

$$\text{Child dose} = \frac{\text{Weight in pounds} \times \text{Adult dose}}{150}$$

BASTEDO'S RULE: Based on age.

$$\text{Child dose} = \frac{(\text{Age in years} \times \text{Adult dose}) + 3}{30}$$

COWLING'S RULE:

$$\text{Child dose} = \frac{\text{Age at next birthday} \times \text{Adult dose}}{24}$$

YOUNG'S RULE: Based on age.

$$\text{Child dose} = \frac{\text{Age in years} \times \text{Adult dose}}{\text{Age in years} + 12}$$

STANDARD PEDIATRIC DOSAGES (NOT FOR PREMATURE, NEWBORN, OR YOUNG INFANTS)*

ANALGESICS

Acetaminophen (Tylenol)

Elixir (120 mg/5 ml): under age 1 year, ½ teaspoonful; age 1-3 years, ½-1 teaspoonful; age 3-6 years, 1 teaspoonful; tablets, 120 mg chewable and 325 mg scored age 6-12 years, ½-1 scored tablet, or 2 chewable tablets every 4-6 hours.

Aspirin

65 mg/kg/24 hr orally or rectally divided into 4-6 doses
Maximum dose: 3.6 grams/24 hr

*Reader is advised to consult other sources for dosages for premature and newborn infants.

Codeine

For pain: 3 mg/kg/24 hr orally, subq, or IM, divided into 4-6 doses or 0.8-1.5 mg/kg as a single dose

For cough: one third to one half of above dose

Dextropropoxyphene hydrochloride (Darvon)

3 mg/kg/24 hr orally divided into 4-6 doses

Meperidine (Demerol)

6 mg/kg/24 hr divided into 6 doses IM, subq, or orally or 0.6-1.5 mg/kg as a single dose

Maximum dose: 100 mg

Morphine

0.1-0.2 mg/kg/dose subq every 4 hr as necessary

Maximum dose: 10 mg

ANTHELMINTICS

Diethylcarbamazine citrate (Hetrazan)

For filariasis: 6 mg/kg/24 hr orally divided into 3 doses for 7-10 days

For ascariasis: 15 mg/kg/24 hr orally as single dose for 4 consecutive days

Gentian violet

For oxyuriasis: tablets, coated, 2 mg/kg/24 hr orally divided into 2-3 doses for 7-10 days; repeated after 7-10 days rest

For oral moniliasis: 0.25% aqueous solution applied topically 3 times daily for 3 days

Piperazine (Antepar, Multifuge, Oxucide, Parazine, Vermizine)

For oxyuriasis:

Up to 7 kg	250 mg	
7-14 kg	500 mg	orally once daily before breakfast for 7
14-27 kg	1 gram	consecutive days
Over 27 kg	2 grams	

For ascariasis:

Up to 14 kg	1 gram	
14-23 kg	2 grams	orally once daily before breakfast for 2
23-45 kg	3 grams	consecutive days
Over 45 kg	3.5 grams	

Note: The above dosages are not for premature, newborn, or young infants.

Pyrvinium pamoate (Povan)

For enterobiasis: 5 mg/kg orally as a single dose; repeat in 3 weeks if necessary

Thiabendazole (Mintezol)

44-50 mg/kg/24 hr orally divided into 2 doses
Maximum dose: 3 grams/24 hr
For cutaneous larva migrans: 2 consecutive days of treatment
For enterobiasis: 1 day of treatment; repeated in 7 days
For trichinosis: 2-4 days of consecutive treatment

ANTIBIOTICS AND CHEMOTHERAPEUTIC AGENTS
Amphotericin B (Fungizone)

Test dose: 0.1 mg/kg/24 hr IV over a 6-hr period
0.25 mg/kg/24 hr IV over a 6-8 hr period; daily increase 0.25 mg/kg/24 hr until levels of 1 mg/kg/24 hr are reached or alternate day dosage of 1.5 mg/kg/24 hr

Bacitracin

For enteric infections: 2,000 units/kg/24 hr orally divided into 4 doses
For systemic infections: 1,000 units/kg/24 hr IM divided into 2-3 doses (50,000 units maximum/day)

Cefazolin (Ancef, Kefzol)

25-50 mg/kg/24 hr IM or IV in 4 divided doses

Cephalexin (Keflex)

25-50 mg/kg/24 hr orally divided into 4 doses; double dosage for severe infections

Cephaloridine (Loridine)

30-50 mg/kg/24 hr IM or IV divided into 3-4 doses; double dose for severe infections
Maximum dose: 4 grams/day

Cephalothin (Keflin)

80-160 mg/kg/24 hr IM or IV in 4 divided doses

Chloramphenicol (Chloromycetin, Amphicol, Mychel)

50 mg/kg/24 hr orally or IV every 6 hr; dose may be doubled for severe infections

---

Note: The above dosages are not for premature, newborn, or young infants.

Colistin sulfate, polymyxin E (Coly-Mycin)

2-5 mg/kg/24 hr orally in 3 divided doses for bacterial enterocolitis
2.5-5 mg/kg/24 hr IM or IV divided into 2-4 doses for systemic infections

Demethylchlortetracycline (Declomycin)

6-10 mg/kg/24 hr orally divided into 2-4 doses

Doxycycline (Vibramycin)

If 45 kg or less, initially 4.4 mg/kg/24 hr orally divided into 2 doses; maintenance dose is ½ initial dose; if over 45 kg, 100 mg orally for 2 doses, then 50 mg every 12 hr, or 100 mg every 24 hr

Erythromycin estolate (Ilosone)

30-50 mg/kg/24 hr orally divided into 4 doses; double amount for severe infections

Erythromycin salts (Erythrocin, Ilotycin, Pediamycin, E-Mycin)

30-50 mg/kg/24 hr orally divided into 4 doses
10-20 mg/kg/24 hr IM or IV divided into 4 doses

Gentamicin (Garamycin)

3-5 mg/kg/24 hr IM or IV divided into 3 doses; IV dose should be given cautiously over a 2-4 hr period

Griseofulvin (Fulvicin, Grifulvin, Grisactin)

20 mg/kg/24 hr orally divided into 1-4 doses; for microcrystalline products, reduce dosage by one half

Kanamycin (Kantrex)

Suppression of gastrointestinal bacteria: 50 mg/kg/24 hr orally divided into 4-6 doses
For systemic infections: 6-15 mg/kg/24 hr IM divided into 2 doses

Lincomycin (Lincocin)

30 mg/kg/24 hr orally divided into 3-4 doses, nothing but water 2 hours before and after each dose; double for severe infections
10 mg/kg/24 hr IM once a day; for severe infection every 12 hours or more often
10-20 mg/kg/24 hr IV divided into 2-3 doses or given in physiological saline or 5% dextrose/water infusion at 8-12 hr intervals

---

Note: The above dosages are not for premature, newborn, or young infants.

Methacycline (Rondomycin)

6-12 mg/kg/24 hr orally divided into 2-4 doses 2 hr pc or 1 hr ac

Neomycin sulfate (Mycifradin, Neobiotic)

100 mg/kg/24 hr orally divided into 4 doses

Novobiocin (Albamycin)

20-45 mg/kg/24 hr orally divided into 4 doses
15-40 mg/kg/24 hr IV or IM divided into 2 doses

Nystatin (Mycostatin, Nilstat)

1,000,000-2,000,000 units/24 hr orally divided into 3-4 doses if over 2 years of age

Paromomycin (Humatin)

For amebiasis: 25 mg/kg/24 hr orally divided into 3 doses for 5 days
For dysentery: twice dose for amebiasis, employed for 7 days

Polymyxin B sulfate (Aerosporin)

Enteric infections: 10-20 mg/kg/24 hr orally divided into 4-6 doses
Systemic infections: 1.5-2.5 mg/kg/24 hr IM or 2.5-3.0 mg/kg/24 hr IV divided into 4-6 doses

Rifampin (Rifadin, Rimactane)

For tuberculosis: 10-20 mg/kg in single oral dose not to exceed 600 mg/24 hr
For *Neisseria* meningitis carriers: use above dose for 4 consecutive days

Streptomycin

20-40 mg/kg/24 hr IM divided into 1-2 doses
Maximum dose: 1 gram/day

Tetracycline group (Aureomycin, Bristacycline, Terramycin, Achromycin, Tetracyn, Steclin, Panmycin, Kesso-Tetra, Sumycin, Tetrex)

25-50 mg/kg/24 hr orally divided into 4 doses
10-25 mg/kg/24 hr IM divided into 2 doses
10-15 mg/kg/24 hr IV divided into 2 doses

Troleandomycin (TAO, Cyclamycin)

25-40 mg/kg/24 hrs orally divided into 4 doses for not more than 10 days

Vancomycin (Vancocin)

40 mg/kg/24 hr continuous slow IV or divided into 2-4 doses

Note: The above dosages are not for premature, newborn, or young infants.

PENICILLINS
Penicillin G

Sodium penicillin G and potassium penicillin G:
    100,000-400,000 units orally 5 times daily, ½ hr ac
    20,000-50,000 units/kg/24 hr IM in 4 divided doses
    20,000-100,000 units/kg/24 hr IV in 6 divided doses
Benzathine penicillin G (Bicillin, Duapen, Neolin, Permapen):
    600,000-1,200,000 units IM as single dose every 15-30 days
Procaine penicillin G:
    100,000-600,00 units every 12-24 hr IM

Penicillin V

Phenoxymethyl penicillin (Pen Vee, V-Cillin, Compocillin):
    25,000-50,000 units/kg/24 hr orally divided into 4 doses

Semisynthetic penicillins

Ampicillin (Alpen, Amcill, Omnipen, Penbritin, Polycillin, Principen, Tota-
    cillin):
    50-100 mg/kg/24 hr orally divided into 4 doses
    150-400 mg/kg/24 hr IM or IV divided into 6 doses
Carbenicillin (Geopen, Pyopen):
    50-200 mg/kg/24 hr IM or IV divided into 4-6 doses
    For severe infections, 250-500 mg/kg/24 hr IM or IV divided into 4-6 doses
Cloxacillin (Tegopen):
    If 20 kg or less, 50 mg/kg/24 hr orally divided into 4 doses
    If 20 kg or more, 1-2 grams/24 hr orally divided into 4 doses
Dicloxacillin (Dynapen, Pathocil, Veracillin):
    12.5-50 mg/kg/24 hr orally divided into 4 doses, 1-2 hr ac
Hetacillin (Versapen):
    20-40 mg/kg/24 hr orally or IM or IV divided into 4 doses
Methicillin (Staphcillin):
    100-150 mg/kg/24 hr IM or IV divided into 4-6 doses
    Double the dose for severe infections
Nafcillin (Unipen):
    25 mg/kg/24 hr orally divided into 4 doses, orally 1-2 hr ac
    50 mg/kg/24 hr IM divided into 2 doses
    Double above dose for severe infections
Oxacillin (Prostaphlin, Resistopen):
    50 mg/kg/24 hr (up to 40 kg) orally divided into 4 doses 1-2 hr ac
    60 mg/kg/24 hr IM or IV divided into 4-6 doses
    Double above amount for severe infections

Note: The above dosages are not for premature, newborn, or young infants.

SULFONAMIDES

Acetyl sulfamethoxypyridazine (Kynex, Acetyl, Midicel)

Initial dose: 30 mg/kg orally in single dose
Maximum dose: 1 gram
Maintenance dose: one half of initial dose once daily pc

Salicylazosulfapyridine (Azulfidine)

Initial dose: 75 to 150 mg/kg/24 hr orally divided into 4-8 doses
Maintenance dose: 40 mg/kg/24 hr divided into 4 doses

Sulfadiazine (or sodium salts)

120-150 mg/kg/24 hr orally divided into 4 doses (maximum dose: 6 grams/
24 hr; initial dose: one half of 24 hr dose)
100 mg/kg/24 hr divided into 4 doses IV or divided into 3 doses subcutaneously (as 5% solution)

Sulfadimethoxine (Madribon)

Initial dose: 25 mg/kg orally
Maximum dose: 2 grams
Maintenance dose: one half initial dose once daily orally

Sulfamethoxazole (Gantanol)

Initial dose: 60 mg/kg orally as single dose
Maximum dose: 2 grams
Maintenance dose: one half of initial dose every 12 hr

Sulfisoxazole (Gantrisin)

Initial dose: 75 mg/kg orally
Maintenance dose: 150 mg/kg/24 hr orally divided into 4-6 doses
Maximum dose: not more than 6 grams/24 hr

MISCELLANEOUS AGENTS

Nalidixic acid (NegGram)

40-50 mg/kg/24 hr orally in 4 divided doses

Nitrofurantoin (Furadantin, Macrodantin)

Up to 7 kg weight: 6 mg/kg/24 hr orally in 4 divided doses
7-11 kg weight: 50 mg/24 hr orally in 4 divided doses
12-21 kg weight: 100 mg/24 hr orally in 4 divided doses
22-31 kg weight: 150 mg/24 hr orally in 4 divided doses

Note: The above dosages are not for premature, newborn, or young infants.

32-40 kg weight: 200 mg/24 hr orally in 4 divided doses
Maintenance dose: over 10 days reduce to one half of above doses

ANTIHISTAMINES
Chlorpheniramine (Chlor-Trimeton, Teldrin)

0.35 mg/kg/24 hr orally or subq divided into 4 doses
0.2 mg/kg single dose orally (long-acting preparation)

Cyproheptadine (Periactin)

0.25 mg/kg/24 hr orally in 3-4 doses

Diphenhydramine hydrochloride (Benadryl)

5 mg/kg/24 hr orally or IM divided into 4 doses
Maximum dose: 300 mg/day

Promethazine (Phenergan)

0.5 mg/kg/dose orally, IM, or rectally
Nausea and vomiting, one half to full dose every 4-6 hr

Tripelennamine (Pyribenzamine)

3-5 mg/kg/24 hr orally divided into 4-6 doses
Maximum dose: 300 mg

ANTIPROTOZOAN DRUGS
Diiodohydroxyquin (Diodoquin)

For amebiasis: 30-40 mg/kg/24 hr orally divided into 3 doses for 21 days
(Maximum dose: 1.95 gram/24 hr)

Quinacrine (Atabrine) hydrochloride

For giardiasis: 8 mg/kg/24 hr orally divided into 3 doses
For tapeworm: 15 mg/kg orally divided into 2 doses, 1 hr apart; saline purge
2 hr after second dose (Maximum dose: 800 mg)

ANTIVIRAL DRUG
Amantadine hydrochloride (Symmetrel)

Age 1-9 years: 4-8 mg/kg/24 hr orally divided into 2-3 doses (Maximum
dose: 150 mg/day)
Age 9-12 years: 200 mg/24 hr orally divided into 2 doses
Known exposure: 10-day course; prophylaxis for A_2 influenza only

---

Note: The above dosages are not for premature, newborn, or young infants.

CARBONIC ANHYDRASE INHIBITORS
Acetazolamide (Diamox)

Glaucoma: 8-30 mg/kg/24 hr orally divided into 3-4 doses

Dichlorphenamide (Daranide, Oratrol)

1.6-6 mg/kg/24 hr orally in 3-4 divided doses

Ethoxzolamide (Cardrase)

4-15 mg/kg/24 hr orally in 3-4 doses

Methazolamide (Neptazane)

2-8 mg/kg/24 hr orally in 3-4 divided doses

CORTICOSTEROIDS AND ACTH
Betamethasone (Celestone)

One fortieth of cortisone dose
0.06-0.25 mg/kg/24 hr orally divided into 3-4 doses

Corticotropin (ACTH, Acthar)

1 unit = 1 mg
Aqueous: 1.6 units/kg/24 hr divided into 3-4 doses IV, IM, or subq
Gel: 0.8 unit/kg/24 hr single dose or divided into 2 doses

Cortisone (Cortogen, Cortone) acetate

2.5-10 mg/kg/24 hr orally divided into 3-4 doses
One third to one half the oral dose IM every 12-24 hr

Dexamethasone (Decadron, Deronil, Dexameth, Gammacorten, Hexadrol)

One thirtieth of cortisone dose
0.07-0.33 mg/kg/24 hr orally or IM divided into 3-4 doses

Fludrocortisone (Florinef, Alflorone, F-Cortef)

One twentieth of hydrocortisone dose
0.1-0.4 mg/kg/24 hr once a day for treatment of Addison's disease

Hydrocortisone and salts (Cortef, Cortril, Hydrocortone)

Four fifths of cortisone dose
2-8 mg/kg/24 hr orally, IV, or IM divided into 3-4 doses

Note: The above dosages are not for premature, newborn, or young infants.

Methylprednisolone (Medrol)

One sixth of cortisone dose
0.4-1.6 mg/kg/24 hr orally, IM, or IV divided into 3-4 doses

Prednisone (Deltra, Deltrasone, Meticorten, Paracort, Metasone, Lisacort)

One fifth of cortisone dose
0.5-2 mg/kg/24 hr orally divided into 3-4 doses

Prednisolone (Delta-Cortef, Hydeltra, Meticortelone, Paracortol, Prednis, Sterane, Sterolone)

One fifth of cortisone dose
0.5-2 mg/kg/24 hr orally, IV, or IM divided into 3-4 doses

SEDATIVES
Chloral hydrate

Hypnotic: 50 mg/kg/24 hr orally or rectally divided into 3-4 doses
Sedative: 25 mg/kg as single dose
Maximum dose: 1 gram

Pentobarbital (Nembutal)

Sedative: 2 mg/kg/24 hr divided into 4 doses orally or rectally
Anticonvulsant: 3-5 mg/kg IM as a single dose

Phenobarbital

Sedative: 0.5-1 mg/kg orally every 4-6 hr
Anticonvulsant: 3.5 mg/kg IM as a single dose

Secobarbital (Seconal)

Sedative: 2 mg/kg/24 hr divided into 4 doses orally, IM, IV, or rectally
Anticonvulsant: 3-5 mg/kg IV, IM, or rectally as a single dose

TRANQUILIZERS
Chlordiazepoxide (Librium)

0.5 mg/kg/24 hr IM or orally divided into 3-4 doses; not recommended for children under age 6 years

Chlorpromazine hydrochloride (Thorazine)

2 mg/kg/24 hr orally divided into 4-6 doses

Diazepam (Valium)

For preoperative sedation or status epilepticus: 0.1-0.3 mg/kg IM or IV as a single dose

---

Note: The above dosages are not for premature, newborn, or young infants.

For anxiety or muscle spasm: 0.12-0.8 mg/kg/24 hr orally divided into 3-4 doses

Hydroxyzine (Atarax, Vistaril)

1-2 mg/kg/24 hr orally divided into 4 doses
Preoperatively, one half of oral dose IM

Prochlorperazine (Compazine)

0.25-0.4 mg/kg/24 hr orally or rectally divided into 3-4 doses; one half of oral dose IM; not recommended for children weighing less than 10 kg

Promethazine hydrochloride (Phenergan)

For nausea and vomiting: 0.5 mg/kg IM, orally, or rectally; may repeat one half to full dose every 4-6 hr

Triflupromazine (Vesprin)

Not used below 2½ years of age
For preoperative sedation and for nausea and vomiting:
1 mg/year up to 10 years of age IM
1-2 mg below 7 years of age ⎫
2-3 mg 7-14 years of age   ⎬ IV

MISCELLANEOUS DRUGS
Aminosalicylic acid (PAS)

250-300 mg/kg/24 hr orally divided into 3 doses, after meals

Atropine

0.01 mg/kg/dose orally or subq; may repeat every 4-6 hr
Maximum dose: 0.4 mg

Digoxin (Lanoxin, Saroxin)

Under 2 years of age (after newborn period):
Digitalizing dose:
0.06-0.08 mg/kg orally
0.04-0.06 mg/kg IV or IM
Maintenance dose:
One fifth to one third of digitalizing dose ⎫ divided into 3-4 doses
orally   ⎬ with 6 hr or more
One tenth to one fifth of digitalizing dose ⎭ in between doses
IV or IM

Note: The above dosages are not for premature, newborn, or young infants.

Over 2 years of age:
   Digitalizing dose:
      0.04-0.06 mg/kg orally
      0.02-0.04 mg/kg IV or IM
   Maintenance dose:
      One fifth to one third of digitalizing dose orally ⎱ divided into 3-4 doses with 6 hr or more in between doses
      One fifth of digitalizing dose IV or IM

Edrophonium (Tensilon) chloride

Myasthenia gravis test: 0.2 mg/kg IV—give one fifth of dose slowly IV in 1 minute; if tolerated, give remainder
Premature infants: 1 mg single dose (IM or subq)

Glycerol

1-1.5 grams/kg orally as a single dose; may be repeated in 6-8 hr

Heparin

Initial dose: 50 units/kg IV drip
Maintenance dose: 100 units/kg added and absorbed every 4 hr (IV drip)
Titrate dose to yield 20-30 minutes clotting time or 2-3 times preheparin clotting time

Ipecac

15 ml orally followed with water; repeat once within 20 minutes if necessary

Isoniazid (INH, Nydrazid)

10-20 mg/kg/24 hr orally divided into 2-3 doses or 5-10 mg/kg/24 hr IM every 12 hr
Maximum dose: 300 mg/24 hr

Isosorbide (Hydronol)

1-2 gm/kg orally

Levarterenol (Levophed)

1 ml of 0.2% solution (0.1% base) in 250 ml diluent; IV drip at 0.5 ml/minute to give $2\mu g$ (base)/M^2/minute
Titrate dose with blood pressure

Mannitol

Infants: 10% solution IV; 1.5 grams/kg over a 30-45 minute period
Older children: 20% solution IV; 1.5-2 grams/kg over a 30-45 minute period

Note: The above dosages are not for premature, newborn, or young infants.

Mechlorethamine (Mustargen, nitrogen mustard)

0.1 mg/kg/day for 4 days IV in concentration of 1 mg/ml of water

Neostigmine (Prostigmin) methylsulfate

Myasthenia gravis test:
0.04 mg/kg/dose IM
0.02 mg/kg/dose IV

Pseudoephedrine hydrochloride (Sudafed)

4 mg/kg/day orally divided into 4 doses

Pyrimethamine (Daraprim)

For toxoplasmosis: 1 mg/kg/24 hr divided into 2 doses at 12-hr intervals; then 0.5-1 mg/kg/day for 30 days; combined treatment with sulfonamides is usually prescribed; daily dose should not exceed 25 mg

Triethylenemelamine (TEM)

For retinoblastoma: 0.082-0.1 mg/kg IM, 1 dose before x-ray therapy and a second dose after x-ray treatment is concluded; dosage dependent on blood count
0.06-0.08 mg into carotid artery as single injection
0.03 mg into carotid artery daily for 7-10 days

Trimethobenzamine hydrochloride (Tigan)

15 mg/kg/24 hr in 3-4 divided doses orally or rectally

Urea

1-1.5 grams/kg/dose as 30% solution IV over 30-45 minute period

Vaccinia immune globulin (VIG)

Treatment: 0.6-1 ml/kg IM repeated as necessary
Prophylaxis: 0.3-0.5 ml/kg IM
Larger doses may be divided

Vitamins

Table 26 shows the daily requirements of vitamins A, B_1, B_2, niacin, C, and D

Vitamins in deficiency states

Vitamin A:
20,000-50,000 IU daily for 1-2 weeks

Note: The above dosages are not for premature, newborn, or young infants.

Table 26. Vitamin daily requirements

	Daily requirements					
	A (IU)	Thiamine B₁ (mg)	Riboflavin B₂ (mg)	Niacin (mg)	C (mg)	D (IU)
2 months	1,500	0.3	0.4	5	35	400
6 months	2,000	0.5	0.6	8	35	400
9 months	2,000	0.7	0.8	9	35	400
1 to 3 years	2,000	0.7	0.8	10	40	400
4 to 6 years	2,500	0.9	1.1	13	40	400
7 to 9 years	3,500	1.0	1.2	16	40	400
10 to 12 years	4,500	1.0	1.4	18	50	400
13 to 15 years	5,000	1.5	1.8	20	50	400
15+ years	5,000	1.5	1.8	20	50	400

Vitamin B (thiamine hydrochloride):
    10-50 mg daily orally or parenterally for several weeks
    Dried yeast tablets, 5-30 grams three times a day
Vitamin B₂ (riboflavin):
    3-10 mg three times a day orally for several weeks
Niacin (nicotinamide):
    50-300 mg daily orally
    25-150 mg daily IM
    Dried yeast tablets, 5-30 grams three times a day
Vitamin C (ascorbic acid):
    200-500 mg daily orally
    Na ascorbate, 0.2-0.5 gram IV or IM daily in divided doses for 1 week
Vitamin D:
    10,000-50,000 IU orally every day for 7 days
    2,000-5,000 IU daily thereafter for several months

Note: The above dosages are not for premature, newborn, or young infants.

REFERENCES

AMA drug evaluation, ed. 2, Chicago, 1973, American Medical Association.
Gellis, S. S., and Kagan, B. M.: Current pediatric therapy, ed. 7, Philadelphia, 1976, W. B. Saunders Co.
Kagan, B. M., editor: Antimicrobial therapy, ed. 2, Philadelphia, 1974, W. B. Saunders Co.
Kempe, C. H., Silver, H. K., and O'Brien, D.: Current pediatric diagnosis and treatment, ed. 3, Los Altos, Calif., 1974, Lange Medical Publications.
Shirkey, H. C., editor: Pediatric therapy, ed. 5, St. Louis, 1975, The C. V. Mosby Co.
Silver, H. K., Kempe, C. H. and Bruyn, H. B.: Handbook of pediatrics, ed. 11, Los Altos, Calif., 1975, Lange Medical Publications.

Index

269

67145